Darwinian Dominion

Darwinian Dominion
Animal Welfare and Human Interests

Lewis Petrinovich

A Bradford Book
The MIT Press
Cambridge, Massachusetts
London, England

This book was set in Sabon by Northeastern Graphic Services, Inc., and was printed and bound in the United States of America.

Library of Congress Cataloging-in-Publication Data

Petrinovich, Lewis F.
  Darwinian dominion : animal welfare and human interests / Lewis Petrinovich.
    p. cm.
  "A Bradford book."
  Includes bibliographical references and index.
  ISBN 0-262-16178-8 (alk. paper)
  1. Animal welfare. 2. Animal rights. I. Title.
HV4708.P48 1998
179'.3—dc21   98-5036
                                                                   CIP

Contents

Preface

This book is the third in a trilogy that applies evolutionary principles to understand the nature of human morality. The first two books, *Human evolution, reproduction, and morality* (1995), and *Living and dying well* (1996), considered the permissible use of humans by humans. Basic philosophical issues were discussed and an evolutionary approach was developed and applied to problems regarding human existence, including conception, birth, living a satisfactory life, and dying.

This book completes this phase of the inquiry by asking questions regarding the permissible use of animals by humans. Philosophical positions concerning animal welfare, rights, and liberation are discussed within a utilitarian framework that stresses the importance of a cost-benefit analysis of values. Attention is paid to the philosophy of science, especially the nature of explanation, the relationship of evidence to theory, and ideas regarding how to evaluate scientific change and progress. Special attention is devoted to the biological conception of species, because it looms large in philosophical discussions regarding the use of animals in research and to consume. The value and necessity of animal research to advance biological and medical science, and to the development of applications of those advances is a dominant concern.

A word of explanation is in order regarding the title, *Darwinian dominion*. The first book had a rather ordinary descriptive title—*Human evolution, reproduction, and morality*—while the second was a bit better in terms of moving beyond mere description—*Living and dying well*. While musing at my desk one evening about a title for this book, I thought of a favorite poem I had heard read by the author Dylan Thomas (1971, pp. 49–50), "And Death Shall Have No Dominion." I played his recording of that poem, and was caught by the last three lines of the first stanza: "Though they sink through the sea they shall rise again;/ Though lovers be lost love shall not;/ And death shall have no dominion." If not Death, what, then? Of course, neo-Darwinism; hence Darwinian dominion. The word dominion I find appropriate; dominion refers to a sovereign entity in one sense of the word, and a rule of authority in another. Darwinism is a powerful disciplinary entity in the first sense, and it provides outstanding power to understand all organic systems in the second. Of course, suffering from a bit of the colon problem that inflicts academics I had to add some descriptive words: *Animal welfare and human interests.*

I must round up the usual suspects who have suffered early drafts of much of the material in all three books. A. J. Figueredo and Patricia O'Neill, both my PhD students and now professional collaborators, criticized the drafts of several chapters, contested some of my ideas, and once again forced me to greater (and briefer) clarity of exposition. In addition I owe much to Marc Hauser, who challenged some of my views, provided valuable references, and suggested radical reorganizations here and there. The MIT Press commissioned a reading of the penultimate manuscript by Michael Ruse, and I profited greatly from his comments, as well as those by some anonymous reviewers. Martin Day also read that draft and whipped me into shape on several aspects, just short of questioning my sanity in a couple of places. Curtis Hardyck, a friend and collaborator since graduate school, with his usual acerbic comments helped me appreciate where I should tighten the argument and writing.

My executive editor at The MIT Press was Betty Stanton. She coaxed and cajoled me through one major revision and then persuaded me to cut the final manuscript by 120 pages. The book is far better as a result: crisper, the logic tighter, and some tangential material deleted. Of course, some good stories were lost; they were interesting and often funny, even though they added nothing to the flow of the discussion except to amuse me during a day's writing. Betty also negotiated the paperback rights to the first two books, and they should now appear, thanks to her efforts.

Katherine Arnoldi, Senior Editor, did a superb job shepherding the copyedited manuscript though the various stages of production. She and the copyeditor, Sarah Jeffries, were magnificent; they nailed me on awkward constructions and repetitious use of favorite words. The little slips attached to the manuscript that indicate a query to the author were often fun to deal with—not my usual experience when dealing with copyeditors. I am very well served by a highly gifted, understanding, and professional group of people at The MIT Press.

So, there you have it. Looking back on the past few years of my life that these books consumed, a comment by Edward Tolman (1959, p. 152), one of several great people I was privileged to study with at the University of California, Berkeley, catches my present spirit: " . . . the best that any individual scientist . . . can do seems to be to follow his own gleam and his own bent, however inadequate they may be. In fact, I suppose that actually this is what we all do. In the end the only sure criterion is to have fun. And I have had fun."

I

Basic Principles

1

Evolutionary Issues

The thesis I develop in this book is a simple one (and probably will be maddening to some). Humans have a set of cognitive abilities that develop from a suite of emotional attachments that mark them unique compared with all others not members of the species *Homo sapiens*. This avowedly speciesist belief is grounded on a complex bundle of characteristics that only humans possess. Humans have language sufficient to support a degree of complexity and level of abstraction that enables us to develop rules of law, theories of nature, principles of philosophy, and codes of conduct. We have minds capable of appreciating the minds of other beings, capable of empathy, and (unfortunately) able to perpetuate evil of unsurpassed enormity. We benefit from a developmental process that equips us to respond to human caregivers and to appeal to those caregivers from the moment of birth onward. When the human infant emerges into the human community it is recognized as a person belonging to that community, and is due respect and succor from members who have full moral standing—what philosophers call moral agency.

Other animals can suffer, can enjoy, can think, and have needs that are necessary to their good welfare and best interests. They, as are human infants, are classed by philosophers as moral patients, and as such are due respect and care for their basic needs. However, by no stretch of the imagination can their welfare interests be considered comparable with those of members of our species. I maintain that, when push comes to shove, the interests of members of our species should triumph over comparable interests of members of other species. This position does not imply that any human whim should take precedence over essential needs and deep welfare interests of nonhuman animals. It only means that human interests should be read as high cards in any game where costs and benefits are taken into consideration. So, with this declaration, let me proceed to the task of supporting these assertions, with the hope that you will take them under serious advisement, even if you fail to be completely convinced of their infinite wisdom.

This book extends arguments begun in two previous ones concerned with the morality of various actions that affect the birth, life, and death of humans. These discussions brought to bear principles of biology, evolutionary theory, neurophysiology, medicine, and cognitive science to develop a logical, consistent, and universally applicable view of bioethics.

Moral philosophers have considered these issue for many years and have developed careful pro and con positions regarding various theories of morality. One major class of bioethical theory is utilitarianism, which considers the costs and benefits of different actions. This approach has several variants, such as the classic utilitarianism that aggregates the good over all individuals concerned, a form that meets with strong objections because of the harm it could permit to individuals. Another form is a preference utilitarianism, in which that good must be considered in terms of an individual's preferences, interests, or desires. One problem with utilitarian theories is how costs (harms) and benefits (goods) should be defined and estimated. Some suggested pleasure and pain as the currency, and others believe it should be the pursuit of life's goals, interests, and preferences.

The other major class of theory is deontological, which argues certain basic values must prevail. These values typically are couched in terms of rights, duties, or freedoms, which are offered as a system of absolute constraints that protect individuals from harm. The problem with this class of theory is that it is not clear what rights and freedoms should be recognized and established as fundamental. This is a major difficulty when rights or freedoms of different individuals come into inevitable conflict; which ones should prevail and for whom.

The philosophical concept of a social contract between individuals should serve as a major factor to constrain the actions of individuals. These social contracts are founded in aspects of biology that enhance the success of individuals to continue the process of transmitting genes to future generations. They lead to the development of tendencies that favor kin, as well as members of one's community who can assist and reciprocate assistance given them. Social bonds between members of a family and community enhance cooperation and communication, but also can lead to distrust and enmity toward those who are not members of the community.

It has been held that a pluralistic moral philosophy honoring both utilitarian concerns and basic rights and freedoms of individuals is preferable to either monolithic view. Pluralism is an appealing position, but in many ways it runs the risk of buying into the problems of both the utilitarian and deontological camps. I propose a pluralism: I am convinced that the web of influences that impel behavior and the outcomes produced are multifaceted, that interactions among different values are highly complex, and that all actions must be considered in terms of the context within which they occur, with an allowance for the nature of all individuals involved.

In my two previous books, *Human evolution, reproduction, and morality* (Petrinovich, 1995), and *Living and dying well* (Petrinovich, 1996), I developed a bioethical thesis to provide an adequate perspective within which to consider the permissible use of humans by humans. These two books considered important issues in human life and death, basically from the perspectives of moral philosophy, evolutionary biology, cognitive science, and social psychology. There were four critical steps in the argument. One dealt with the biology of reproduction, which centers on the ultimate value (in terms of differential reproductive success) of the proximate mechanisms of cooperation and communication. A second level involved philosophical and biological bases for this differentiation between human moral agents and moral patients. I maintained that one of the most important events determining the moral status of an individual occurs at birth. At that point, a third emotional level comes into play at which attachment occurs—the organism attains the status of personhood. The neonate is recognized as a member of the human moral community, which entitles it to respect from all moral agents who, from that point on, must assume duties and responsibilities toward this moral patient. The status of personhood is the biological embodiment of the social contract that molds the family and community. It represents the end point of fetal development, and signals the successful progress of the reproductive process that drives evolution and connects us with all of nature.

The fourth step was the attainment of the status of a moral agent. It held that only some humans have the characteristics that signal agency. These characteristics are cognitive, including the ability to understand rules, causation, and intentionality, all of which depend on the possession of language that is capable of supporting a complex syntax.

In *Human evolution, reproduction, and morality* the basic points were developed and applied to moral issues involved in reproduction—contraception, abortion, infanticide, and issues forced on us by development of new reproductive technologies, such as artificial insemination, in vitro fertilization, and surrogate motherhood. In *Living and dying well* the arguments were applied to moral issues regarding genetic screening and manipulation, especially those involved in the Human Genome Project, whose goal is to locate all genes of the human genome and establish the base sequences of all its DNA.

Attention was then turned to criteria for death, because it is now possible to keep individuals in a persistent vegetative state for long periods of time. When death should be considered to have occurred is of intense ethical concern, because organ transplantation is becoming more refined and successful, and donor organs are in desperate need; but to be of use they must be taken as soon as possible after death. Questions regarding the permissibility of suicide and euthanasia raise difficult issues that affect medical practice. These issues regarding the creation of life and prolongation of death have made it necessary to establish review boards to consider matters of medical ethics in hospitals, especially in the management of intensive care units, and indeed in all areas of health care. Questions concerning the level of health care to which all members of human society should be entitled raise many difficult bioethical issues, and it is here that moral philosophers have made strong contributions to continuing debates. Philosophers have insisted that practical medical decisions and their economic implications should be considered with a steady concern for basic moral principles that define a just society. Proactive discussions of the moral implications of developing technologies must take place before political, commercial, and legal imperatives force society to seek quick moral fixes.

The Scheme of this Book

I extend the theme in this book to develop a concept regarding life and death that is adequate to encompass a complete range of moral problems regarding the permissible use of animals by humans. In chapter 1, evolutionary issues crucial to the concepts that follow are reviewed. Chapter 2 contains a discussion of primate societies based on prehistorical archaeological data, the characteristics of two nonhuman primate societies, and human hunter-gatherer societies. The nature of early hominids and what is known of the social organization of hunter-gatherer societies are discussed. This material provides a perspective within which to consider the nature of human societies compared with communities of other animals. Chapter 3 reviews the philosophical positions alluded to above, which provide the essential background to understand the extension of bioethical concerns to the animal realm. Chapter 4 consists of a brief presentation of philosophy of science, and a discussion of research methods. The former is intended to make it possible to understand the value of specific research studies; the latter centers on the nature of theory, relationships between evidence and theory, and the nature of scientific progress.

Chapter 5 contains an extensive discussion of human fetal development and neonatal capabilities. This discussion is important because it highlights the incredible number of physiological and behavioral developments that guarantee successful entry of the neonate as a member of human society, entry that enhances the likelihood it will receive the care necessary to survive. The process of social bonding is of central importance to theories developed here, because it is essential to the elements that determine moral standing as a human moral patient. In chapter 6, infant sensory and cognitive development are addressed, as well as animal and human cognition, theory of mind, and intentionality. Critical differences exist between humans and other animals in their ability to understand and manipulate the complex symbol systems that make it possible to understand rules and the concept of causality, and to have a future orientation, all things that are required to function as a moral agent.

A direct consideration of issues involved in the permissible treatment of animals by humans is joined in chapter 7, where the views of Tom Regan regarding animal rights are discussed. That chapter includes an extended discussion of the concept of value, because both Regan and Peter Singer wrestle with questions of how to determine the relative value of animals and humans; I do not believe that the solutions proposed by either of them are adequate to the task. The chapter concludes with a review of the legal status of animals. Chapter 8 is a continuation of these matters, wherein Singer's views regarding animal liberation are addressed. They are considered within the framework of evolutionary principles, and strong exception is taken to his statements regarding speciesism.

The book then moves to specific issues regarding the use of animals by humans, especially in experimental research. In chapter 9, the views of the research abolition and reform movements—antivivisectionists, animal rights, and animal liberation movements—are presented, followed by reactions of the scientific research community. Chapter 10 examines selected issues regarding the permissibility of research of several kinds using animals. This is done in light of considerations introduced in the preceding chapter; evidence is marshaled to speak to critical issues, and a defensible bioethical position is suggested. In chapter 11, the use of animals in basic research that is nonapplied in its original intent is discussed. A decision model is described that can be used to consider the ethical nature of such research. Specific objections to psychological research using animals are brought forward and found to have little merit. The permissible use of animals for educational purposes is also approached in light of moral principles that were developed when issues arose regarding the regulation of research practices.

The procedures used to raise animals and kill them for food raise issues that have been discussed at length by animal rights and liberation advocates. In chapter 12, whether and under what circumstances it is permissible to eat humans are addressed, followed by questions regarding the permissibility of eating animals. Arguments against factory farming and in favor of vegetarianism are considered.

Chapter 13 is concerned with ideas regarding the importance of species preservation to maintain biodiversity, as well as the permissibility of maintaining animals in zoos and as pets. Chapter 14 is a brief epilogue that concludes the long journey taken in these three books.

Although I do not consider the detailed fabric of basic evolutionary theory in the present chapter, I highlight aspects that are critical regarding the permissible treatment of animals by humans. These address the questions of what is a species, and what is the importance of the species concept when considering taxonomic differences and their development? The species is of utmost importance when the process of reproduction in nature is concerned, because it represents the taxonomic limit within which reproduction normally occurs, and reproduction is the evolutionary engine. Because speciation is an important event, factors concerning the role of adaptation in the process of natural selection are discussed at length.

Archaeological evidence regarding the evolutionary origins of the primate series is considered in chapter 2, because it has been maintained that special regard should be accorded those nonhuman primates that are the closest phylogenetic relatives of humans. That discussion is followed by speculations regarding the probable nature of early human societies, because it was within those societal structures that much of what we consider to be a universal human nature evolved. Attention is directed to prehistoric and present-day hunter-gatherer societies to provide insights regarding the essential characteristics and further developments of human societal structures.

Humans have been built of the same stuff following the same natural regularities by which the stuff of other animals was developed. To obtain a full picture of differences and similarities between animals and the way humans should treat them, it is necessary to consider basic processes of evolution as well as the distinct qualities of different species. The natural moral sense people have is built on sympathy, fairness, self-control, and duty, and is formed out of the interaction of innate dispositions with external familial experiences. The maternal sentiments on which parental affection is based are universal in humans, and are fostered by the earliest experiences a neonate has with its caretakers, rather than being some late product of civilization.

Basic Principles of Neo-Darwinism

Several basic principles constitute the core of Darwinian theory as it has developed since *The origin of species* was published (Darwin, 1859). Ghiselin (1969, p. 232) was on the mark when he stated, "To learn of the facts, one reads the latest journals. To understand biology, one reads Darwin." Rapid advances have been made in Darwinian theory since that remark. They are based on increased understanding of primate origins provided by recent archaeological findings, intensive studies of the behavioral ecology of a number of animal species (including insects, fish, birds, and mammals), refinement of the theoretical network of evolutionary theory, better understanding of relationships between structures and functions of organisms (the phenotype) and its underlying gene structure (the genotype), and better integration and understanding of the role of molecular biological processes in evolution.

Advances in development of the fundamental core of contemporary Darwinism support the belief expressed by Dennett (1995, p. 20): "It unifies all of biology and the history of our planet into a single grand story. Like Gulliver tied down in Lilliput, it is unbudgeable, not because of some one or two huge chains of argument that might—hope against hope—have weak links in them, but because it is securely tied by hundreds of thousands of threads of evidence anchoring it to virtually every other area of human knowledge."

Dennett (1995) identified Darwin's great idea (which he dubbed "Darwin's dangerous idea") to be evolution by natural selection. Darwin's major breakthroughs were achieved because his approach embodied at least four methodological advances, as well as several substantive ideas that provided the basis for what is now called neo-Darwinism (Petrinovich, 1973). The first advance was to view members of a species in populational terms that emphasized the importance of variability in the distribution of characteristics, rather than applying the typological thinking of the day that emphasized essential characteristics every member of a species was considered to possess.

The second advance was Darwin's reliance on the deductive method throughout his research and writing. He was a careful observer, gathered as much evidence as he could on whatever question was under consideration, and used a wide range of methods to evaluate the principles he was developing. Contrary to the view of some detractors, he did not merely amass facts in an inductive manner. Darwin used the hypothetico-deductive method in all of his studies—on the formation of coral reefs, orchids, and barnacles; his classic studies on worms; and the study of emotions in human and nonhuman animals. He applied the theory of evolution through natural selection to all of these endeavors to organize his observations and bring them to bear on the central hypotheses (Ghiselin, 1969). Mayr (1991) observed that, although Darwin used the hypothetico-deductive method extensively, he was methodologically pluralistic, making extensive use of evidence from a wide range of sources to refute opposing ideologies.

A third methodological nicety was Darwin's insistence on a style of deduction that allowed for the probabilism required to deal with organism-environment interactions. He used probabilism both in terms of analyzing multiple causative factors, and recognizing the vicariousness of contingent evolutionary outcomes. Finally, he viewed the complex interplay of variables in a way that emphasized the flux of evolutionary processes and the complex nature of those manifold factors that influence organismic development. A given end point can be reached through mechanisms involving different classes of factors, such as natural selection, sexual selection, or genetic drift produced by mutation. The same selection pressures could produce different outcomes, any one of which might be a satisfactory solution to environmental demands. If there is only one efficient solution to a specific functional demand, very different gene complexes may come up with the same solution, albeit by different pathways. As Mayr (1970, p. 366) expressed it: "The saying 'Many roads lead to Rome' is as true in evolution as in daily affairs."

Evolution is driven by a mechanism of natural selection, similar to the Malthusian notion of competition for survival in the face of limited natural resources. Dennett (1995) argued that this idea was a purely logical one and had nothing at all to do with political ideology; it can be expressed totally in abstract and general biological terms. Dennett took pains to note that Darwin was certainly an ordinary mortal, and as such was the inheritor of modes of expression, attitudes, and biases that were part and parcel of his station in Victorian society. However, the economic metaphors that characterize evolutionary thinking today are the source of much of the power of evolutionary analyses, and one of the deep features of Darwin's discovery.

At the end of *One long argument*, Ernst Mayr (1991, p. 162), Alexander Agassiz Professor of Zoology at Harvard and the leading authority on the progress of ideas in biology, wrote: "The basic theory of evolution has been confirmed so completely that modern biologists consider evolution simply a fact." He considered this basic theory to be a fact as much as the observation that the earth revolves around the sun, and noted that evolution provides the factual basis for the fundamental theory of natural selection on which the four additional Darwinian theories rest. These additional theories are that of common descent (that all organic beings have descended from one primordial form), that development of diversity is a critical component in the evolutionary process, the theory of gradualism (discussed below), and the theory of natural selection (including sexual selection). Mayr emphasized the critical importance of the probabilistic nature of selection, which acknowledged the role of chance in evolution. Evolution is not a monolithic theory that rises or falls depending on the validity or invalidity of a single idea, a point also made in the statement quoted above by Dennett. Dennett (1995) remarked that anyone today who doubts that the variety of life on this planet was produced by a process of evolution is "simply ignorant—inexcusably ignorant," and I strongly endorse that statement.

Species

The theory of natural selection specifies a breeding population of individuals as the unit of interaction in nature. A populational view embodies the theory that individual organisms of a given species vary in the distribution of their characteristics. This is in stark contrast to a view in which all members of a species are considered to have the same essential, static characteristics that typify and define all individuals belonging to the species. The idea of a variable distribution of characteristics leads to the conception of a systematic underlying variability in the phenotypes (appearances) of different individuals who make up the species, and it is these appearances on which natural selection operates directly. The essentialist view that every individual has the defining characteristics typifying its species leads to the mistaken belief that if an individual establishes a new population by colonizing a previously unoccupied area, that individual's descendants will all be typical representatives of the species. A populationist stance emphasizes that no two individuals are the same, and no individual is ever a typical (essential) representative of a species. If pioneers establish colonies, dominant characteristics of the new population could be quite different from those that are most prevalent in the parent population.

The currency that constitutes the payoff in the process of natural selection is differential reproduction. Traits possessed by individuals who succeed in reproducing viable young, who are themselves reproductively successful, will come to be the most common traits in the population. Darwin reasoned that if these traits were heritable, they will be passed on to succeeding generations, and those reproducing individuals can be said to have been the fittest, given the particular environmental demands. Darwin did not know the mechanism of inheritance, because the role of the gene was not appreciated when he was writing. His solid observational base, however, made it easier for later theorists to develop what is known as the modern synthetic theory of evolution—a stage that Mayr (1991) dates to have occurred between 1936 and 1947—that introduced genetic mechanisms into the evolutionary process.

The critical unit to consider is a population of organisms capable of interbreeding (which is part of the definition of a species); individuals in the population vary in the genes each possesses; these genes are expressed in the structure and functioning of different organisms; and they are heritable. The major mode of transmission of genes from one generation to the next is, for most species of plants and animals, accomplished through sexual reproduction. In this process, a conceptus receives one-half of its genes from the mother and one-half from the father, one function of which is to maintain a desirable level of variability of genotypes and phenotypes in the population of interbreeding organisms. The centrality of the process of sexual reproduction for birds and mammals has been discussed at great length in the biological literature, and I reviewed critical steps in the argument elsewhere (Petrinovich, 1995).

Speciation Another central aspect of Darwin's theory concerns the relationship between breeding groups and their ecology. Mayr (1970) stated that geographic isolation is the most important mode of speciation among animals. He wrote (p. 179): ". . . in sexually reproducing animals a new species develops when a population that is geographically isolated from the other populations of its parental species acquires during this period of isolation characters that promote or guarantee reproductive isolation after the external barriers break down."

New species often develop when pioneers from an established colony move into a habitat not previously inhabited by the species and found a new colony. A high proportion of the founder population might, by chance, have a gene or complex of genes that is rare in the parent population. These genes, especially if they adapt the animals to peculiarities of the new habitat, may replace those that were the more frequent ones in the parent population, and this replacement can be accomplished quickly. This sequence of events may be the most important process by which rapid evolution occurs in small speciating populations (Mayr, 1970).

Rapid speciation would be expected whenever the size of the founder population is small (favoring chance sampling variability in gene frequencies), environmental pressures favor an unusual genotype that might be present, and the founder population becomes geographically (or behaviorally) isolated, which reduces or stops gene flow between it and the parent population. If the new gene arrangement has a high selective value in the homozygous condition, it will have a good chance of becoming established, even if only 2 among 100 or 1,000 offspring survive. Large populations tend to be evolutionarily stable. Mayr considers population size to be the most important factor contributing to rate of speciation; small breeding populations are more likely to undergo speciation (and perhaps extinction) than large ones.

Three points are important. First, the process driving evolution works on the phenotype, and in that sense is not primarily a genetic event, although the characteristics selected must be heritable. Mutation supplies the gene pool with one source of genetic variation, but natural selection induces evolutionary change. As Cronin (1991) remarked, it is selection that does the "thinking" in speciation, even though that thinking is the result of random selection processes. Second, because physical and behavioral characteristics are not normally the product of a single gene, any single mutation usually will not result in a character change; such change depends on major or minor reconstruction of the genotype. Third, the selective value of a gene is not absolute, but in any individual case is largely determined by the external environment and the developmental system within which the gene operates. When these points are recognized it is understandable why considerable evolutionary inertia exists, because pronounced changes in a trait usually require evolutionary change of considerable portions of the genotype. Large numbers of genes contribute to the shaping of any phenotypic trait, making it less likely that polygenetically based traits will be modified easily by natural selection.

The species concept is important because it plays a key role in the process of evolution by natural selection. Each species represents a different aggregate of genes that controls a unique developmental (epigenetic) system, occupies a unique environmental niche that imposes its own demands, and is usually polymorphic and polytypic, making it possible to adjust to changes and variations in the total environment. When the population becomes large enough, the species sends out pioneer populations that explore new niches and possibly become founders of a new community. Although members of each species share a set of unique characteristics, the individuals that constitute the species differ from one another. It is as Cronin (1991, p. 352) wrote: "Admittedly, we are unique. But there's nothing unique about being unique. Every species is in its own way."

Each species can be considered to be a biological experiment, and it is highly probable that the experiment will end up in an evolutionary dead-end street, with extinction the likely outcome. However, Mayr (1970, p. 374) wrote, "Without speciation there would be no diversification of the organic world, no adaptive radiation, and very little evolutionary progress. The species, then, is the keystone of evolution."

Darwin proposed that evolutionary change usually takes place through a gradual change in populations, rather than by a sudden production of new individuals that represent a new type. He considered this gradual change to occur through the production of variations among individuals in every generation, with evolution taking place because only small numbers of the variants survive to reproduce. There is, therefore, a continual generation of variability, and a differential rate of reproduction by those individuals who reproduce—variation is followed by selection.

This idea of gradualism was challenged by Eldredge and Gould (1972), who proposed that evolution proceeds through stages of punctuated equilibria; periods of changelessness (equilibrium) are interrupted by sudden and dramatic brief periods of rapid change (punctuation). Rapid speciation takes place during these short bouts of punctuation, and when a successful new species becomes widespread and populous, another period of static equilibrium is entered. This stasis could last for millions of years, during which only minimal change is observed.

According to Mayr (1991), whenever speciational evolution occurs in large populations it is basically gradual, in spite of the sudden appearance of new species, and this suddenness is not in conflict with the Darwinian paradigm. The interesting questions are how often such major changes in founder populations occur, and what percentage of new species enter a subsequent period of stasis.

Addressing the issue of punctuated equilibrium, Dennett (1995) held that much of the dispute regarding gradualness depends on the scales used to represent evolutionary change, by which both time and change of characters are represented. The issue turns on whether speciations appear at a constant rate over time or whether at certain periods evolution is at a dead stop. If a species is successful, if it becomes large, and if there are no sudden and extreme changes in the environment, then little evolution would be expected; at least until the population exceeds the carrying capacity of the environment, which would violate the environmental change *if*. A species that has adapted successfully would not be expected to change much until one of the above *ifs* became inoperative. By definition, this makes it necessary for at least some of the variants in the population of individuals making up the species to adapt to new pressures if the species is to avoid extinction. When some are able to adapt, changes might take place in gene frequencies for some of the successfully breeding individuals; some might be pioneers and found new colonies that become isolated and speciate, and others might not survive. The picture could be construed to be a single genealogical line that passes through a bottleneck (produced by radical environmental changes that diminish the gene pool) and continue as the same species, or two or more species that pass through the bottleneck and continue as distinctly different species entities, or a species that does not meet the challenges and becomes extinct.

Dennett (1995) expressed concern that Eldredge and Gould suggested no alternative mechanisms that could produce the sudden changes they proposed. Most experts reject explanations that depend on sudden mutations that would produce "hopeful monsters." If no alternative mechanism is specified, both Dennett and Mayr prefer explanations based on the standard mechanism of gradualistic micromutations and natural selection. New lineages appear on the scene as candidates to be selected as species following a period of stasis. If a species succeeds as an interbreeding group, this period of evolutionary change will be followed by another period of evolutionary stasis. It does not appear that the concept of punctuated equilibrium is as non-Darwinian as it has been characterized.

Most animal species have a range of general strategies to cope with environmental demands, and they also have a set of specialized mechanisms to deal with specific circumstances encountered while trying to make a living. One evolutionary principle that holds across animal species concerns those aspects of morphology, physiology, and behavior involved in reproduction. The reproductive episode is of profound evolutionary significance because it provides the coin of the evolutionary realm that must be cashed in to perpetuate the genes of the reproducers. A high differential reproduction rate means that characteristics responsible for that high rate will allow organisms bearing them to occupy available environmental niches more successfully than their competitors.

Adaptation

Evolutionary theorists devoted careful attention to problems of diversity and emphasized the importance of speciation. Major emphasis is on problems of phyletic evolution, which involves the process of adaptation. Evolution is not merely a change in gene frequencies, but is the result of twin processes producing diversity and adaptive change (Mayr, 1991). Classic Darwinism emphasized benefits brought about by adaptation, but underestimated the costs (Cronin, 1991). Modern Darwinism, in contrast, emphasizes that benefits of adaptations involve inevitable costs, which leads to a more flexible view, leaving room to recognize that mixed tactics can be used by different members of a species.

Both multiple simultaneous causation that influences the course of evolutionary development, and pluralistic solutions different organisms and species can make when confronted with a similar evolutionary challenge should be considered. Mayr (1991, p. 148) wrote: "In short, there are several possible solutions for many evolutionary challenges, but all of them are compatible with the Darwinian paradigm." He construed evolution as a process similar to that of a tinkerer who makes use of whatever is most readily available in a given situation.

Natural selection can seize on any advantageous characteristic, no matter how little it has been used in the past, how small and insignificant it is, or however deeply buried it might seem. The organism exploits whatever is available and tries it. If it works, fine; if it does not, then it loses, but another one that tried a different option might succeed.

Because natural selection is such a critical concept, the processes it involves have received considerable attention, especially the role of adaptation. Considerable controversy surrounds the necessity and sufficiency of adaptations. Some worry that it is easy to claim an adaptive significance for almost anything if one tries hard enough, to spin what Stephen J. Gould called a "Just So Story." The problem with applying this caution uniformly is that much evolutionary theorizing must be done after the fact. Changes evolved over time, and the puzzle is to decide how they occurred and why. As Cronin (1991) posed it, Mother Nature herself could have been oblivious of the brilliant moves she had made until she stumbled upon them, and Dennett (1995) added that adaptationists should hardly be faulted for being unable to predict those brilliant moves.

Gould considered it important to be sure that presumed adaptations are not in reality what he called exaptations (Gould & Vrba, 1981). An exaptation refers to structures or functional characteristics that developed to serve other purposes than those served at present, or were functionless concomitants of developments that were adaptations for other purposes. These exaptations can become secondary adaptations through the force of natural selection. This terminological distinction stresses the fact that all organismic change did not come about to serve the single, particular function of interest at the moment, and it avoids teleological implications of considering all changes to be preadaptations for that function.

It is necessary to evaluate critically all adaptationist arguments because we usually must engage in what Dennett called "reverse engineering": One looks at an existing entity to figure out why it is structured as it is, given the functions it serves. Because evolution can work only by selecting and discarding existing structures, certain things might have been used;

not because they originally developed as adaptations (they could be exaptations), but because natural selection will seize on whatever is available to adapt the organism to increase its level of differential reproduction (through secondary adaptation). Again, the metaphor of the tinkerer is apt. The analyst is placed in the difficult and problematic position of affirming the consequences based on presumed antecedents. Most often this is the only way evolutionary reconstruction can be done.

George Williams (1966) succinctly identified the problem when he counseled that the concept of adaptation should not be invoked if lower-level physical or chemical processes are sufficient to explain a set of events. Yet, it can be argued that adaptation is a central concept in ecology, ethology, and evolution, and that its proper use has led to many discoveries and insights. All adaptive characteristics are the result of natural selection, but all characteristics are not adaptive (Cronin, 1991). It is crucial to appreciate the concept of adaptation if we are to understand evolution, but it must be invoked with caution to have heuristic value and lead to increased understanding of organic systems.

Phylogeny

A few general remarks are in order regarding phylogenetic development. Matters regarding the relationship of humans and the other primates are of concern to those who question the permissibility of research using some of the primates, especially chimpanzees. The concept of a branching phylogenetic tree is important, and should be kept in mind when comparing any two phyla, families, or species. Although the quantitative difference between a pair of species in the percentage difference in DNA structure (as indicated by DNA hybridization estimates) is astonishingly small, profound differences can exist in terms of morphology, physiology, behavior, and cognition. Humans differ from chimpanzees only in about 1.6% of their DNA, and from gorillas in about 2.3%; monkeys differ from humans and apes in about 7% of their DNA (Diamond, 1992). Yet, these small quantitative differences are responsible for tremendous qualitative differences between our minds and those of any other species. It can and will be held that the differences between our minds and those of other species create a wide enough gulf to make a moral difference, and I pursue that argument in depth in chapter 6.

Humans differ vastly from all other species because we are the only one that has an extra medium of design: A culture based on a complex language system. Wrangham, de Waal, and McGrew (1994) adopted this position, citing the absence of experimental evidence to support a hypothesis of cultural transmission of behavioral variants to an extensive degree for other species. With chimpanzees, the cultural transmission observed is at best inefficient and is usually absent, and those social traditions that are found are similar to those found in species of birds, species that are radically different from primates. Their conclusion was that cultural traditions for nonhuman animals arise through repeated inventions, with succeeding generations copying the recognition of opportunity, rather than the specific technique. It is this process that could explain the behavioral traditions of chimpanzees and the closely related bonobos.

Prior to Darwin, the dominant view regarding phylogeny was that of Aristotle, who proposed the *scala naturae*—the great chain of being. According to this view all organisms are part of a single linear scale of ever-growing perfection. Animal species are arranged along this ladder, going upward from lower, simpler organisms at the bottom, moving up through worms, insects, and fish, continuing to mammals (rats, cats, and dogs), ascending to the primates, and reaching the top rung of the ladder at humans. This concept was based on the belief that God created the world for the sake of humans who only stood below the perfection of the angels and God, and animals were less perfect copies of God, created for the sake of humans.

As more became known about the world of life and the diverse characteristics of different species, the unity symbolized by the *scala naturae* began to disintegrate (Mayr, 1982). By the time Darwin published the *Origin* he no longer required God as an explanatory feature, because every aspect of creation described in the Bible was contradicted by his construal of the natural world. In fact, Mayr (1991) considers Darwin's comments against special creation to be his "one long argument." One of the major triumphs of Darwinism is that it alone explains how the organic world has the appearance of deliberate design without the intervention of a deliberate designer.

The modern conception of phylogeny is that species are genetically different, with these differences having been selected in response to ecological and behavioral pressures. There is not a sequential ladder, but a divergent, treelike structure with each organism's time line beginning when it is born and stopping when it dies. Either the offspring line continues or, if no offspring, the line suddenly halts. The tree of life has been spreading its branches for 3.5 billion years, and the usual mode of representing that branching is to plot time on the vertical axis, spreading the branches out along the horizontal axis, with newer, continuing branches spreading farther as phyla and species become more diverse.

Tattersall (1995) proposed that the evolutionary tree should be considered in terms of a "scenario," including information about such things as adaptation, ecology, behavior, ancestry, and time. The danger with this approach is that, because of its complexity, the compellingness of the story comes to depend too much on storytelling abilities. He concluded that analyses should begin with and proceed from simple considerations of branching diagrams (called cladograms) that indicate how closely a taxon is related to others. A tree can be developed, justified by evidence, only then moving to the level of a scenario. This approach makes it possible to identify testable elements at each step, and to arrive at a complex scenario through a series of falsifiable hypotheses.

It is not proper to conceive that any fish, for example, was the ancestor of any reptile, bird, or mammal, even though the fish line branched off first and the others branched later. The fish line continued to develop separate branches from the others, and these in turn became established on their own and continued their separate and different identities. Although the primate line split off into Old World monkeys about 25 million years ago, the main line continued branching, developing into the rest of the primates, with the monkey line continuing its separate course to the present. The branching primate line also continued its separate course to the present, with orangutans diverging about 13 million years ago and gorillas about 10 million years ago; the human line branched off about 5 million years ago (Wrangham & Peterson, 1996, p. 261, top diagram). The primate line continued to the common chimpanzee, with the pygmy chimpanzee (bonobo) diverging about 3 million years ago.

Wrangham and Peterson (1996) used recent genetic evidence to summarize primate phylogeny. The gibbon line split off early, followed by the orangutan and then the gorilla. Another line branched off and split into the human, then the bonobo, and last the chimpanzee. They interpreted this to mean that chimpanzees *(Pan troglodytes)* and bonobos *(Pan paniscus)* are our closest living relatives and we are theirs, and chimpanzees are more closely related to humans than to gorillas *(Gorilla gorilla)*. The two most closely related species are chimpanzees and bonobos, which became separate species 2.5 to 3 million years ago. Next to this pair is humans, then gorillas, followed at a distance by orangutans. The common ancestor of chimpanzees and humans lived about 5 million years ago. *Homo sapiens* is only about 150,000 to 230,000 years old, and is considered to have evolved particularly fast, although not as fast as cichlid fishes (Goldschmidt, 1996). During this 5 million-year period immense behavioral evolution occurred within the humanoid line.

Now that a few basic concepts in evolution, important for later discussions, have been presented, it will be useful in the next chapter to examine the structure of two nonhuman primate societies, the chimpanzee and the bonobo. Their behavioral tendencies are quite different, even though they are closely related phylogenetically. Chimpanzee social organization is similar in some respects to that of humans, and that of bonobos is quite different. It will be of interest to consider what is known of prehistoric human societies that can be gleaned from archaeological data, and revealed by study of human hunter-gatherer societies that might be organized along lines that could have prevailed in the environment of evolutionary adaptation (EEA) of humans.

Similar or Different Enough?

An issue that is important to keep in mind throughout this book concerns the nature of continuities that might exist between individual members of different species. On the one hand, humans are animals who evolved in much the same way as other animals, a fact used to justify the belief that the behavior of all animals should be explained in much the same way as that of humans. On the other hand, an impeccably Darwinian approach could lead to the opposite conclusion—that concentration on psychology rather than behavior could make the study of humans markedly different from that of other animals. Similarities might be based on the sameness of strategic principles that belong ultimately to genes, with specific behavioral outcomes being quite discontinuous, in the sense of there being different proximate mechanisms that attain the same ultimate goal.

It is difficult to determine when animals are so similar to humans that they provide adequate models to understand humans, and when they are so different that it is pointless to use them to gain such understanding. If animals to be used for experimental purposes are comparable with humans, is it permissible to subject them to any treatment that would not be permissible with humans? Singer (1990a, p. 52) considered the matter: "So the researcher's central dilemma exists in an especially acute form in psychology: either the animal is not like us, in which case there is no reason for performing the experiment; or else the animal is like us, in which case we ought not to perform on the animal an experiment that would be considered outrageous if performed on one of us." Russell and Nicoll (1996, p. 119) considered this remark to be as clever as it is unsound: "The fact is that animals are like us in some ways that we can study for potential human benefit and unlike us in other ways that allow for their use by ethical human beings." Their statement takes the opposite spin, that all research is permissible, whereas for Singer, none is. Russell and Nicoll noted that experiments are also done for the sake of learning about animal biology and behavior—knowledge for the sake of knowledge—and it is never known when such experiments may later prove to have relevance for human or animal health or well-being.

All organisms have similarities, certain conservative tendencies persist in all organic systems. Humans and chimps share about 98% of their genetic material, which some take to indicate almost complete similarity between the species. However, that 2% makes all the difference; humans are not only physically different, but they scale the cognitive heights to a level that is qualitatively different from any other species.

Even a 1% difference in DNA is not small (Pinker, 1994). The information content in DNA is ten megabytes, big enough for a universal grammar with room left over. In fact, the 1% difference could make all the difference because DNA is a discrete combinatorial code; one could change one bit in every byte and produce an organism that is 100% different from another.

Another cautionary tale is suggested by the fact that the tiny organism known as yeast shares about 20% of its genes with humans, and at least one of these genes is intersubstitutable in humans and yeast. This preserved genetic similarity undoubtedly represents conservative characteristics involved in the basic functions of life, such as cellular metabolism and reproduction within the organic medium shared by yeast and human cells. Is 20% overlap enough for us to respect yeast rights (at least 20% of them), or should the cut-off be 50%, or 98%? Small quantitative differences can have immense importance, or not mean much at all in terms of determining qualities of similarity and difference that are physiologically, psychologically, and morally relevant.

The small percentages of genetic difference between humans and chimpanzees produce important differences between them (Diamond, 1992). We have an upright posture, large brain, ability to speak, sparse body hair, and peculiar sex lives. All of these differences must be concentrated in the 2% or less genetic difference between these species, two evolutionary lines that diverged about 6 to 8 million years ago. It is interesting to consider the 2% difference between humans and chimpanzees in light of the estimated 0.1% difference in genetic bases between individual humans, an estimate that was attributed to Dr. Eric Lander, director of the Whitehead Institute/M.I.T Genome Center (Hilts, 1996). This 0.1% seems quite small, but it represents the total difference in inherited qualities involved in the tremendous individual differences between peoples in terms of the natural lottery.

Tooby and Cosmides (1995) called attention to a basically different perspective that different people have regarding evolutionary processes, noting that these perspectives have general implications for the meaning of similarities and differences. One perspective is a phylogenetic one focusing on the similarities between species in terms of the inheritance of homologous features from common ancestors. A radically different perspective focuses on the evolved functional designs that adapt organisms to demands of their environment. From the phylogenetic perspective that emphasizes linearity, it is convenient to assume that few qualitative differences exist between the human brain and that of other primates or mammals. At the level of neural architecture and cellular function, gross continuities are obvious, and similarities can be used to argue that humans are just more elaborate animals from a continuous series, therefore making it morally impermissible to experiment on our phylogenetic relatives.

The adaptationist perspective emphasizes the uniqueness of each species in the ways they adapt to their particular environmental niche. With this approach it is important to investigate adaptive functional differences in such things as information-processing strategies, language ability, tool use, and coalition formation. This perspective emphasizes the importance of investigating the uniqueness of each species, suggesting it is morally permissible to understand all of these different species.

It may be that both approaches are essential and correct because they are complementary ways to view the evolutionary process (Tooby & Cosmides, 1995). Similarities should be established to understand general evolutionary tendencies, and differences should be studied to understand these tendencies in evolutionary terms.

A host of dissimilarities between human and nonhuman animals determine the treatments commonly considered permissible. Humans have kept other humans as slaves, and also keep pets. However, human slaves (at least in the United States) were treated in a different manner from animals, and laws reflected that difference. In general, it is permissible to eat animal moral patients (at least those that are not common house pets), but not human moral patients. If a band of devotees defended the practice of cannibalism on the grounds that they restricted their practice to anencephalics and the newborn, even the most dedicated carnivores among us would be unimpressed with that justification, and no doubt the strongest legal action would be taken against those individuals.

Moral Implications

In most Western slave-holding societies, humans kept as slaves, although considered property, were entitled to a considerably higher standard of care than other objects of property. In the United States, slave owners could be punished for behavior that was considered extremely cruel, at least in the eyes of other slave holders, and it was not permissible to eat slaves or kill them for trivial reasons. One reason for the protection of slaves was that humans are different from other animals—all humans have a sense of future and are therefore capable of experiencing terror to a degree not possessed by other animals (Hare, 1979). Hare also noted that slaves (and prisoners, I might add) could be subjected to atrocious punishments for the purpose of striking terror in them and their peers. Such punishments would be ineffective, and hence not justifiable, when applied to animals.

It is permissible for me to destroy my car if I decide to, as long as I do not create a nuisance, but it is not permissible for me publicly to beat my dog to death. The reason I can beat my car and not my dog is that the dog suffers pain and has welfare interests that a car does not have. I can kill my old dog if it is suffering, but not my aged parent. This difference is maintained for complex reasons, one of which has to do with the idea of the human community and the interest in honoring social contracts.

Even though some humans (e.g., slaves, blacks, children, Native Americans, Latinos, and women) are treated badly, they still are able to argue for their place in the world in a way that is not possible for animals. Slaves could work harder to earn money and thereby purchase their freedom (Francione, 1995), a privilege that is not possible for nonhumans, who always remain property and are not able to understand the concept of freedom.

Numerous obvious differences in status between humans and animals justify different permissible treatments. Animals are seldom punished for kinds of wrongdoing that a human would be, and people are encouraged to respect an animal's nature. If a squirrel takes peanuts from a young girl's plate at a picnic and she then throws stones at it, she would likely be rebuked by a parent on the grounds that the squirrel is only doing what is necessary to survive and provide for its family (Leahy, 1991). However, if another child had stolen the nuts it would be considered proper to urge the girl to defend her property and her moral right of ownership. If the thief was an adult, the parents would most likely become involved in the defense.

Leahy observed that it is permissible to run over a dog with a car to avoid wrecking one's car, but it would not be permissible to run over a human for that reason. One can kill an animal that attacks or trespasses on one's properly, but not a child or adult human. Animals can be "put down" when they are old, but not humans, even though the animal has been a member of the family for many years. All these differences indicate a major distinction that is drawn between humans and members of other species.

Carruthers (1992, pp. 108–110) described a fantasy in which Astrid has left earth on a space rocket and is on an irreversible trajectory that will take her forever out of contact with her fellow human beings. In her rocket she carries a cat and the original *Mona Lisa* painting. Carruthers proposed two cases: In one case Astrid becomes bored and begins to use the painting as a dart board; in the other she becomes bored, ties the cat to the wall, and uses it as a dartboard. Carruthers suggested that most would intuitively agree there is a great moral difference between the two cases. He thinks that Astrid does nothing wrong in throwing darts at the *Mona Lisa*; no one will ever see the painting again (even though he allows she acted wrongly in taking it with her in the first place, because it denies earthlings the pleasure of seeing it). However, it is wrong to throw darts at the cat out of idle amusement, even though no person will ever be distressed at what she has done. He concluded that contractualism alone cannot accommodate what common sense tells us about the moral treatment of animals. Although animals are owed respect due to a respect for legitimate concerns of animal lovers, that is not enough. Throwing darts at the cat is wrong, because cruelty to an animal is wrong since the animal can experience pain and suffering. What Astrid did in both instances is bad because it manifests and expresses bad character.

There is an ordering of objects and moral patients in terms of the respect they are due, and moral agents are obliged to behave in ways that honor it. Machines and other inanimate natural objects are at the low end of the dimension, with plants receiving more consideration, many species of animals more, with pets and those beings that appear the most human-like (nonhuman primates) even more, and human moral patients the most. As Rollin (1992) humorously expressed it, animals are morally more like children than like wheelbarrows. A line is crossed when the individuals is a member of the human species, and these distinctions, too, are graded. Leahy (1991) suggested a diminishing ordering of obligation that makes sense evolutionarily: Immediate family, relations, friends and colleagues, fellow countrymen, one's racial group, people at large, animals, and natural inanimate objects. Incidentally, this ordering not only makes sense evolutionarily, but it is found in studies of human moral intuitions (e.g., Petrinovich, O'Neill, & Jorgensen, 1993; Petrinovich & O'Neill, 1996; Wang & Johnston, 1995; Wang, 1996a, 1996b).

Plous (1993) considered psychological mechanisms that are related to the human use of others. People are likely to help other humans whose race, nationality, appearance, religion, and political views are similar to their own. They also favor animals whose appearance is similar to humans, and support those endangered species that are biologically more similar to *Homo sapiens.* Animal activists rated the capacity of animals to feel pain much higher than did nonactivists, although ratings of their overall similarity to humans was similar for the two groups. It has been noted that people not only like those who are similar to themselves, but tend to befriend and marry them as well. Plous found that people would be significantly more uncomfortable eating chimpanzee meat than zebra meat, which suggests some revulsion to eating those more similar to us, a topic that is considered in chapter 12.

Attribution of degrees of similarity and higher cognitive functions to different animals corresponded to their phylogenetic group membership, with pets and primates accorded special consideration (Eddy, Gallup, & Povinelli, 1993). The ordering in terms of both similarity and cognitive function was humans, cats and dogs, nonhuman primates, other mammals, birds, reptiles, amphibians, fish, and invertebrates. Important factors that influenced the judgments were familiarity with the animals in question and the existence of an attachment bond, especially with dogs and cats.

Another complexity regarding degree of human similarity and difference to a given animal is introduced by the fact that its moral status can change depending on the perspective within which it is viewed. Herzog (1988) discussed a typology of mice: Good mice, bad mice, and feeders. In a laboratory, good mice are used for research purposes; they were bred to the purpose, and their existence depends on their utility. Their status as good mice entitles them to protection by the Institutional Animal Care and Use Committee (IACUC), and they are placed under Public Health Service (PHS), and United States Department of Agriculture (USDA) regulations.

Bad mice are free-ranging animals seen scurrying along the corridors of the laboratory. These pests are considered a threat in a lab facility, where it is important to prevent contamination between rooms. They are to be eliminated as quickly as possible. Poison is not used for fear of contaminating the good mice. Snap traps are ineffective, so the preferred method is the "sticky trap," which essentially is a rodent form of flypaper. When a mouse steps on the trap, its fur becomes bound to the trap, and about half the animals are dead when found during daily rounds. These mice suffer a miserable death that most animal care committees would not permit in an experiment. Because the building did not have a problem with wild rodents, these bad mice must be good mice that escaped. Herzog (1988, p. 474) concluded, "Once a research animal hits the floor and becomes an escapee, its moral standing is instantly diminished."

The feeder mice are quite different: They are raised as food for snakes used for research. They are in an anomalous situation. Although protected by USDA regulations because they are mammals, they are used to feed snakes that are specifically excluded by those regulations. The situation is further clouded in the case of research on predation and antipredator tactics. Herzog proposed the following rationale. A scientist conducting research on snakes does not need to get approval of the animal committee to feed research animals a diet of live mice. Because these snakes eat only live prey, not providing them with an adequate supply of live rodents would result in their starvation and could be considered cruel. Herzog asks us suppose that the investigator is interested in the ethology of antipredator behavior in rodents. If the researcher wants to introduce live mice into a snake's cage to study the encounters, the procedures would fall under jurisdiction of the IACUC, whereas if the mouse is simply snake food its use does not have to be approved by the committee. Herzog (p. 474) concluded, "Thus, the moral (and legal) standing of the mouse depends on whether it is labeled *subject* or *food*."

Herzog's point is that moral judgments about other species are neither logical nor consistent, but are the result of both cerebral and visceral components of the human mind. As discussed when the status of pets is considered in chapter 13, the roles that animals play in our lives and the labels we attach to them deeply influence our sense of what is ethical. Herzog believes that such labels are the result of the role the animal typically occupies relative to humans—labels that influence the behavior and emotions directed toward that animal. I add that certain biologically instated moral boundaries are imperatives—children, kin, neighbors, and species, and these are influenced less strongly by other considerations than is the case when the evolutionary imperative is not involved.

2

Primate Societies

Human Archaeology

In his book *The fossil trail*, Tattersall (1995) presented a clear and compelling discussion of the difficult issues involved when considering fossil evidence for human evolution. This evidence is extremely important because it provides information regarding the physical structure of individuals as well as types of artifacts that can be used to make inferences about daily activities of community members.

Evidence regarding human evolution is based primarily on a less-than-perfect fossil record, which is, however, being rapidly improved by new archaeological discoveries. Such evidence is interpreted using data obtained with several dating methods, including fluoride dating (which is not too reliable, but can establish contemporaneity of objects), radiocarbon dating methods (useful as far back 40,000–50,000 years ago), potassium-argon dating of rocks (effective between 100 thousand and 1.3 billion years ago), DNA dating, analysis of mitochondrial DNA which can estimate ancestries as recent as 1,000 or so (Cann, 1995), electron spin resonance (from the present to more than 1 million years ago), thermoluminescence, and uranium-series dating (from 5,000–350,000 years ago). Although each of these techniques has limitations, data derived from a combination of them make it possible to date fossils, artifacts, and the sediment layers in which they were found with considerable accuracy. Some techniques can be performed on relatively small samples of material, most rely on different physical assumptions, are effective with different kinds of materials, and are accurate for different preceding periods of geological time (see Stringer & Gamble, 1993, for a brief discussion of dating methods).

The evolutionary tree showing the possible line of ancestry and descent among species belonging to the human family was illustrated by Tattersall (1995, p. 234). The *Homo* line split from *Australopithecus africanus* (A) into *H. rudolfensis* (about 1.9 million years ago, which disappeared) and *H. habilis* (about 2.1 million years ago; brain volume about 500 ml), from which *H. ergaster* split (about 1.9 million years ago), which in turn split into *H. erectus* (about 1.5–2.0 million years ago which disappeared) and *H. heidelbergensis* (about 600,000 years ago), which split into *H. neanderthalis* (about 500,000 years ago; brain volume about 1400 ml, which disappeared) and *H. sapiens* (about 300,000 years ago, according to the fossil and archeological records; brain volume about 1400 ml), which continues as the modern human line. Analyses of mitochrondrial DNA indicate that the human and Neanderthal lineages diverged even earlier— 550,000 to 690,000 years ago—with the Neanderthal lineage being four times as old (Krings et al., 1997). The Neanderthal disappeared as recently as about 30,000 years ago. It is unlikely that *H. sapiens and H. neanderthalensis* hybridized: no hybrid fossils have been found in locations where evidence for long-term cohabitation is best (Tattersall, 1995), and analysis of mDNA evidence also indicates no interbeeding occurred. It appears that, although *H. erectus* dispersed from Africa into virgin territory, early *H. sapiens* moved into regions already occupied by hominid relatives, with these others displaced in the process.

Recent evidence (Swisher et al., 1996) supports the conclusion that *H. erectus* was alive in Indonesia as recently as 27,000 to 53,000 years ago, at least 250,000 years after it was thought to have been extinct in Asia. If these conclusions are correct, three species—*H. erectus, H. neanderthalensis,* and *H. sapiens*—could all have been on earth at the same time.

Given that *A. afarensis* is the major contender as a critical node in human evolution, its characteristics should be considered. Members of this species were fully bipedal, and males were bigger than females, being about four and a half feet tall. Both sexes were powerfully built, their arms were longer in proportion to their legs than ours are today, their hands were humanlike only a bit longer and more curved, their brains were small (about 460 ml, compared with 400 ml for chimpanzees, 460 for gorillas, and 1,400 for us), and their canine teeth were conical as in apes, but resembled human teeth in their reduced size. There is no evidence they were tool makers, a characteristic that did not appear for another million years. The time lag before tool making existed led Tattersall to suggest that bipedalism did not develop in response to the need to free the hands to make tools and carry them around. Rather, early hominids likely spent a good deal of time in trees where they would be sheltered from predators and able to forage safely in the daytime.

Tattersall (1995, pp. 156–158) endorsed a theory developed by Owen Lovejoy in 1981. The transition from ape-style quadrupedalism to upright posture probably took place in stages, each accompanied by increased reproductive success. Females could not increase their rate of reproduction much because their offspring needed extensive care and required years to become independent. It would be to the advantage of females to co-opt males into feeding and protecting the family. Males would still be free to roam about, not being the primary caregivers, and if bipedal, they would have their hands free to carry food home. The male's interest in assuring his successful paternity would be expected to increase his interest in establishing a pair bond and assisting the female. A system of prominent sexual signals developed to reinforce this bonding, including secondary sex characteristics such as prominent breasts and facial hair in females and males, respectively.

Homo—From Then to Now

Rather than discuss data bearing on specific cultures, I develop a "big picture" based on my reading of the literature. I relied heavily on Tattersall (1995) and on the theoretical overview presented by Bettinger (1991) in his book, *Hunter-gatherers*. The intent is to come up with an idea regarding the structure of the first human societies, and to consider how this structure might have changed in response to ecological pressures. This might make it easier to understand how early human societies could be similar to, and differ from, other animal societies. Evidence for cultural associations led Leakey to place *habilis* in the *Homo* family (Tattersall, 1995). Archaeological evidence indicates that, by 2 million years ago, tool-using hominids were cutting up the carcasses of large mammals, probably after scavenging the kill of other carnivores. *Homo Habilis* probably were scavengers, were able to chase away animal killers of other species, and dismembered carcasses with stone tools. In these scavenger-gatherer societies, meat provided only a minor proportion of the diet (Tattersall, 1995).

At about this same time (2–2.5 million years ago) a critical period in human evolution occurred during which there was a remarkable shift in the fauna in various parts of Africa, probably due to a climate shift as a result of polar glaciation that produced drastically lower temperatures, resulting in dry, open savannas in place of extensive woodlands. The animal types changed from those such as forest antelopes to species that grazed in the open. Glacial and preglacial climates made vast areas of northern Eurasia periodically uninhabitable by hominids, presumably spurring major migrations and causing local extinctions (Tattersall, 1995). Sea levels also would have risen and fallen, alternately creating islands and producing land bridges. These changes in flora and fauna would cause a fragmentation of formerly continuous populations of humans, which would provide ideal conditions for speciation to occur. Thus, the variety seen among later Pleistocene hominid fossils is exactly what would be expected. At about this time stone tools appeared, and the hunted *Australopithecus* was replaced by the hunting *Homo*.

About 1.5 million years ago *H. ergaster* appeared, as well as the first clear evidence for hand axes and cleavers, manufacture of which required complex mental machinery. Tools were abundant and consistent in size and shape, represented a highly successful technology that spread widely throughout the world, and remained in production for well over a million years. They were used by the later *H. erectus* as well. Hominid dentition and stone tools were found in China that are at least as old as known Indonesian *H. erectus* specimens (Wanpo et al., 1995). They are estimated to be over 2 million years old, which would mean they were coincident with the earliest diversification of *Homo* in Africa. The Chinese findings might be from a species that existed at the same time as the African *H. erectus* and possessed a stone-based technology. This could mean that stone tools were in use in Asia at the same time the genus *Homo* diversified from Africa. Therefore, *H. erectus* may have evolved in situ in Asia at the same time they existed independently in Africa.

Systematic group hunting of large-bodied mammals may have first appeared with modern *H. sapiens,* and although there is only one hominid species in the world at present, more than one could have existed contemporaneously in earlier times (Tattersall, 1995), an assumption supported by the archaeological findings discussed above. With the appearance of *H. sapiens*, the others disappeared, and *sapiens* attained a high degree of reproductive cohesiveness. Current variation among individual members of the species is not large, with the various human races being less different from each other than are subspecies of many polytypic species of animals (Mayr, 1970). No genetic isolating mechanisms separate any of the races of mankind, and even social barriers to reproduction function inefficiently in places where different races come into contact (Mayr, 1970). Humans occupy more different ecological niches than any other known animal, and *sapiens* have "specialized in despecialization."

Mayr also observed that isolation mechanisms in hominids develop so slowly they never last long enough to become perfected, and this lack of isolation is the result of both mobility and the ability to be relatively independent from the environment. These characteristics make true geographic isolation impossible in recent times. With the steady improvement of communication and means of transport, geographic isolation becomes more and more unlikely.

The structure of society at the time *sapiens* appeared consisted of relatively small groups of individuals, most of whom were kin who survived primarily by gathering and processing plant materials, with these provisions supplemented increasingly by meat provided by male hunters. Most food processing was done by women, with men collecting at ever greater distances and devoting more and more time to hunting. The one constant factor throughout this period of evolutionary adaptation is the mother-infant bond. This bond was important given the extreme vulnerability of neonates and young infants who had to be nursed for a considerable period if they were to survive. Women would prosper more in terms of survival and reproductive success if aided by men, who assisted in the care and provenance of young, and would want to ensure that the offspring they were providing for were theirs. The community was probably based on cooperation among members of the nuclear family and its network of kin.

Two Nonhuman Primate Societies

Similarities and differences in characteristics of societies of different primate species provide insights regarding differences between human and nonhuman animals. Comparisons among chimpanzees, their sister species the bonobo, and humans are interesting because chimpanzees and bonobos both evolved from the same ancestors that gave rise to humans. The bonobo is one of the most unaggressive species of mammals. In contrast, human and chimpanzee males were characterized as "demonic" (Wrangham & Peterson, 1996), potential brutes, because they conduct deliberate searches for both alien and conspecific victims, and kill and mutilate helpless neighbors despite appeals for mercy. Only for these two species does the loser's death seem to be part of a plan. Both species also dominate and batter females and force copulations, and males commit infanticide occasionally, behaviors not typical of bonobos.

Chimpanzees

In the early days of primate study, chimpanzees were thought to live peacefully in stable social organizations with little intra specific or inter specific aggression—an Eden of prehistory. As more investigators conducted intensive studies of groups whose members were known, the picture began to change. Male chimpanzees were observed to kill other males with whom they had been close companions, but who now were members of another community due to a split of the larger community into two.

Wrangham and Peterson posited that distribution of food, especially roots, was an important factor influencing the distribution, social organization, and behavioral tendencies of primate societies. Their theory is that 5 million years ago our ancestors crossed from tropical rainforest to woodland. The teeth of the new woodland apes *(Homo* progenitors) were modified to eat roots, which were abundant in their ancient habitats and provided the key fallback food when preferred fruits and seeds were out of season.

Chimpanzees still live in African tropical rainforests, which probably have changed little for 5 to 10 million years. These apes display knuckle-walking, hang by their arms, and are large-brained, heavily built fruit eaters. They can stand erect and walk upright, but do not have the skeletal and muscular structure to make this posture easy. Chimpanzees live only in areas where there is enough damp rainforest to provide several square kilometers for each individual. This old ape lineage continued to rely on the forest, conserving behavior and morphology; whereas a new ape lineage continued to harvest fruits and seeds, but began to walk upright in order to carry the abundant roots to a tree where they could be eaten safely, which kept them from starving during times when other foods were not available. Chimpanzees also hunt and consume meat whenever they can, and meat is a preferred food, although prey (such as the preferred colobus monkey) are not abundant enough to satisfy their nutritional needs.

Wrangham and Peterson characterized chimpanzee society as one in which individuals share a defended communal range, with males living forever in the groups to which they were born, and females moving to neighboring groups at adolescence. The males, who are members of a genetically patrilineal kin group, defend their range with aggressive and potentially lethal violence. The community is male bonded, and the intense, male-initiated territorial aggression includes raiding into neighboring communities to attack and kill other chimpanzees. Victims may be either male or female; aggression is directed more toward adult males, and less severely toward obviously fertile females, who may be forced to travel back to the home territory with the raiding party. Wrangham and Peterson claimed that out of 4,000 mammals and 10 million or more other animal species, this suite of behaviors is known only among chimpanzees and humans. Another similarity they observed is that about 30% of adult male chimpanzees die from aggression, about the same percentage as in human Yanomamo villages.

When a male chimpanzee reaches adolescence he has attained the size of an adult female, and begins to engage in brutal behavior toward each female in the troop whenever the even larger males are not present to take sides. This behavior continues until he has dominated each of the females. When a female becomes sexually receptive (signaled by dramatic anogenital swelling) she attracts a flock of males and favors some more than others, even though most adult males can force copulation regardless of her favor, absent more dominant males.

The frequency of male-male grooming is higher than that between females or between males and females (Muroyama & Sugiyama, 1994). The function of the male grooming seems to be to establish and reinforce bonds between males, bonds that would be useful to form coalitions to gain access to resources and to females, and to compete more effectively against neighboring groups.

Males challenge each other when a receptive female is present, and females can be injured during the course of these fights and chases. A female often disappears for several days from the community circle when she is cycling to avoid such stress. She often leaves with just her offspring and a single favored male, and it is during this time that she is most likely to be impregnated. This system benefits the female: She avoids injury; it also benefits the male: He assures his paternity. Unfortunately, there are costs as well. The female moves into a relationship with a male who dominates and can batter her, and she is separated from male or female kin who could serve as allies. The process of sexual selection would enhance those characteristics that increase the ability of males to be aggressive, enabling them to dominate and batter females. This selection process clearly does not work for the happy welfare of females. Favored males may become reproductively more successful, but at a cost of developing physical and behavioral characteristics that enhance the propensity to engage in violence against males, mates, and females in general.

A chimp foraging party ranges between two and nine individuals, with mother-child groups, and even individuals, often traveling alone. Females spend much of their time alone or with only their young, and female-female grooming is low except between female kin (Muroyama & Sugiyama, 1994). Because chimps must travel a considerable distance to obtain enough food for all individuals, they organize into small parties, and cannot afford to live in large permanent troops all year. Food availability is centered on seasonal items that grow in patches of variable size and density. Such "party-gang" species are territorial whenever economics allow it, and xenophobic as well. Parties sometimes fuse into larger groups, and at other times split into smaller groups to be more flexible in response to the distribution of desirable foods. When they are in small troops they are vulnerable to attack by neighboring troops that happen to have more individuals. One adaptation to this reality is to favor the natural selection of male characteristics that make them good fighters.

Because they often are in small groups, males display fear and suspicion of members of other groups who might do them harm, consume all the food, kill young, and steal females. Intragroup loyalty by social bonded males is beneficial because they are more effectively aggressive against the depredations of other groups. The down side is that this intragroup loyalty will be accompanied by hostility toward any outgroup—them.

Bonobos

The social behavior of bonobos is in stark contrast to that of the closely related chimpanzees as well as of humans. Bonobos were probably descended from a chimpanzee-like ancestor about 1.5 to 3 million years ago. Wrangham and Peterson (1996) suggested that climate change caused the divergence between the gorilla and bonobo lines; gorillas are more extensively distributed, and the less numerous bonobos evolved within southern forests once the ancestral gorillas left. Although originally called pygmy chimpanzees, bonobos are only a little smaller than chimpanzees, their hands are smaller, their bodies are more slender, they have longer legs, shorter arms and clavicles, a more ventrally located clitoris, and smaller ears, mouths, and teeth (Wrangham et al., 1994). The size difference between males and females is the same between bonobos and chimpanzees. Bonobos knuckle-walk and move bipedally with greater ease than chimpanzees, but bipedalism accounts for less than 10% of bonobo movement in the canopy (de Waal, 1989). The animals travel substantial distances arboreally, and locomote and hang under branches, whereas chimpanzees travel terrestrially between feeding and resting sites (Doran & Hunt, 1994).

The range of bonobos is restricted to the lowland rain forest of the Congo basin in equatorial Zaire (now the Democratic Republic of the Congo) (Doran & Hunt, 1994). This range does not contain gorillas as competitors, whereas the chimpanzee range does, a factor that might lead to different foraging patterns for the two species. It is possible that differences in feeding patterns between chimpanzees and bonobos exist because the chimpanzee pattern is constrained by the presence of gorillas

(Malenky, Kuroda, Vineberg, & Wrangham, 1994). Gorillas and chimpanzees both must rely on terrestrial herbaceous vegetation during seasons of reduced fruit productivity. These competitive interactions lead to habitat partitioning, which would affect both foraging patterns and food preferences.

Compared with chimpanzees, bonobos have similar food preferences, habitat, and physiological characteristics, but no gorilla competitors live in the ecological range of bonobos. Their preference for, and consumption of, herbaceous foods is more similar to that of gorillas than chimpanzees. It was suggested that the larger, and more stable foraging party size observed for bonobos, compared with chimpanzees, is due to availability of a reliable food supply not jeopardized by competition. Relaxation of this restriction on food resources in lean seasons could make it possible for them to forage in large and stable parties (Wrangham & Peterson, 1996).

One of the most striking differences in behavior between bonobos and chimpanzees concerns interactions between sexes. There are no reports of bonobo males battering adult females, forcing copulations, or killing infants. As with chimpanzees, males live in communities, share a home range with eighty or more others, travel in various-size (but larger) parties, live within a male kin group, and defend their range against outsider males.

Whereas chimpanzees have a marked dominance hierarchy, with adult males dominating all females, bonobo pairs are codominant. The top male and top female are equal, both dominate the next pair, and so it goes down the line. Males whose mothers are alive tend to rank high because their mother's support is crucial if they are to compete successfully with other males. This enhanced competitive success occurs because the mother usually outranks many males, sons are almost inseparable from their mothers, and females cooperate with one another, while males do not. If a son is attacked by a male and calls for help, and if the mother responds and also calls for help, other females will counterattack in her support. This female support group is established when an adolescent female who has left her own group enters a new community and settles there. Although she is unlikely to be kin with any of the new group, she has to work to develop a support network, and does this by sitting close to and grooming other females. She also has sex with older females, which creates a social bond between them. However, dominant females respect their subordinates and do not display aggression toward them (unlike males), and in case of tension, reconciliation is quick. Female-female grooming is more common than for chimpanzees; for both chimpanzees and bonobos males groom each other, compete for status, and form male dominance hierarchies.

Bonobo males do not engage in fights as often because they risk running afoul of a coalition of mother and friends should they attack a female. Another factor is that it is difficult for males to tell when females are ovulating, unlike the case for chimpanzees, and males and females engage in frequent heterosexual and homosexual sex, from manual genital manipulation to inventive copulation. Bonobos have been reported to mate as often as dozens of times a day, and sexual activity starts long before the onset of puberty—at about one year of age. It was suggested that this higher frequency of copulation decreases concern among males about who mates with females, thereby lessening competition for the favors of females.

Wrangham and Peterson attributed the evolution of this pattern of high levels of sexuality and lack of male dominance to bonobo females' ability to disguise the time of ovulation, making it impossible for males to compete with one another to inseminate the females. This disguised ovulation, combined with a strong mother-son bond and a tendency for females to cooperate with one another, renders males powerless in the face of a determined female majority. Whatever sexual selection takes place will not be for aggressive male characteristics, but for more nurture, more support, and greater lust for life rather than death.

Summary
It is difficult to know what caused the extraordinary differences in social systems of bonobos and chimpanzees. They both developed from a common ancestral form, but evolved in ecological settings that were quite different in terms of types and availability of foods and competitive pressures to attain those foods. Despite both being patrilineal societies, with females migrating from the familial troop, family dynamics and ways of coping with problems of making a living differ immensely.

Chimpanzee males are extremely aggressive; bonobo males are very gentle. Whatever the causative factors, it is interesting to compare these social systems to that of a closely related species, but from another family—*Home sapiens*.

Human Hunter-Gatherer Societies

Anthropologists and evolutionists have had an enduring interest to understand patterns of social behavior of hunter-gatherer societies. This interest is driven by the assumption that knowledge of these patterns could provide insights into modes of behavior existing in the EEA for modern *H. sapiens*. Bettinger (1991) contends that no anthropological theory can lay credible claim to generality until tested against evidence found for hunter-gatherers, evidence he believes provides one of the cornerstones of anthropology. One source of evidence regarding the structure of prehistoric hunter-gatherer societies is based on studies of initial contacts with Western contemporary societies that were isolated from such outside influences until discovered, such as the !Kung San of the Kalahari Desert (Lee, 1979) the Yanomamo of highland Venezuela (Chagnon, 1992), and the Ache of Paraguay (Hill & Hurtado, 1996). Another source is based on archaeological studies of artifacts and their location in camps of prehistoric humans. These findings can be compared with excavations of more recent origin to construct models of similarities and dissimilarities of community organization and lifestyle.

Early anthropological studies were based on the assumption that strict Darwinism had no relevance to the understanding of social evolution. Inheritance of acquired characteristics was considered the important, and perhaps chief, cause of human social evolution, with natural selection of little importance (e.g., Spencer, 1887). It was assumed that there was an evolutionary struggle for existence, whereas humans struggled to secure happiness. It was further assumed that human social change was a natural movement toward inevitable progress. One consequence of this presumed progressiveness was that Social Darwinists justified their opposition to social reform on the basis that it interfered with natural processes; this in turn justified the attitudes of leaders of the British Empire who disparaged primitive peoples, views that served Britain's national program of imperialism and colonial domination. On the other hand, Alfred Russel Wallace noted that "savages," rather than being primitive ignoramuses, were capable of impressive feats of navigation that required intricate knowledge, the pooling of detailed information, acute observational skills, and excellent memory. T. H. Huxley concurred, and suggested that as soon as early peoples started living socially, heavy demands pushed humans to develop advanced mental faculties. Over a hundred years later Nicholas Humphrey attributed the evolution of human self-awareness to the complexities of social living (see Cronin, 1991, for an excellent presentation of these points).

With the accumulation of evidence from intensive field studies, views regarding the nature of primitive societies changed radically. It was originally presumed that "primitives" died young, worked hard and long to obtain a subsistence diet, waged continual war against nature, starvation, and neighbors, and were victims of superstition and ignorance. Accumulating evidence reveals that, rather than being underprivileged and backward, members of these hunter-gatherer societies were highly sophisticated in the use of ecological resources, and compared with agriculturists living in the same environments, they did not die young, often worked less and had more spare time, ate better, and suffered fewer periods of famine. This revised view led investigators such as Bettinger (1991) to develop ecological analyses drawing on principles of optimal foraging theory that were developed by behavioral ecologists to understand animal foraging strategies. An advantage of these models is that they consider the total cultural system, and they have been applied successfully to understand many animal societies. Cultural systems reach an equilibrium in order to cope with variable demands of the environment, and Bettinger believes that people in societies who cope directly with such demands are highly sophisticated, with agricultural practices developing only when circumstances beyond their control irrevocably upset traditional ways of life.

One of the most comprehensive and careful studies of a foraging people is of the Ache of Paraguay (Hill & Hurtado, 1996). Daily life in the forest is centered around the food quest. The men hunt about seven hours a day, pursuing mammalian game with bow and arrow and collecting honey when it is available. Women extract fiber from palm trees and gather assorted fruits and insect larvae for about two hours a day. They also carry the family's possessions, children, and pets, spending about two hours a day moving camp. They care for children and highly vulnerable infants the rest of the time. Hunters share meat and honey evenly with adult members of the band, but less often share other gathered items. The bands, which are composed of closely related kin (as well as "friends"), have a median size of about 50 individuals, varying between 3 and 160 on single days.

A compelling aspect of this study was that the authors employed life history theory, thereby exploiting a theoretical focus adequate to understand critical events in the life cycle of many animal species. This focus led them to do more than gather descriptive demographic data that typify so many studies of primitive societies. When matters are considered within the context of the life history cycle, data are collected because they bear on variables known to be important in regulating characteristics of various species of animals, and they can be placed in a general theoretical context whenever changes occur in such elements as the distribution and types of ecological resources, population density, and community structure.

All organisms have a major problem regarding allocation of energy resources, and face a series of trade-offs between current and future reproduction, and between the number and fitness of offspring produced (Hill & Hurtado, 1996). With the same reproductive effort a parent can produce many cheap offspring who have a low chance of surviving and finding a mate (r-selected), or fewer high quality offspring who have higher survivorship and higher fertility at adulthood (K-selected).

Important variables in life history models include such things as variations in fertility at different stages of the life cycle, variations in nutrition status, age at sexual maturity, optimal interbirth interval, age at which menopause occurs, and environmental hazards. Data collected from the Ache included a complete census of two study populations, and the dates of all births and deaths for seventeen years. These data provided a complete description, not a sample, of fertility and mortality. Living adults were interviewed regarding their reproductive histories, and the interviews included questions regarding respondents' offspring and sibling's reproductive history, as well as those of their parents and grandparents and their parents' siblings.

It was found that Ache women were large in size and had high levels of fertility, compared with the !Kung. Levels of mortality from violence were high, and the juvenile sex ratio was biased toward males. Ritual child homicide had noticeable effects on the sex ratio and on child mortality rates. No member of the group was allowed to shoot an arrow at another member of the group, but members of another group could be shot on sight. Kinship and neighbor loyalty were of profound importance, and coalitions were formed against outsiders. Women tended to evaluate men according to their strength, bravery, agility, and alliances. These social patterns were attributed to the importance of foraging in an environment of variable resources that could be scarce at times, as well as the fact that small foraging bands would have to compete with other bands for the resources.

These patterns are quite different from those reported for the !Kung, whose women are small, have low fertility levels, low mortality due to violence, and strong female-biased juvenile sex ratio. Communities are more egalitarian and conservationist, live monogamously, and share communally. Women are politically equal to men, and do not depend on men economically—more the ideal of the noble savage. Resources for the !Kung are abundant and continuously available throughout the year. Such lack of variability makes it possible to establish a central base camp, and exploit available resources within a two-hour walk around it. When resources within that range are exhausted, the central base camp is moved to a new location. This foraging system allows for greater stability and more communal activities than is possible for the Ache, who must be continually on the move to exploit more unpredictable resources.

Hill and Hurtado observed that neither of these groups is "representative" of foraging peoples; however, by examining patterns of life history variation, the conditions that cause differences are revealed, and within this perspective doubt is cast on any idea that rigid specieswide parameters are at work. They noted that humans are different from apes in critical respects. Human babies are born larger and are weaned earlier; although they grow at the same rate as chimpanzees and orangutans, they grow for several more years, whereas gorillas grow faster, are larger, and have faster infant growth rates and higher adult mortality. Compared with chimpanzees, Hill and Hurtado (1996, p. 471) concluded:

". . . humans have longer life spans, longer reproductive spans, higher fertility, and higher offspring survival than chimpanzees. Chimpanzee populations are often near demographic equilibrium. Most traditional human populations (especially those not being heavily exploited by more powerful neighbors) that have been demographically described are growing rapidly." The annual mortality rate in adulthood was 2% prior to the onset of senescence, which is by far the lowest for any land-based mammal or primate. It was possible to draw these comparative conclusions because the same kinds of data were gathered for the human study populations as are available for other primate species that have been studied using life history theory.

Critical differences between human and chimpanzee life histories are produced by events associated with a reduction in hominid adult mortality rates, as well as the existence of male provisioning patterns. Higher chimpanzee mortality rates are probably due to significant predation from carnivores and hominids, and higher male provisioning was tied to a transition from being frugivores to becoming carnivorous omnivores. Also critical was human social foraging, the development of weapons, pair bonding, predatory behavior, multimale and multifemale social groups, and the ability to engage in complex communication. Development of these characteristics made possible the long life spans, early menopause, and high fertility that characterize humans. Hill and Hurtado's surprising suggestion is that humans are not the archetype K-selected species that many have assumed, but that a host of traits evolved under density-independent conditions, with others being adaptations designed to survive periodic, extreme population crashes.

When considering the foraging and gathering patterns of different societies it is obvious that one must consider the nature of ecological resources and how they impose constraints on behavior patterns different individuals must use to survive. Different ecological factors favor certain kinds of community structures, and evolution by natural selection favors characteristics that enable individuals to exploit available resources more effectively. Agriculturalism supports a tendency toward cooperation and communication, but this cooperative tendency is overlaid on a highly competitive background of human nature, as we will see in the next section.

The Two Faces of Adam and Eve

When the essence of basic human nature is discussed, one of two positions is often assumed: That human nature is beastly, savage, and red of tooth and claw; or that human nature rests on capacities to cooperate, communicate, and trust. As with many polarities truth lies in both views. Human nature could be based both on competitive and cooperative tendencies, just as many transactions in nature have both costs and benefits. Because two opposing forces are at work does not make it impossible to steer a moral course, capitalizing on tendencies that are benevolent, and inhibiting (or using to better purpose) those that would be despicable in a just, moral world.

The idea that basic human nature is benevolent has a long history. Early philosophers and anthropologists spoke of the noble savage who becomes corrupted by living in a society that encourages a style of life that corrupts the noble nature. Rousseau asserted that humans in their natural primitive state were ruled by passions that could be satisfied adequately in a world without cultural institutions involving monogamy and private property; tendencies toward violence would be suppressed by a sense of innate pity and compassion. This notion of peaceful primitive society was enhanced by views of early cultural anthropologists (e.g., Margaret Mead), novelists (Melville), and artists (Gauguin) who evoked visions of tropical paradises where pensive, self-possessed people reproduced with serenity, where open promiscuous sensuality and free-wheeling peace and freedom were the norm. These pastoral paradises were lost through the culturally acquired human evils that typify modern, especially Western, societies. Many observers worried that evolutionists too often seek to explain behavior by appealing to adaptationism—the familiar Just So Story. However, social scientists have been guilty of explaining behaviors that were based on inaccurate descriptions that appealed to cultural processes that fit their general social science model, what can be called Just Ain't So Stories. It is documented (see Wrangham & Peterson, 1996, chapter 5) that idealized accounts of tropical paradises were far from realistic, were based on only brief contacts with the societies and supported by an inadequate data base, and were the product of biased expectations that ignored the darker sides that existed. Be that as it may, the idea of an idyllic pastoral paradise that reflects basic human nature has strong appeal, leading to the acceptance of the idea that human problems are produced by cultural and political developments that weaken the deep sense of equality inherent in all peoples.

This optimistic view of the world is also reflected in ideas of evolutionary theorists who emphasized biological processes that would support the development of cooperation and communication to enhance the reproductive success of parents, stressing the importance of kin who help, and extolling the virtues of other community members who could reciprocate such help. There is the nagging reminder, however, that all of this benevolence and altruism is based on an underlying selfish interest of those individuals who replicate their genes more successfully than do competitors. If the focus is on proximate mechanisms by which this selfish ultimate goal is achieved, a more promising spin can be given to support the development of a just society that leads to a morally desirable egalitarianism. The faces of Adam and Eve produce a warm glow of the possibility of returning to Eden, if only the social evil that has led to emphasis on the accumulation of worldly goods, power, and subjugation can be undone.

Others emphasized the continuities between nonhuman and human animals, concentrating on the basic necessity to survive in a competitive world in order for the fittest to survive. Modern evolutionary theory stresses the necessity to strive for enhanced reproductive success in competition with others of the social and genetic community. It is important for a male to succeed in the competition for females and to defeat rival males. A female must enhance her likelihood to gain a fit male who, after impregnating her, will help raise young so they can enter the breeding community and perpetuate the genetic complement. The emphasis therefore, is on people engaging in continual struggle to best others, cooperating only to achieve their own ultimate success, often at the expense of others.

T. H. Huxley (1894), an evolutionist and ardent defender of Darwin, equated the ethical process with a personalized sympathy he called conscience. This ethical process must overcome evolved processes of what he referred to as "cosmic evolution." He reminded, "The thief and the murderer follow nature just as much as the philanthropist" (p. 30). He believed that cosmic evolution may teach us how good and evil tendencies may have come about, but could not furnish a reason why what we call good is preferable to what we call evil. He also believed competitive processes are greater the more rudimentary a society. The ethically best course is one that replaces ruthless self-assertion with self-restraint; replaces tendencies to thrust aside or tread on competitors with respect and assistance to one's fellows; replaces survival of the fittest with the idea of fitting as many as possible to survive. Huxley's view of the ethical stance was, "It repudiates the gladiatorial theory of existence" (p. 82). A basically evil, competitive human nature is to be restrained and modified by law and custom, "using intelligence to combat the instincts of savagery in civilized men."

Williams (1989), in a sociobiological expansion of Huxley's essay, agreed that natural selection is as bad as Huxley maintained, and that it should be neither run from nor emulated, but combated. The task is to overcome billions of years of selection for selfishness, and he believed that using biology to understand the enemy could help.

The view that primitive societies were more savage than peaceful received support from recent analyses. Keeley (1996) concluded that human warfare is universal, given that 90% to 95% of known societies have engaged in it. Those small-band societies that do not engage in warfare have very high homicide rates. Thus, there is either warfare or homicidal feuding. Keeley's book consists of extensive documentation of the prevalence of violence and warfare throughout prehistoric times and during recorded history. In primitive societies warfare against outsiders ("them") was more relentless and uncontrolled, often without rules, and was aimed at annihilation. Warlike practices of such societies can be just as sophisticated as those of "civilized" ones, and in small-scale societies the matter is one of "my relations, right or wrong," whereas in larger ones it is "my country, right or wrong." War always has been universally condemned, with peace being preferred. Keeley asked why, given this universal attitude, is it universal? The discrepancy between attitude and reality makes it difficult to argue that values and attitudes play a significant role in promoting peace or war; if they did wars should be rare and peace common, instead of the opposite being true. These face's of Adam and Eve acknowledge how difficult it will be to reach Eden, given our basic demonic, warlike nature, but hold out hope that through understanding this evil nature, we shall overcome.

Summary and Conclusions

Based on archaeological findings of H. habilis artifacts, it was concluded that campsites were the focal point of individuals who hunted and scavenged animals. Hunters were principally males because females would be encumbered by offspring, and would mostly have gathered plant foods and maintained camp. When males discovered carcasses they would transport bits of them to the campsite, an activity that would be possible because bipedal locomotion freed hands for carrying. Carcasses were dismembered using stone tools, and food was shared among members of the social group, which implies an ability to engage in complex communication (that could have involved language) as well as reciprocity in social relationships.

Making tools required a degree of forethought on the part of these early hominids that seems beyond that of living apes, whose occasional tool use consists of such activities as stripping twigs picked up on the spot to "fish" for termites. Tattershall (1995) cited an experiment by Toth and his colleagues who attempted to train a bonobo to flake simple stone tools similar to those attributed to early hominids. The trained animal was one of the best from the Yerkes Primate Research Center communication studies. It was able to learn to strike flakes from a core, but after many months of training was nowhere close to making tools at the level of early hominids. They contended that early hominids had a much better cognitive understanding of what tool making is about than a modern ape is able to acquire, even with intensive tutoring.

During the Pleistocene, the population of H. sapiens was large and increasing, and widespread population movement and displacement occurred as a result of population growth and climatic change (Bettinger, 1991). Organized hunting of herd animals took place, perhaps with stockpiling of meat, and people had a bone tool technology to make specialized flake tools. Multiple small groups formed seasonally, and evidence of interregional variation suggests cultural variability. Items of personal adornment, symbols, and art also appeared, as did naturalistic sculptures. All these things appeared at once, and it has been suggested that population growth and climate change created incentives for local technoeconomic specialization, with the development of increasingly sophisticated tactics to procure resources.

It is reasonable to suppose that vocalized language evolved at this time as a direct response to the need to communicate this complex behavioral information. Art, ethnicity, and ritual could be equivalent consequences of a single process that is inherently evolutionary and materialistic; they developed in response to changes in environmental conditions that elicited a variety of adaptive innovations resulting in technological sophistication and specialization, and represented complex forms of cultural transmission. Bettinger concluded that humans are special kinds of animals—cultural animals. They are ultimately subject to the same kinds of laws that govern all organic systems, but are also subject to special processes made possible by advanced mental abilities that facilitated development of linguistic communication.

The material reviewed in this chapter provides reasons to regard the human species as a biological entity possessing special characteristics. Biological species are basic units of nature, and are critical to evolution. Of great importance are characteristics that hold together a social communal species such as humans. Most important are factors that influence the success of reproducing males and females. Mating choices influenced by sexual selection are critical for many species, and some maintain that sexual selection has been a major force in shaping humans. In addition, mechanisms that lead to social bonding between breeding couples, kin, community, and, especially, between mother and infant impose powerful biological constraints on human behavior.

Although absolute differences between humans and other primates in DNA structure are not large, those that exist are accompanied by immense differences in structures, physiological functions, and behavioral abilities. The capacity for complex cooperation and communication that characterizes humans makes us dissimilar to other animals. All human cultures have a complexity of design because they ride on the complexity of the language system.

It is important to understand the nature of environments in which early humans evolved because they provided selective pressures shaping that evolution. A compelling picture of the initial demands on evolving

H. sapiens and early hunter-gatherer societies shows *H. sapiens* to be a genetically homogeneous species with a particular skill at despecialization—humans have radiated into more different ecological niches than any other animal species. Distribution of resources varied at different times and places, and humans developed strategies to cope with this extreme range. Although they share many biological characteristics with other species, their complex array of cognitive capacities resulted in such emergent qualities as systems of morality.

It is a mistake to assume that behavioral plasticity demands an entirely open-ended, all-purpose mind. Cronin (1991, p. 376) wrote, ". . . natural selection can enable us to act adaptively by equipping us with specially-tailored information-processing machinery, with specific content-full rules that will generate flexible behaviour." Evolved rules for behavior need not be rules for behavioral rigidity. We have inherited a bundle of capabilities and propensities, with preferences and taste, powers of discrimination, and certain ways of doing things. This construal enhances our dignity more than would be the case if we came into the world with a sparsely structured tabula rasa awaiting the hand of experience to dictate its future.

3

Philosophical Background

This chapter addresses some philosophical concepts that are important when considering the morally permissible treatment of animals by humans. The intent is not to develop innovative ideas, but to inform readers regarding the serious and complex nature of basic philosophical issues. Too often-discussions of animals rights and social justice are approached in such a cavalier or high-handed fashion that they border on polemics and platitudes invoked to support whatever position the advocate prefers.

Three philosophical positions are central to the concerns of this book. The first involves the concept of rights: What does it mean to claim a right exists, and what implications should this claim have for all members of a community? A second position involves ideas of utilitarianism: Which advocates acting to enhance the good of those in the community. The task is to arrive at an adequate definition of good. Some define it in terms of happiness; some in terms of interests, desires, welfare, or increased pleasure and decreased pain. A third position emphasizes the necessity of respecting a social contract: The rules of morality mandate respect for the terms of an imaginary social contract between community members. The terms of the contract depend on some form of bargaining among moral agents, each of whom may attempt to maximize his or her own individual utility. These three major philosophical positions are addressed in turn, because any discussion of how humans should treat animals requires clear thinking about each of them.

When considering the nature of and the basis for morality, it is important to define welfare, characterize interests, identify desires, and decide how to recognize and scale values. It is necessary to consider these issues because they represent the properties that theories of rights are intended to guarantee. Many rights have been proposed, and as will be shown when rights and values are considered at length, the major problem is to decide which ones are paramount, and which are to be given the most weight when several are involved. The latter is especially difficult when the postulated rights are incompatible with one another.

The importance of beginning the study of morality by considering the structure of nature has been stated often. Griffin (1993) suggested a list of what he called prudential values: Enjoyment, basic components important to human existence and agency (autonomy, essential material provisions, and liberty), understanding, recognition of accomplishment, and deep personal relations.

Griffin believes the ways we are taught in childhood sets us on a moral path "pretty much for life." These moral dispositions are deep, and it is difficult to go against them. In this view *ought* implies *can*, and any system of morality must meet a requirement of psychological realism, meaning that rules must mesh with underlying natural human nature: "One cannot ask for what the human frame cannot deliver" (Griffin, 1993, p. 162). Evolution entrenched in us both self-interest and limited altruism, and similar to members of other species, we defend ourselves with a tenacity that we do not display regarding most others of our own or other species.

James Q. Wilson (1993) maintained that moral and political philosophy must begin with a statement about human nature. Whereas we may disagree about what is natural, we cannot escape the fact that we have traits and predispositions that set limits on what it is possible to do, and these provide constraints and guides to what we should do. Although our moral sense is sophisticated, it has evolved, nonetheless.

Brink (1993) cited the importance of an individual person's self, but suggested that sacrifice by an individual can benefit other people. This conflict between the two faces of Adam and Eve was posed in chapter 2; some tendencies lead us to act from the well-spring of selfishness, whereas others compel beneficence toward others, leading to acts of unspeakable kindness. Recipients of beneficence are likely kin or members of one's social community who can reciprocate a moral agent's sacrifice, and the cost of missacrifice can be considered as a possible utilitarian benefit.

In *Human evolution, reproduction, and morality* (Petrinovich, 1995) I developed a theory that is the foundation for much of what will be discussed here: A basic distinction between moral agents and moral patients is crucial to moral standing. Moral agents have full standing in the moral community, and as such they have direct moral duties to one another and must assume burdens of moral responsibilities toward moral patients. Moral patients lack abilities that make them accountable for the outcomes of their actions. I distinguish between two classes of moral patients. The first is composed of humans, such as neonates, infants, mental defectives, and the senile. The second includes most if not all nonhuman animals. The reason for this division is to point up the critical nature of personhood—an idea that is discussed next—and to emphasize the importance of species membership.

Organisms that are incapable of reasoning or understanding abstract concepts cannot be held responsible for acts that injure others, because these moral patients are unable to understand concepts of right and wrong, or to comprehend ideas of causal relationships between their actions and the resulting effect on others. Moral agents, on the other hand, are considered to understand moral rules and the expectations of society, and are held culpable when violations of these rules and expectations occur as a result of their actions.

An event significant to moral standing is the point in development when an organism can be considered to have attained the status of personhood. I believe that the standing of personhood is achieved at birth, when a public and responsive entity, the neonate, first appears (Petrinovich, 1995, chapter 9). It is at this point that a biologically mandated social contract is struck between the neonate and members of that particular species community. The social bonds forcing such a contract have been demonstrated for most species of animals in which extended parental care is necessary for infants to survive. These social bonds are struck, and in many species provide the basis for community organization. Bonds between the human mother and her infant are especially important, and interactions between the two are critical to normal child development. This attachment leads organisms to develop in ways that are compatible with traditions of the society into which they are entering, and also encourage tendencies of members of the community who must take responsibility to foster the development and care of new members of society. In the ultimate sense it is important that the genes they share with others be perpetuated into future generations.

This evolutionarily mandated social contract makes human infanticide intuitively unacceptable, even though the neonate is not yet developed beyond the stage of a human moral patient. Although infanticide occurs under certain circumstances in many cultures, it requires explicit or implicit justification, just as do murder, incest, and war. The contract fosters cohesive elements that advance community reproductive interests, and as a result of successful enforcement of its terms it enhances the ultimate reproductive success of community members. These ideas are developed further when social contracts are discussed. It is important to draw philosophical distinctions carefully, because failure to consider the niceties of distinctions often clouds discussions of the responsibilities of humans toward humans and toward animals of other species.

Rights

The idea that individuals have rights that should be respected by everyone has considerable intuitive appeal. The case for animal rights was argued at length by Tom Regan (1983), and his treatment of the issue (considered in chapter 7) is referred to frequently in debates regarding the permissible treatment of animals by humans. Mackie (1984) characterized rights theory as an attempt to develop and clarify the popular notion that "everyone should have a fair go". A large number of positive rights have been claimed by different people, ranging from those involving basic aspects of existence to ones that reflect narrow specific interests. Among positive rights suggested are to life, to reproduce, to die with dignity, to privacy, to be wanted, to freedom, to pursue projects, to liberty, to respect, to control one's own body, to bear arms, to free speech, to freedom of association, to freedom of the press, to freedom of religion, to justice, to medical care, to a minimum income, to a job and housing, to sexual expression, and to private property. Several negative rights also have been suggested, including freedom from harm, torture, arbitrary arrest, imprisonment, execution, suffering, and hunger. These lists could be extended almost indefinitely, with people including and emphasizing their particular beliefs. When rights are considered as natural (see next section), care must be taken to ground them in some set of basic terms of existence, "Otherwise we may find that our proclamations have turned into platitudes, ritualistically carted out to excite a hoped-for emotional response, but bereft of substance" (Lomasky, 1987, p. 9).

Qualities of Rights

According to Almond (1993), rights have five basic qualities that must be explicitly recognized if the concept is to have any meaning: Who has them; what is their content; on what are they based and justified; are they inalienable; and are they absolute? In addition, rights are of different kinds. For example, active and passive rights include claims that generate a duty on a debtor, powers that endow one with a right to act to affect others, liberties that give one a privilege not to act, and immunities that protect one from the actions of others.

If rights are considered in terms of powers, the people who have them must be capable of making choices free from interference by others. There is no simple answer to the question of who or what has rights. Some suggest that the ability to reason satisfies the necessary and sufficient conditions to have the capacity for choice. This would include most adult humans and members of some other animal species, although Frey (1980) would exclude animals categorically on the grounds that they are unable to reason. Some contend one must be a person, which restricts rights to humans. Still others define the critical condition to be the capacity to suffer, which includes animals, but excludes comatose humans, and to have interests, which includes animals, human fetuses, and perhaps trees and plants, which could be construed to have a biological interest to reproduce. If the criterion adopted is too wide, the concept loses force, because it applies to everyone and everything; if it is too narrow it could omit categories of individuals that many desire to include.

It is necessary to define needs, desires, beliefs, and interests if they are to provide the criteria to determine who has the inherent value that some (e.g., Frey) state are necessary to provide a grounding for rights. Frey developed a philosophical position against granting animals moral standing based on his belief they do not have the necessary mental capacities. The position is extreme and defended with energy, but many (e.g., Regan,

1983; DeGrazia, 1996) consider it largely to be mistaken because it rests on an outmoded theory of mind and an inadequate appreciation of behavioral evidence. However, it is worth examining because it represents one of the extreme poles in the controversy.

Frey (1980) proposed that interests require beliefs, beliefs require minds, and animals have no minds in the sense of having what he called mental states. Because these terms are used almost universally, often without clear definition or with only a narrow stipulated meaning, it will be useful to consider what each of means.

Frey denied animals rights because they have no interests. He denied the broad concept of rights to humans as well, on the grounds that the only rights that should be recognized are legal ones that flow from the codes, rules, and laws society has developed to reflect the basic structure of natural morality. He found the concept of moral rights to be superfluous and difficult to ground, and nothing would be lost by giving up claims to them altogether. I will puruse this last point later in the chapter.

Needs, desires, beliefs, and interests are discussed to examine the conception of rights as a necessary factor. A basic concept is that of a *need*, which can be specified objectively and applied to most objects, and it can exist with or without a cognitive component. One can say that, to run satisfactorily an automobile needs gas. The auto does not know or experience this, but the need exists, as a prospective driver would soon find out. In this sense, a need refers to an objective state of a being. Animals need (among other things) food, water, and a balanced diet; their behavior might not reflect the need for a balanced diet, however, when, for example, a rat overindulges in food rich in sugars but lacking other dietary essentials. The rat persists in eating the sugar food, and might even die from a lack of essential dietary elements that are available but not consumed. The existence of needs can be determined through analysis of an organism (or machine) as a machine, looking at the way the system is built, how it operates, and how it is powered.

Desire is more difficult to understand because it implies the existence of mental components that cannot be observed directly. An animal might have a need, but no corresponding desire. If a desire exists there must be an object of the desire, which implies the animal has a concept of an object or action toward which the desire is directed. Often the existence of a *belief* is implied to the effect that an action will lead to a state satisfying the desire. With humans it is relatively simple to determine whether they have a belief; you ask, and if you want to check the veracity of the statement you observe the individual's behavior in an appropriate context. If behavior is consistent with the stated belief, all is well. With animals it is more difficult because they cannot respond to your question.

Research literature supports the conclusion that animals display behaviors that make it reasonable to assume beliefs and desires exist for them. For example, one can create an "expectancy" (which can include both a desire and a belief) for a highly palatable food and devise a task for an animal (say, a rat or a monkey) that, if solved will provide the food—a food that would be preferred over all others. If the hungry animal solves the problem and obtains the food it readily consumes it. However, if unbeknownst to the animal, a less palatable food had been surreptitiously substituted, when the animal solves the problem it will reject the less palatable food, even though it would normally have accepted it. Not only will the animal reject the food, monkeys were observed to even throw the cup at the experimenter when they received the less desirable food with the expectation they would get better stuff (Tinklepaugh, 1928). Tolman (1932) used the Tinklepaugh experiment to provide an operational translation of the concept of expectancy, and it embodies the characteristics sufficient to draw the inference that an animal has a desire, as well as the belief, that solving the problem will result in fulfillment of the desire for a highly palatable food object.

Frey (1980) insisted that beliefs cannot exist without language, because it is necessary to believe a given sentence is true; because animals lack linquistic proficiency they cannot believe any sentence is true. Hence, they are unable to believe anything, and because it is necessary to have a belief in order to have a desire, animals cannot have desires either. He based this theory on a behavioristic analysis that runs as follows: ". . . animals cannot have beliefs unless they have minds, and they cannot have desires unless they have beliefs; but they can and do have needs whether or not they have beliefs, whether or not they have minds, whether or not they are aware of their deficiencies in particular respects, and whether or not they are even conscious," (p. 73).

Interest is defined in terms of welfare: The individual has an interest in its well-being. To serve this welfare interest, animals should have an interest in a variety of things that contribute to their good or welfare. On the other hand, interests can also be considered in terms of preferences: Individuals have an interest in pursuing and obtaining what they prefer, they take satisfaction in this activity, and their preferences may serve their welfare interests. Of course, individuals might have a preference (as with the Sophisticated Lady, for "smoking, drinking, never thinking of tomorrow") that does not serve their good welfare. In Feinberg's (1978) view, to act in another creature's interest is to act for its good, and this thought is extended to include plants and "mere things," which, although they might not have interests of their own, might have a good or welfare we can promote or retard.

A question can be asked whether moral patients, such as babies, animals, and comatose persons can have interests, because they lack a coherent cognitive structure and even the construct of "things." It has been argued that interests can exist if the idea of an interest holder is extended to include community members who are moral agents, who have an interest in seeing that interests of moral patients are respected. Feinberg (1978) believes a mute creature can make claims only by means of a vicarious representative speaking for it. However, having no interests of its own, that creature has no good or welfare of its own, apart from those of the representative speaking for it. The concept of interest is compounded of wants and aims, which presupposes rudimentary cognitive equipment—"the ability to recognize and distinguish, to expect and believe, and to adopt means to ends" (p. 56). I engage this point in chapter 8 when the issue of marginal cases is considered. Interest is construed in terms of welfare interest throughout this discussion, because protecting the welfare of moral patients is one of the duties and responsibilities moral agents must assume.

Questions regarding the criteria for rights cannot be resolved until an answer has been provided to the question of who has rights (Almond, 1993). If the appropriate criterion is the capacity to suffer, then rights are passive claims by individual organisms against the infliction of pain by others. If the capacity for choice is the criterion, some individuals will have rights to act in certain ways, and their freedom of action will be protected from interference by others. It is the behavior of other people that is relevant to secure a right: It would be meaningless to claim a right in the face of physical events beyond the control of humans; it is meaningless to insist that we have a right not to experience an earthquake, unless we are imploring a wrathful deity. Must an individual be able to claim a right for that right to exist? For example, babies and comatose humans are not able to claim rights, but many consider them to have some, if only because of the responsibilities of moral agency other members of society must assume.

It is said that some rights are inalienable, whereas others can be waived if a person so decides. I could decide to relinquish my rights to my personal property and wealth and give it to some charitable organization, even though members of my immediate family might object. However, I am not permitted to forfeit my right to life and give you permission to murder me in cold blood. Some rights are absolute, such as the right to life, liberty, and not to be tortured, whereas others might be relaxed, subject to individual needs, concerns, and beliefs.

Questions regarding the relative importance of rights become serious when conflicts arise between people who champion different sets of rights. A classic instance is seen in the context of the abortion debate. Some feminist, pro-choice advocates argue their position by evoking the right of a woman to control her own body, and opponents insist that the right to life of the fetus is of paramount importance and must be protected at all costs. Each insists on the priority of the particular right they hold as basic, absolute, and inalienable, and there seems to be little hope that either side will convince the other. Another instance is when individuals insist that the right to free speech allows them to hold forth wherever and whenever, whereas others insist that the expression of free speech should not invade their personal right to privacy or threaten their collective safety. In cases such as the latter, it is possible for third parties to adjudicate the differences, and the likelihood is great that reasonable compromises can be reached: You insist on free speech, but agree to relinquish the freedom to yell "fire" in a crowded theater.

In many cases it is not possible for opposing parties to reach compatible agreement. One party prevails through force, it successfully obtains majority approval from the community, or it obtains a legal judgment on its behalf. This problem of evaluating the priority and relative importance of different values will be met once again when we consider the utilitarian position. One central problem for the utilitarian is to establish the relative good or harm of different possible outcomes of decisions.

The problem of justification is serious enough to lead me to suggest that rights should not be used at all, because it is difficult to arrive at more than arbitrary decisions regarding which ones have moral priority. If rights are justified as stipulated primitives, it is difficult to understand how they can serve a useful function as fundamental elements in moral discourse when different individuals stipulate different basic principles. For example, Dworkin (1977) does not ground his ideas of rights in human nature, but simply offers them as "fundamental and axiomatic," basing them on stipulation rather than argumentation. The use of stipulation, recommendation, intuition, and natural law to ground rights is open to attack. I believe that natural law can be used properly and profitably to ground human morality in evolutionary biology, with no loss to the richness of the concept of morality and without the attendant arbitrariness regarding content that the idea of rights entails.

Human Rights According to Lomasky

Ideas of the moral philosopher Loren Lomasky are worth examining because he developed a compelling and coherent theory of rights emphasizing individualism within the context of the social community. In this section I discuss his conception of human rights, and in the next section I recast it in terms of evolutionary principles that avoid the concept of rights, applying it only in the narrow legal sense. The biological conceptions sacrifice none of the power of rights arguments, avoid the arbitrariness involved in identifying the quality and content of rights, and use biological principles that have universal value in leading to understanding of the actions of sexually reproducing organisms throughout a range of animal and plant species.

Lomasky (1987) classified rights into three basic types. The most determinate and explicit are legal rights, defined by a body of law and institutional regulations. They are established by the community and designed to achieve specific practical goals. On the second level are moral rights, which assume different forms given the norms that characterize specific cultures, and they develop spontaneously in society. These moral rights are culturally relative, open ended, and mapped onto a more basic third level—natural rights. This level is morally regulative at the most general and basic levels of life. In my opinion this level is grounded in evolutionary biology, with its force being to enhance successful reproduction of individuals, which results in transmission of genes to succeeding generations. Natural rights are independent of any particular social structure, but presuppose some sociality whenever any moral community is involved, as inevitably it is. Lomasky accentuated the importance of sociality because he considered rights to be interpersonal. I will develop the implications of this view, but suggest that the idea of rights is not necessary to discuss moral principles. The most basic level—the natural—is discussed first, because the moral level is considered to map onto the natural, and the legal level is a codification of the moral level.

Lomasky began by stating that difference rights claims can be made at different life stages; once a child is born it enjoys the right to be wanted, a right it does not have before birth. Mackie (1984) contended that to maximize aggregate utility, the well-being of individuals should be considered at successive phases of life, and this perspective is more sensible than one focusing on maximizing the aggregate over a person's entire life. If a great deprivation is suffered at an early stage of life it might make no difference how many further goods are experienced—they might well be of little use. Brink (1993) held that it is important to recognize what he called the "separateness of person" stages, and insisted that one should be concerned with the way goods are distributed among the temporal stages of one's own life and among the lives of others. A biologically based theory of morality emphasizes the importance of such life history stages, and is based on the assumption that experiences at biologically significant stages are critical throughout the course of development. Congruent with my philosophy is the idea that birth signals the start of one of the most important stages ushering the neonate into the social community. At this point the human neonate is moved to a different status from that of moral patients of other species, because it is, for the first time, recognized as an individuated member of the human species.

Rights depend on a recognized individualism, and individuals have sovereignty over their own lives, in Lomasky's view. The hallmark of a person is to have a persistent attachment to ends that allows him or her to pursue projects free from interference by others. This emphasizes the importance of a biographical life, rather than a mere biological one. One problem with Lomasky's formulation is that young children do not hold rights because they do not yet have the critical characteristics that would allow them to pursue persistent projects. This same problem bedeviled Michael Tooley (1983), who used properties of neurophysiological development to ground moral agency. In his view, the requisite neurophysiological development required to support a unified consciousness over time (and to have thoughts) is not present in infants, and this development must occur to support the characteristics that establish the status of personhood with its attendant moral agency. Thus, personhood could not reasonably be said to occur before an infant was three months of age. If this criterion is accepted, infanticide would be permissible up to that age, a conclusion that Tooley and I (Petrinovich, 1995) both find intuitively unacceptable.

Lomasky worried that his ideas regarding infants were dubious because they lead to the conclusion that neonates merit no further moral attention than need be paid to a "piece of cheese or a puppy." To avoid such a conclusion he adopted the equally dubious one that embryos and infants possess rights because they are *potential* persons, and should be accorded moral rights because of this potential. Several objections can be made to positions based on potentiality. Harris (1992) contended that it is just as reasonable to maintain that, at conception, we are all potentially dead; yet, that would not be a sufficient reason to treat us as if we are already dead. In fact, the likelihood that we will be dead is much higher than the likelihood a neonate will live long enough to become a moral agent. Such weak arguments that individuals should be treated *as-if* they were something else than what they are should be avoided.

Feinberg (1980) identified what he called "the paradoxes of potentiality"; almost anything has potentiality to be something else, given appropriate circumstances. For example, dehydrated orange powder will be orange juice if water is added, or lemonade if we add a lot of lemon juice and sugar to the mix, or poisonous if we add arsenic, or a poisonous orange cake if we add cake ingredients and bake, or an orange-colored building block if we add cement and let it harden. It is best to focus on what *is* rather than *as-if*.

Kleinig (1991) agreed there is a paradox because anything at all can almost be anything else, making it absurd to appeal to potentiality as a basis for moral assertions. I discuss these and several other theories in chapter 10 of *Human evolution, reproduction, and morality,* where potentiality is rejected as it has been developed to oppose the permissibility of abortion.

Lomasky suggested young children are holders of rights because of their social relations to the community's project-pursuers (moral agents). This moves the argument regarding rights from one that is *internal* to the rights holder to one that is *external.* This change emphasizes mutual and reciprocal relations to others with whom one is involved in "complex recognition patterns," and it is critical because it provides the lever to avoid difficulties encountered when attempting to establish the moral status of children.

At the outset, the fetus is the private experience of the mother and it exists in relative anonymity. It is clear that *some* fetus is being carried, but little distinguishing information marks it as a *particular* fetus. Should it be instantaneously annihilated and another miraculously substituted in its place, the event would be undetected by community members. No one would either realize or appreciate that a distinct individual had been lost. Mother and fetus have a special relationship, and the mother's body responds privately to many of the events of pregnancy. At birth, however, mother and neonate undergo a transition from anonymity to public standing, and it is this event that signals the onset of personhood.

Richards (1996) objected that the presence of the fetus is known to others besides the mother, and that technology can detect the presence of a fetus even before the woman knows she is pregnant. Also, the father and relatives detect the fetus kicking prior to birth, "even with the first thump against the belly." At this point "plans will be laid for a contract with the Chicago Bears" (p. 560), and the parents realize that the fetus carries as an inherited legacy those social capacities that would make it possible for him or her to enter the social world of organized sports. Richards prefers the view that an individual becomes a person over a period of time during which biological development and social interaction advance, a process that begins in the womb. I discuss those developments in chapters 5 and 6.

It might well be that I overstate the case when I propose that interests and welfare of the existing person, the mother, trump those of the potential person, the fetus. The matter might better be considered by letting the mother's welfare play as a higher card than that of the fetus, with the value of the fetal card increasing as development proceeds. If this suggestion is taken seriously, the specific characteristics that confer increasing value must be specified if the argument is to bear meaningful weight.

I believe the welfare of the mother will always take precedence over that of a fetus whenever the mother's life is at stake. This belief is based on theories regarding the higher value of actuality over potentiality, as set forth in this section. The sequestered reality of the fetus is broken at birth, and the individuated human moral patient—the neonate—is now public. Its terrestrial appearance influences and determines the important qualitative change in the moral standing between it and fetus, and forges the social contract.

Infants can have rights even though they are not project pursuers, and they should be accorded the respect due rights holders, because at birth they become recognizable members of the social community—human moral patients. Lomasky considers rationality and the ability to reason as necessary conditions for one to have rights.

Lomasky (1987) appealed to the affection moral agents in the community have toward infants, noting that the community's moral agents suffer injury if an infant is harmed. He concluded, "Common morality ascribes rights to the child because it recognizes rights in the adult it will become. . . . To damage an infant is to damage the project pursuer it will be" (p. 160). Although one's own projects have first call on one's efforts, they need not have exclusive call, and it is important to have a stable morality that responds to the calls and needs emanating from others. His position can be recast in terms of a biologically evolved social contract, as explained below.

According to Lomasky, only a sentimental regard for young places them within the moral community, and it is the emergent potential of developing young to become project pursuers in life that provides this standing. He considered children's rights to be welfare rights; they need food, shelter, and emotional and intellectual stimulation. These, together with freedom from harm, are their basic natural rights.

At birth, the neonate enters a family, and that event is a ubiquitous aspect of human development. Having children is an integral component of a person's projects, and the family normally includes the mother and father (at least this would almost certainly have been the case in the EEA, if the infant was likely to survive). The parental pair, plus siblings and kin, continually nurture the infant; nurturance is required for it to survive, and care is often provided by unrelated members of the social community.

An Alternative Construal of Lomasky's Views

The evolutionary ideas I discussed at length elsewhere (Petrinovich, 1995) are compatible with many of those outlined by Lomasky, but have the added feature of being grounded by processes involved in biological development, and avoid problems encountered when the idea of potentiality is used to avoid approval of infanticide.

I discuss next mechanisms that evolved to promote emotional attachment between infants and caregivers (particularly the mother) and to enhance the likelihood young will be accepted by the community, which in turn would enhance the likelihood of survival. It is within the family that the earliest and most enduring patterns of intimate associations are established, and the family network of social relationships provides the raw material from which the moral community is fashioned.

The primary role of family members as caregivers entitles parents to a substantial guarantee of noninterference in a just society. Parents are accorded wide discretion in the specific ways they raise their children, with restrictions being placed only to guarantee the child is not harmed. Civic institutions prohibit abusive treatment and enforce laws protecting children, with considerable latitude permitted regarding parents' wishes in such matters as lifestyle, education, and medical care. In general, it is allowable to meet a child's welfare requirements in alternative ways, as long as they are considered adequate to prepare the child to live as an independent project pursuer.

I developed what Summer (1984) referred to as a natural rights theory, but avoided introducing the concept of rights. I believe it more useful to appeal to natural powers of the biological universe as they are understood by evolutionary biologists, ethologists, and, increasingly, psychologists.

Sumner expressed surprise that in modern debates only scant attention has been given to the question of what characteristics would make rights natural. He proposed that natural rights theory must satisfy four conditions: It contains some rights; it treats rights as morally basic; it ties possession of rights to possession of some natural property; and it accepts some form of realist epistemology. Feinberg (1978) suggested that a human right must be held equally by all human beings, unconditionally and unalterably. He extended this definition to include animals, as long as there is respect for a basic right not to be treated cruelly; a creature capable of suffering should not have to endure unnecessary pain or torment.

Sumner included two overriding basic requirements: Possession of properties that define the rights of an individual must be empirically demonstrable, and possession of those properties by an individual requires the existence of no particular institution or convention. He added the caveat that, whereas certain properties may be logically independent of social institutions, they could be causally dependent on such institutions. It is through institutions that these properties are expressed, and basic natural principles cannot be grounded on additional moral principles—individuals possess them by virtue of natural (evolved, biological) properties that are matters of empirical fact.

Lomasky was wise when he suggested critical stages in the development of moral standing should be considered from an external rather than an internal perspective. The advantage of the external view is that it stresses the interaction of an individual with members of the social community within which it is embedded: Morality is essentially interpersonal. The major problem with theories focusing on the individual's developing internal properties is that the social nexus receives little emphasis, and appeals have to be made to such things as sanctity of life or the developing sentience of the organism (viewed either neurophysiologically or psychologically). When one relies on the criterion of sanctity, there is little to discuss if the essentially theological grounds are not accepted. It is difficult to apply neurophysiological or psychological criteria consistently to give moral standing to human infants early enough without arbitrarily excluding animals of other species and decertifying comatose humans.

Lomasky's conception of the fetus as private and anonymous leaves the primary moral focus on the mother. The initial interaction with the fetus mainly is the private experience of the mother. A conceptual problem is that if one relies on potentiality as the critical factor, why should it not be pushed back to the individual sperm and egg before they are united, as each has the potential to combine to form an individual. I find that construal discomforting.

Lomasky concurred that a critical step in moral development occurs at birth, and it is generally agreed that something of profound developmental and social significance occurs then, even though some theorists have taken pains to discount its moral significance (see Petrinovich, 1995, chapter 9, for a detailed presentation of these arguments). At birth the neonate is no longer anonymous, but has a recognizable individual presence responded to socially by caregivers, especially the mother. These individuated behaviors evoke responses from the neonate, and caretakers interpret them to be social. The neonate is able to react to certain stimulus configurations (such as the voice tone used in the "motherese" spoken to the infant by almost all people, and to the configuration of the human face) with motoric activity and smiling. The research bearing on the infant's sensory, motor, and social capabilities is discussed in chapters 5 and 6.

Neonates and infants have innate tendencies to establish an immediate social bond between themselves and primary caregivers at the earliest possible moment. Visual components reinforce vocal components that are active prenatally and appear almost full-blown at birth. Such redundancy is important when the function being served—social bonding—is of extreme importance to guarantee the infant receives the special consideration that enhances the likelihood of being nurtured during a most critical time. Bonding will occur, and even through the infant might be blind or deaf, it will be capable of responding to other channels of input with a proper motoric response, usually through smiling and limb movement.

James Q. Wilson (1993) considered the family to be a universal human institution. Through the process of natural selection individuals are produced who are not simply skilled at reproduction, but skilled at parenting. Kinship ties are the essence of a family, and they sustain child care obligations, both economic and noneconomic, accompanied by mechanisms that restrict who has sexual access to whom. Virtually every society defines the family through a marriage that is a publicly announced contract, making the sexual union of a man and a woman legitimate, establishing explicit responsibilities for child care, and enunciating extensive provisions regarding the possession and distribution of goods.

These evolved patterns of interaction initiate a social bond admitting the neonate as an individuated member of the human species, and as such, provide it with the status of personhood. This status does not depend on the neonate's level of rationality (for it undoubtedly has little) but on an emotionally based bond established between the neonate and its community. Because the human infant requires an extended period of intensive care, this emotional bond is based on evolved behavioral processes that enhance the likelihood it will survive. This is necessary if the neonate is ultimately to contribute to the reproductive success of the parents.

This degree of moral standing entitles the neonate to have its welfare protected, and confers duties and responsibilities on parents as well as the social community. The mother is the primary caregiver, the father and immediate kin have both biological and social involvement, and the community at large is responsible to ensure the infant's welfare. The social bonds have an emotional basis, they do not depend on the infant's rational state, and they impose duties on all who are considered moral agents within the human community. These aspects of human nature develop in the normal course of existence, and in the EEA would have bonded infants with their kin, who would have lived near the infant. In modern times we usually live as close to nonkin as to kin (other than parents and siblings), so now the mutual advantage can be greater among friends and neighbors than among far-flung kin. Yet, because of their adaptive significance in the EEA, kinship ties continue to exert a powerful influence.

Considering matters this way emphasizes the importance of strong biological tendencies, extends moral standing to impaired neonates as well as to those who develop normally, and confers a personhood unique to the human animal—the child is recognizably one of us. We should show respect for a newborn puppy and be concerned with its welfare, but that concern has a different emotional base and tone from that enjoyed by the human neonate because of the processes of emotional bonding occurring immediately between it and its mother.

At this stage, the child has the standing of a moral patient, a standing also enjoyed by animals, but the infant displays specifically human emotional responses evoking the attribution of emotional capacities that set it apart from those other beings entitled to welfare respect. This special standing is due not merely to an infant's potential, but is based on the continuing evolved social dynamics among humans.

The next critical stage in moral development is when the individual moves from the status of moral patient to that of a moral agent with a full moral standing that confers several freedoms and duties: Freedom from harm and freedom of welfare and respect, and duties and responsibilities to extend those freedoms to others. The criteria on which the stage of agency are based are those rational and cognitive ones that make it possible to have the sense of a continuing autobiographical self, ability to understand rules, causation, and intentionality, and ability to reason. Learning is important in social development because it is the pivotal phenomenon permitting cultural transmission (Dennett, 1995). It makes it possible to encode information, think about it, and transmit it to others. With the advent of a written record, ideas can be transmitted to countless unseen generations of people now and in the future.

It is proposed later that it is important to understand indicators of these cognitive abilities when considering individual organisms, to avoid the oft-made charge of speciesism. These indicators are based not on typological assignment, but on the characteristics of individual organisms, and constitute the necessary and sufficient requirements to be a full member of a moral community. These aspects of cognition are discussed in chapter 6.

As noted when discussing Lomasky's ideas, an emotional bond establishing the initial social contract does not depend on mere sentimentality, but represents a biologically evolved social contract that enhances the ultimate evolutionary payoff—the inclusive fitness that contributes the currency of reproductive success in evolutionary systems. In one sense, these evolved dispositions are what Mackie (1984) called "spontaneous premoral tendencies," because they exist in many nonhuman species as well as in humans. They are fostered genetically, serve to resolve problems of survival, mimic the appearance of calculation and purposiveness, and, if internalized, become adapted normative conventions in behavior. When these tendencies are present they enhance cooperation, reciprocation, and legal norms that secure various explicitly identified legal rights. Within this perspective it is not necessary to grapple with qualities, content, or justification of rights, or determine where they came from. By viewing things from an evolutionary perspective, nothing of the power of Lomasky's theory has been lost, many confusing and complex issues that arise when rights are invoked have been avoided, and the concept can be justified on the basis of well-understood and generally accepted biological principles involved in the evolution of all sexually reproducing organisms.

The intent is to avoid problems arising when it is asserted that this and that kind of natural right is involved. Feinberg (1984) considered a right to be a valid claim against another's conduct, with the cogency of the claim being the reasons proffered in its support. The rights claim, in his view, becomes valid when its rational support is not merely relevant and cogent, but decisive. Theory based on evolved behavioral traits avoids the necessity of seeking rational support for the scope, content, quality, and power of rights, because these traits depend on social bonds evolved to serve the ends of successful reproduction.

I suggest a Benthamite position, assuming there can be no rights without duties and powers, and no duties and powers without laws. This position leads to the conclusion that rights should be constricted to the legal sense, accepting the view that the point of law is to abridge liberty for the sake of making remaining liberties more useful by restraining individuals from interfering with other individuals. It follows, as Midgley (1983) construed the matter, that rights have to be conferred explicitly by a particular society, and they can be given only to its own consenting members, with no one having a right who cannot understand and claim it. If this view is accepted, the tasks of philosophers are to identify rights under the law, to specify the duties and responsibilities the rights entail, and to make provisions for what ought to occur when actions suggested by those duties and responsibilities are violated.

The concept of rights should be restricted to the realm of laws and institutional regulations that are the codified norms and rules developed by each moral community within its cultural milieu to further the interests of its members. Institutions are natural entities that continue to grow throughout our lifetime; reforms to remove human suffering might not yield to changes external to a particular culture, because they require internal reform of basic institutions such as systems regulating property use and ownership.

The legal system within which laws are framed insists that those to whom rules are applied accept them. Laws depend on the independent existence of biologically developed natural moral factors that, while independent of the laws themselves, provide grounding for legal principles.

The concept of rights is a valuable construct and, contra Thomson (1990), they are assertions about privilege under the law. Thomson contended that it is not useful to consider legal and moral rights as two distinct territories within the realm of rights. I suggest we not use the term rights in the moral realm at all, but restrict them to the legal realm, believing nothing necessarily is lost in the process, while clarity is gained. This general position regarding the advisability of dropping the language of moral rights and restricting the term to legal rights was also set forth within the realm of environment ethics (Taylor, 1986).

Utilitarianism

Philosophical utilitarianism offers a distinct alternative to rights theories and is preferred by some who find too many problems when rights are extended to nonhumans. One of the major philosophers identified with the animal liberation movement is Peter Singer, who developed a utilitarian position. Singer (1990b) is explicit that when he speaks of rights it is only a convenient political shorthand that is in no way necessary to his position; however, he is not always consistent. When considering the moral standing of great apes, he just as explicitly wrote (Cavalieri & Singer, 1993, p. 1): "They have basic rights that are denied to those outside this sphere." The present discussion develops the basic ideas of utilitarianism in chapter 8, with Singer's arguments considered in detail.

Utilitarianism is one variety of the larger framework known as consequentialism, a position that stresses the general importance of considering the consequences of actions in order to address the issue of whether they are right or wrong. A critical problem is to define the relative goodness and badness of different actions. One can be a consequentialist and define good and bad in a number of ways, for example, in terms of one's own hedonic pleasure or pain, satisfaction or dissatisfaction, happiness or despair (ethical egoism), or one can use the classic ideal of establishing an objective characterization of pleasure and pain.

It is not a simple matter to evaluate the goodness of outcomes, because they vary not only along some qualitative affective dimension, but also in terms of the probability that an action will produce a given outcome, a probability that must be considered in context of the world in which the action is embedded. People consider the probabilities of various outcomes as being variable from time to time and place to place, rather than treating them as fixed, static quantities (Pettit, 1993; Wang, 1996b; Wang & Johnston, 1995).

The classic utilitarian conception of utility is formulated around attaining pleasure and avoiding pain. Some talk of aggregated levels of pleasure and pain across individuals. One disadvantage of this is that individuals become replaceable. Frey (1984a) noted that what matters when an individual is killed is the loss in total pleasure in the world produced by the loss of that individual's pleasure, even though the killing is done painlessly. However, if the killed person is replaced by another with an equal amount of good, the killing would not be wrong, because the world has experienced no total loss in aggregated pleasure. This position runs afoul of the compelling intuition that it is not permissible to harm (e.g., kill or torture) one innocent individual to increase the good of many others. Some philosophers reject such a monolithic utilitarianism, preferring a liberalism that accords an irreplaceable value to each individual, emphasizing that the worth of each individual must be protected—and I agree.

All utilitarian positions encounter problems when the relative goodness of different kinds of outcomes for an individual must be determined: Is being well fed better than being well sheltered; is enjoying pleasant companionship better than doing things that move one toward career goals; if such things do differ in goodness, how much better is the one than the other? Even more difficulties are encountered in determining relative goodness for different people: Is my experience of pleasure and contentment attained through writing books more or less than your pleasure in climbing mountains? The problem of determining the strength of different outcomes is pernicious, and is encountered whenever attempts are made to assess the relative strengths of different needs, desires, values, or preferences for a given individual, or across individuals. According to Pettit (1993), every moral theory invokes values in a manner making it sensible to recommend, in a consequentialist fashion, that they be promoted, or in a nonconsequentialist one, that they be honored. In the ultimate evolutionary sense, there is no problem, because we have an underlying metric that can be tuned to the value of various actions to enhance relative reproductive success, and this metric is reckoned in terms of relative contributions to inclusive fitness.

To avoid problems encountered by classic utilitarianism, a major variant, act utilitarianism, is often endorsed. Hedonistic and ideal varieties attempt to identify what one ought to do to produce the best consequences. Act utilitarianism is a conjunction of consequentialism (given its standard of intrinsic goodness and badness) and a range component, which means that right and wrong are determined by consequences affecting everyone (Frey, 1984b)

It is possible to evaluate action because people are likely to agree most of the time regarding states of affairs representing better consequences (Smart, 1973). Most agree that satisfaction of basic needs for food, shelter, clothing, and health are minimal conditions that all must have to enjoy any higher level of contentment. Once these minimal conditions are satisfied, Smart held that it is possible to evaluate the goodness of various types of contentment and enjoyment, and to grade them in terms of happiness defined in terms of the ability to attain enjoyment "at various times." This view considers welfare interests to be primary and other interests such as liberty as being less so, although Smart acknowledged that humans have an intrinsic preference for more complex and intellectual pleasures, a point emphasized by J. S. Mill as well.

Copp (1993) believed that meeting one's basic needs is of central importance to achieve good, and these needs might differ from an individual's preferences from time to time. There are objective needs: If a person has a basic need for something, he or she has a reason to secure it or keep it; if doing a certain act might prevent a person from meeting a basic need, he or she is not rationally required to do it. People have common fundamental needs, and they are not due to peculiarities of individual preferences. Finally, derivative needs are peculiar to background circumstances of particular contexts. For example, if one is in a continually dark environment (artificial or natural), one has is a derivative (but vitally important) need for light. Copp spoke of the necessity to "ground" a need in terms of what "the need is needed for." If a person needs something because of desire, preference, or value, it is merely occasional and not on the same level as basic needs required to survive and live an optimific life. Such things as a need for friends, companions, and a sense of self-respect, as well as freedom from harassment and continual fear, can be basic needs. A person who is deprived of these basic things is leading a blighted and harmed life.

Brink (1993) suggested that attention should be directed to the size of an individual's complaint (although it is difficult to understand what complaint adds beyond what is implied in that of need), and priority should be given to individuals who have most serious complaints. It might be possible to classify needs or complaints in terms of levels of urgency and aggregate them to obtain the best outcome within each level. In this way, one might be able to satisfy the aggregate needs of those who are worst off and still maintain non aggregation across levels. Such an approach might avoid the undesirable aggregative features involved in resource allocation, and would speak to Mack's (1993) objections regarding the lack of justice involved in aggregative forms of consequentialism. This issue is addressed further when justice is discussed within the framework of social contracts.

Lurking in the context of these viewpoints is the idea of preference utility, which some considered to be a weak concept on which to base a utilitarian theory. A preference utilitarianism is concerned with the maximization of desire satisfaction. Certainly, one desires not to be killed, and invoking that desire would bar replacement of one person that is to be killed by another in a comparable state, a replacement that could be considered permissible by classic utilitarianism. Although it is appealing to consider each person's preferences, it is difficult to accommodate all the various ideas of good that people might embrace in order to decide how to equate all "goods" within and across individuals to arrive at decisions regarding the moral permissibility of actions.

Goodin (1993) noted that J.S. Mill chafed at the conclusion that good is equivalent to desire because things such as truth, beauty, love, and friendship might not be desired by many people; Mill insisted these things are good, irrespective of an individual's desire. Whereas one person's list of necessary basic resources would be expected to be similar to anyone else's, when preferences, pleasures, and even pains are considered they can be highly idiosyncratic. Such variability makes it difficult to recognize and understand the preferences of others. It has been suggested that interest welfarism (which is similar to Copp's ideas regarding the importance of meeting basic needs) provides a better conception because it directly involves the satisfaction of welfare needs, abstracting welfare interests from expressed wants, giving the notion of utility practical content.

Social Contractarianism

The idea of a social contract is usually cast in either a legal sense or in one of honoring the promises an agent makes to others. Respect for contracts is critical to establish and maintain a just society, according to the theory developed in depth by John Rawls (1971), a theory that has received careful attention by the philosophical community (see Daniels, 1989). Social contracts are used here in a broader sense to involve behaviors of individuals who make up a community, and are grounded in evolved tendencies that promote the ultimate reproductive success of those individuals. Certain proximate behaviors evolved because they increased the likelihood of successful mating, reproduction, and nurturance of young, characteristics that enable them to reach the reproductive stage that continues propagation of genes in the family line. These behavioral tendencies are cooperation, communication, and reciprocation, and they are the behaviors that bind a society together.

The social contract is difficult to understand, because there is no inherent reason for such a theory to be individualistic, or to consider it as based on reasonable and free agreements of any kind (Kymlicka, 1993). The Kantian contractualism of Rawls (1971) is one of the most prominent theories of morality and provides the basis for his theory of justice. Rawls accepts the basic Kantian assumption that people should not be treated as means, but as ends in themselves. This moral equality entitles each person to equal consideration, which Kymlicka maintains gives rise to a natural duty of social justice that requires the promotion of just institutions; justice is not based on consent or on a desire to gain mutual advantage, but is simply owed to persons as such.

Feinberg (1989) construed Rawls' theory to fall within the social contract tradition because it emphasizes the importance of doing one's part if one accepts the goods provided by social institutions. It is not permissible to change rules in the middle of the game of life because that would disappoint honest expectations, and defeat welfare interests of those whose commitments and life plans were made with the assumption that the rules would be continued.

Instead, one should develop the idea of a social contract to embody a basic principle of impartial deliberation, with each person taking into account the needs of others as free and equal beings (Rawls, 1971). This contract gives equal consideration to everyone and is negotiated from a position of equality. Rawls refers to this as the original position in which people are asked to disregard knowledge of their status in society, to ignore the levels of their natural talents and endowments and their role in the social structure. It is inescapable that some people will be better off than others because of natural and social advantages they enjoy through the draw in the natural lottery, a factor that is beyond anyone's direct control.

It is hoped that by disregarding one's original position, all people are treated similarly, because no one knows what hypothetical position he or she occupies in society due to what Rawls calls the veil of ignorance. Although everyone might be trying to do the best they can for themselves, they do not know whether they are in a hypothetical favored or unfavored position in society. They may be better able, if they are well-intentioned, to decide impartially what is best for everyone who will be influenced by a decision. This mechanism is employed with the hope it will enhance the likelihood that people identify sympathetically with every person in society, and take the interests of all individuals into account as if they were their own interests—a bit of the Golden Rule. One presupposition is that individuals have a sufficiently developed imagination to form an adequate notion of the possibilities for themselves and for others, as well as the emotional flexibility to have empathy for feelings of others.

Rawls invoked a difference principle when considering how surplus resources should be distributed: The position of the better-off is to be improved only if necessary to improve the position of the worst-off. Decisions should not allow lesser life prospects for some to produce a greater sum of advantages for the aggregate.

The distribution of surplus goods is of major interest in Rawls' theory of justice. It is assumed that each individual should be motivated to demand what is due, and that each is disposed to expect and to favor demands by others for their due, while refraining from actions that would deprive anyone. All persons may be expected to pursue individual self-interests, with special (evolved) deference to interests of friends and relatives, but with safeguards against favoritism or free riding. To make social cooperation possible, it is necessary to prevent free riding (Gauthier, 1993). Although it could be selfishly advantageous for an individual to be a free-rider, as well as to show undue partiality toward friends and relatives, it could also be advantageous for people to cooperate with strangers to receive fair deals for themselves and to detect when others are cheating. James Q. Wilson (1993) considered the norm of reciprocity to be universal, and that virtually everyone who has looked has found it in every culture for which information is available. He considered the rule requiring reciprocity to be as strong as the incest taboo, and that it is instilled to detect backsliders.

A number of research studies support the view that people have special evolved cognitive mechanisms to detect cheaters. These studies investigated modes of solving logic problems involving social interactions that included an element of trust to the effect that others were honoring the rules of the system compared with problems not involving trust, but with the same logical form (see Gigerenzer & Hug, 1992; Tooby & Cosmides, 1992). Formal logic problems that were seldom solved when presented in a neutral setting were figured out quite easily when framed to detect cheaters.

Social cooperation is necessary if humans are to survive, reproduce, and flourish. We can suppose each person would want other members of the community to possess a sense of justice, would prefer to interact with those who possess it, and would find a sense of justice desirable insofar as it increases the willingness of others to interact with them to enjoy fuller realization of their own concerns. This desire to conform to societal norms that promote justice can be viewed as the outcome of an evolutionarily developed social contract, even though it may not have a rational foundation.

Gauthier (1993, p. 197) commented, "A community of persons each possessing a sense of justice may be expected to exhibit both greater stability and greater success in capturing the potential fruits of cooperation than a comparably sized group of persons lacking that sense. Competition between the two groups should favor the former. A sense of justice is thus functionally useful at the social level." Individuals would be expected to survive and flourish if they cooperate with other members of their community, and the sense of justice that fits them for such cooperation is valuable no matter what their particular aims and concerns. This account of justice establishes a link between the rational acceptance of emotional bonds forged to enhance social cooperation, considered at the ultimate evolutionary level, and the use of these bonds to promote the individual proximates realization of utilitarian goals.

Baumeister and Leary (1995) conducted an extensive review of psychological research concerning the desire for interpersonal attachments as a fundamental human motivation. They concluded this desire is one of the most far-reaching and integrative constructs available to understand human nature, because the need to belong satisfied all of the criteria for a motivation to qualify as fundamental and innate. These criteria were as follows: They readily produce effects under all but adverse conditions; have affective consequences; direct cognitive processing; when thwarted, lead to ill effects (such as on health or adjustment); elicit goal-oriented behavior designed to satisfy them; are universal, in the sense of applying to all people; are not derivative of other motives; affect a broad variety of behaviors; and have implications going beyond immediate psychological functioning.

This attachment motivation could be based initially on bonding between mother and infant, as I believe. The authors suggested these tendencies would be selected because they enhance reproductive success by motivating people to seek frequent, affectively positive interactions within the context of long-term, caring relationships. Their conclusion (p. 520) was: "People form social bonds readily, even under seemingly adverse conditions. People who have anything in common, who share common (even unpleasant) experiences, or who simply are exposed to each other frequently tend to form friendships or other attachments. Moreover, people resist losing attachments and breaking social bonds, even if there is no material or pragmatic reason to maintain the bond and even if maintaining it would be difficult."

A contractarian moral system was developed by the evolutionary biologist, R. D. Alexander (1987) in his book, *The biology of moral systems*. He held that individuals seek to further their ultimate reproductive interests in ways involving both direct and inclusive fitness involving kin, mates, and others in the community, and that it is important to maintain status and a good reputation within the community to enjoy the fruits of reciprocation. This interest in community status restrains unbridled self interest that might be deleterious to the interests of others. He stressed the importance of considering pleasure and comfort within the context of reproductive interests. These are not trivial refinements because they ground contractarian and utilitarian models of moral philosophy in modern evolutionary biology.

Moral Pluralism

When a hierarchy of different needs is involved, it is possible that a moral pluralism must be applied that emphasizes different kinds of needs and desires that make the lives of different people good. Kekes (1993) identified three basic philosophical conceptions that have been proposed. The first is monism, arguing for one and only one reasonable system of values that is always the same for all humans everywhere. The task in applied ethics, according to this view, is to create institutions, formulate principles, and educate people to enhance the likelihood they will live according to the one reasonable system of values.

The second is relativism, in which all values are the result of conventions developed within the context of political, cultural, economic, and religious influences. There cannot be, according to this view, a uniquely reasonable system of values because no one value can be justified on objective grounds; all are culturally relative and affected by contextual realities.

The third position, which Kekes accepts, is moral pluralism, taking into account the relationships between different sets of primary and secondary values, and considering a life good only if it is both "personally satisfying and morally meritorious." Humans have a plurality of primary values that include basic physiological needs (e.g., having food and not being tortured), psychological needs (e.g., for love and freedom from humiliation), and social needs (e.g., for respect and freedom from exploitation). In addition to these primary values, a plurality of secondary values includes things that allow one to derive personal satisfaction from connoisseurship, artistic pleasure, peak physical condition, sense of humor, artistic creativity, and cultivation of style. These are important contributors to the good life, but would not necessarily be involved in leading a moral life. This concept of the good life is broader and more inclusive than that of the moral life. Certain things could be impediments to a good life—ignorance, stupidity, and impoverished imagination—that would prevent people from making use of their possibilities. These could result from the bad luck of the draw within natural or social lotteries, or from inadequate nurturance even though the initial draws were satisfactory. These ideas raise problems regarding what should be done when a conflict arises between moral (primary values) and nonmoral (satisfaction promoting) components.

Perhaps the best way to encourage a personally satisfying and morally meritorious life is to adopt a moral pluralism respecting what individuals wish for themselves. This pluralism emphasizes the realization of possibilities that may make lives good. Pluralists should set their own conception of the good life as merely one possibility among many reasonable options, understanding that there is no absolute basis to prefer one particular set of secondary values over others. Individual differences are fostered, and experiments in different ways of living are encouraged as long as actions neither harm others nor deny their interests and liberties. The assignment of weights to such incommensurate and incompatible secondary values is a serious problem when seeking to develop pluralistic moral principles that provide an appropriate basis to decide proper courses of action.

A pluralistic moral system insists that primary needs must be guaranteed to all, but realization of primary needs might still be worth very little to people if they cannot enjoy secondary values that are peculiar to their idea of the good life. It is possible to respect the primary value of liberty, but still maintain that an individual can voluntarily give up one's liberty, by joining the army, for example. Thus choices must be reasonable and voluntary, and the focus is on those possibilities the realization of which might make lives good. As Kekes (1993, p. 14) wrote: ". . . it thereby wishes for us what we wish for ourselves."

This view acknowledges that one value might override another when the two come into conflict—what is called a "trump"—and a particular value might always take precedence over all others when it is present. Kekes considered a value to be overriding if and only if it has five characteristics: It is the highest, thereby taking precedence over all conflicting values; it is universal, meaning it holds for all human beings; it is permanent, holding for all times; it is invariable, holding in all contexts; and it is either absolute, meaning it ought not to be violated under any circumstances, or prima facie, meaning it holds normally, but may be violated in a specific circumstance if and only if the violation is required by the value in general.

Moral pluralism can be sensible evolutionarily. One enduring fact of biological adaptations is that it is desirable to preserve variability in the distribution of phenotypic traits in a breeding population. Too much homogeneity in population characteristics could be detrimental to the survival of individuals whenever external conditions change quickly and radically. It might be desirable, therefore, for the moral ideal to have a framework that fosters realization of plural, conditional, incompatible, and incommensurate proximate values, rather than one that establishes some specific value that always trumps. We should always remember, however, the one overriding ultimate value in the evolutionary view—differential reproductive success.

The Concept of Value

Much of the discussion in this chapter dealt with issues that arise when it is necessary to determine the relative moral value of different courses of action. If a society is to be moral, the principles developed to promote morality have to respect basic values that define it. The concept of value is of paramount importance when cost-benefit analyses are involved, and a number of difficulties arise when estimating the strength of different values. It does not matter whether a theory is based on deontological rights or utilitarian outcomes. It is necessary to assign values to possible outcomes in terms of either the respect of rights or outcomes of cost-benefit calculations; it is necessary to estimate how to determine the relative good and bad of various states of being and outcomes of actions.

Macklin (1988) believed philosophers have a major responsibility to clarify the logical aspects of moral theories and to explicate their metaphysical aspects. There are epistemological problems, and she blamed shortcomings in social science theory and practice for difficulties encountered in attempts to determine the critical facts required to apply moral theory. I suggest the basic problem is that philosophers are not aware of the progress social scientists have made to measure qualitative subjective states, coupled with a tendency to view moral quandaries as so complex they will not yield to objective measurement.

Macklin was correct when she remarked that a theory that cannot be applied, or one that is exceedingly difficult to apply in practice, is a flawed theory. It will never be possible to decide which of a set of competing theories is correct. However, clarifying the nature of underlying theories can provide a deeper understanding of the conflicts regarding morally relevant considerations, making it possible for reasonable opponents to agree to disagree. The relationship between ethical theory and action is the same as the relationship between scientific theory and empirical data. Nagel (1979) agreed, noting that ethics is not a science, but that the relation between ethical theory and practical decisions is analogous to the relation between scientific theory and beliefs about the world.

It is difficult to estimate relative strength when deciding which of qualitatively different values are the more important, and which should be brought to bear to support a decision. It is especially difficult when decisions regarding which value is the strongest involve two or more values that belong to different dimensions. It is even difficult to decide whether two different values should be considered to belong to one or two dimensions: Do pain and pleasure represent qualities that are not directly comparable, or can they be scaled along a single affective dimension? In either case the problem is to determine how much of the one is equal to the other. If it were possible to estimate degrees of pain and pleasure using some comparable unit, we still have to determine the number of units on the pain scale that equal a certain number of units on the pleasure scale, and whether this comparability should be established in biological, moral, or psychological units. In the qualitative sphere, decisions involve questions such as what degree of ill health is equivalent to how many years of life, and how each of these should be valued in light of costs to provide them.

Although it can be argued these questions are merely interesting conceptual niceties, they arise whenever the priority of different rights is raised, and whenever it is necessary to determine the utilitarian outcome of different decisions. Questions regarding the strength of relative values and estimation of their relative importance are major stumbling blocks for most ethical theories when they are applied to decide the morality of one course of action versus others.

When discussing philosophical concepts regarding important values that should be used to decide morally permissible treatment, deciding relative value is a central concern. For Griffin (1993), it was how values are to be recognized and scaled (see p. 54). Almond (1993) identified five different qualities involved in the idea of rights, including who has them, their content, and how to distinguish between active and passive rights (pp. 57), and asked, when different people champion different sets of rights as basic, which should prevail to determine social policy (pp. 60–61). Frey (1984a) worried about the difficulty and propriety of aggregating pleasure and pain across individuals. Lomasky (1987) rejected any aggregated utilitarianism, preferring liberalism stressing the necessity of protecting the worth of each individual (pp. 63–64). Goodin (1993) acknowledged strong arguments regarding the list of goods so necessary they would be desired by all (e.g., freedom from pain and hunger) as well as idiosyncratic preferences that various individuals would value just as highly (e.g., freedom of speech, religion, being honest, and keeping promises); p. 77. Kekes (1993, pp. 81–83) held out for a moral pluralism, with different primary and secondary values. He suggested plurality of primary values, including basic physiological, psychological, and social needs, as well as secondary values, such as personal and artistic pleasures, humor, style, and creativity, generally respecting what people wish for themselves.

In addition to general expressions of philosophical concern, specific questions refer to relative values that move to the forefront when the welfare of animals is compared with that of humans. The relative value of an action has to be considered whenever questions involve the permissibility of using animals for the benefit or enjoyment of humans. Not only are these difficult issues, but the procedures used to estimate the strength of competing values often are not consistent, nor are they applied universally, especially when choices involve different kinds of creatures.

One of Regan's (1983) central concerns was over equal inherent value (chapter 7); Feinberg (1978) said that human's duties to animals should rank below the greater claims due family, friends, and other humans (chapter 7); Singer wrestled with the problem of how to equate the pain of animals with such peculiarly human interests as enjoying a longer and vigorous life and enriching the human condition, and suggested that beings able to live fuller lives might have more moral value (Chapter 8).

When discussing basic concepts of moral philosophy in *Human evolution, reproduction, and morality* (Petrinovich, 1995) attention was devoted to estimating relative value. Brandt (1987) questioned how it can be decided that the value to speak freely on political matters might be stronger than the value to own capital goods, and how both can be considered weaker than the right not to be tortured. It is intuitively obvious that the right not to be tortured ought to be stronger than the other two and that it should trump them. What of the relative value of free political speech and owning goods? Here, considerable differences of opinion arise, and it is important to resolve such differences amicably if society is to function reasonably.

There are several ways to estimate relative values. One would be to assign all values to an explicit category according to their overall moral relevance. Kagan (1988) suggested that clusters of value should be identified, the assignment of an action to one cluster should be based on sound fundamental moral theory, and cluster assignment should justify actions. Several schemes to form clusters have been suggested: Natural rights and liberty rights (Lomasky, 1987); basic, fundamental, and derivative needs (Copp, 1993); urgent and less urgent needs (Brink, 1993); a plurality of primary and secondary values (Kekes, 1993); and welfare and secondary interests (Feinberg, 1989).

If a series of qualitative categories is established, it would not be difficult to let those values that are assigned to the basic category trump ones in the lesser categories. This would be a satisfactory process if only the world presented us with simple, uniform, one-dimensional alternatives. Unfortunately, it usually does not; several values might be involved at the same time, and they all must be considered to determine a proper course of action. It might be necessary to consider some values as high cards rather than as trumps, and this brings us back to the problem of how to assign relative worth to each. Although the problems of estimating relative strengths of different values are difficult, they are not insurmountable and if a reasonable practical ethics is to emerge from sound ethical theory, they must be faced squarely.

Kagan (1988; discussed in Petrinovich, 1995, pp. 127–128, 148–150) pondered how to decide to combine different values. One intuitively appealing method is, once the elements have been identified, to add up the strengths of those values in each of the actions and choose the one that has the most positive points. Even if it were possible to make these identifications and assign proper strengths (a couple of big ifs), it is by no means obvious that an additive principle will be sufficient. Some things might trump others, meaning that certain actions would be demanded (or prohibited) whenever one of the trump utilities is in the ledger, no matter what the alternatives. If such is the case, a multiplicative rule would be appropriate: The critical utility would assume a zero quantity if the action is to be prohibited (always resulting in a product of zero for that action); if the value is of vast importance, it could assume a quantity many times that of any other utility in the equation (which would swamp the product of any other set of utilities that did not include the critical one).

Another problem is the possibility that a value might have different strengths depending on the context in which it appears (Becker, 1973). A value might take a large number of different legitimate quantities depending on the setting and the effect it has on other individuals who are not considered in the equation. Therefore, a value could be distributed in different ways in different circumstances. Sumner (1981) thought it was not possible to devise a formula to weight the various factors involved in many moral decisions because the relevant variables display too many variations and combine in too many novel and unexpected ways.

Whenever the situation is so complicated that neither a simple additive nor multiplicative rule leads to intuitively adequate outcomes, the sets of values must be considered in terms of complex, higher-order interactions. The point of going into this number stuff is not to support the conclusion that the matter is hopelessly complex, as many would have it when they face a set of variables. Measurement, scaling, and analytic procedures were developed by social scientists to find order and rationality when underlying reality is extremely varied. I suggest that closer collaboration between philosophers, measurement and statistical specialists, and those in applied disciplines (such as social and biological scientists, engineers, educators, and medical experts) would represent an important step toward resolving some of the epistemological problems that concerned Macklin.

These abstract niceties are fine, but what happens when reality is examined (see Petrinovich, 1996, pp. 78–81, 130, 156–157)? Kamm (1993) examined the problem of establishing relative value in the context of organ donation, posing the question of how one should determine the relative value of living an additional five years at the end of life, compared with completing a work in philosophy. If it is decided the work in philosophy is sufficiently valuable, one might, on utilitarian grounds, give the organ to enable the author to live the five years required to complete the work, rather than allocate it to someone who will live the five years but not complete any particular project. The problem involved in seeking a neat solution in this case is that an impermissible elitism could be promoted that would violate the equal right to life of the two individuals. The critical question is, should such a weight be used to tip the balance in favor of one versus the other? Although no easy solutions are at hand, at least the relevant philosophical principles can be recognized, and the decision can be debated and decided on the basis of some logical conclusion from an identifiable set of basic premises.

The importance of the general and specific views as discussed can be illustrated by actual situations in which systematic scaling procedures were use to solve difficult problems in the distribution of scarce medical resources (Petrinovich, 1996, chapters 5, 8, and 10). Kilner (1990) developed a scheme to allocate scarce organs for transplantation to needy recipients based on socio-economic, medical, and personal criteria. Each criterion was evaluated in terms of its utilitarian value, emphasizing two principles: The most good for the most people and individual well-being. Following this analysis, policy recommendations were drawn up that included important values from the list. Although this method is considerably subjective, it is a valuable step because it brings the values applied into public view, and suggests ways to make the moral choices demanded within the scope of medical and financial realities.

More formal procedures were used by the state of Oregon, which faced severe economic problems due to a desire to provide universal access to health care for all its citizens. To do this on an unlimited basis was not possible economically. Therefore, a rationing plan was established based on a model of informed decision making (Kaplan, 1993, 1994). Groups of citizens developed standards of care that Oregonians determined to be important to their communities. This step provided a list of possible condition-treatment pairs that concerned citizens. When thirteen standards were identified, the citizens arranged them in a list by priority, thus capturing the relative values of community members. At this point a committee of experts from a variety of medical specialties evaluated the services using a quality of well-being scale (QWB) constructed by Kaplan and his group. They estimated the expected medical value of treatments for various conditions, thus capturing values of the medical community.

The QWB was then used to obtain opinions from a sample of Oregonians regarding the relative desirability of treating various health conditions to capture the values of citizenry. Up to this point the issue of financial costs was ignored in the interest of determining the medical value of treatments without having financial realities impose explicit constraints. In light of financial realities, the treatment list was reduced to 568 high priorities the state could afford to provide. Conditions not covered were those for which treatment is ineffective because they just run their course, a home remedy exists that is just as efficient, treatment is cosmetic, or treatment is futile. The plan covered all effective preventive medical care, visits to physicians for diagnosis and treatment, psychological treatment for conditions ranging from psychosis to substance abuse, gynecological care, noncosmetic surgery, physical and occupational therapy, dental services, prescription drugs, and hospice care. The plan was put in place, over objections by some of the conservative elements of the public, and now enjoys widespread support by Oregonians.

Other formal and informal approaches to allocate scarce resources have been successful, several of which I described in *Living and dying well* (1996). It is possible to use instruments developed by social scientists, along with information regarding effectiveness of treatments developed by medical scientists and practitioners, combined with estimates of financial costs developed by medical economists, to provide factual bases to demonstrate the reasonableness and practicality of moral positions delineated by moral philosophers. Because differences exist in basic values people use to ground the premises of their beliefs, complete agreement will never be possible. Clear understanding of such differences, however, should make it possible to recognize them as well as reasons for points of agreement. This represents the first step in developing mutually acceptable policies by well-intentioned persons. Resulting policies will have a bit of the reality of utilitarian cost-benefit and equal respect for individual freedoms that should be respected in a just society.

Points made by Nagel (1979) provide a good summary of this section. Human beings are subject to moral and motivational claims of very different kinds because they are complex creatures who view the world from many perspectives—individual, relational, impersonal, and ideal. Each perspective results in different claims, and these claims might be difficult to resolve when they conflict with one another. Because of these conflicting and incommensurable claims, something (or nothing) must be done, but a unitary action does not mean justification is also unitary.

Good judgments might not be completely justifiable—they are satisfactory, the best that can be done given the circumstances. The hope is that general principles can be discovered and codified by understanding patterns embedded in the decisions people make and in their intuitions. Nagel emphasized that this analysis is not a method of decision making; it is one way to understand the ethical considerations involved in reaching responsible and intelligent decisions. This discovery process might reveal that general principles in practical, ethical reasoning have to be restricted to one aspect of the subject (e.g., one specific component of rational motivation) rather than be comprehensive. What is proposed is a method to analyze practical problems to discover what evaluative principles are relevant and should be applied. A simple description of basic methods that can be used to discover and codify principles that guide decisions can be found in Petrinovich (1981). It might be possible to create a domain-specific ethic that is comparable with domain-specific cognitive principles developed by cognitive scientists using insights provided by evolutionary theory. I have suggested throughout this book that ethical theory might profit if the same vein of evolution is mined.

This excursion through philosophical issues involved in rights, utilitarianism, social contractarianism, moral pluralism, and the concept of value should provide an adequate basis to consider moral positions regarding the ethical treatment of animals. More philosophical issues are discussed in chapter 4, together with matters relating to the philosophy of science. These issues become critical when questions regarding the permissibility of research using animals arise. Often they ask how it is possible to know the value of following a line of research before the results are known, and how it can be decided what changes constitute progress in science. Problems address how general conclusions can be drawn from specific observations, and how widely experimental results can be generalized to animals of the same species and to those of other species. Questions regarding the worth of various kinds of research projects are among the most hotly debated when discussing the treatment of animals, and they are addressed directly in later chapters. Too often important matters regarding research methods and philosophy of science are badly understood and willfully misused by those on different sides of the debates. The intent of chapter 4 is to clarify them to bring the discussions of research presented in chapters 9, 10, and 11 closer to the point of reasonableness.

4

Research Methods and the Aims of Science

The use of animals in biological and behavioral experiments has been discussed extensively. One polar position is that such use is never permissible whenever it would not be permissible morally to subject humans to the same procedures. The opposite pole is that any research with animals is permissible whenever it is possible to improve the human condition, and even in the interest of reaching a better abstract understanding of the workings of the universe. Often great passion is evident in these debates, similar to that surrounding abortion or physician-assisted suicide.

To approach the question of whether and under what circumstances animal research is permissible, abstract points regarding the nature of science in general should be considered, to understand the relationships between data and theory. Scientific progress also is important—how it can be decided that something is worth knowing, and if knowing it represents an advance in knowledge that warrants research time and effort. Generalization of data to theory is another central issue, especially generalizing on the basis of data obtained in one species, with one testing procedure, or a single situation. Specifically, how broadly can results be generalized to arrive at general laws of biology, behavior, or psychology, or be applied to alleviate suffering?

Conceptual Frameworks

The most critical aspect of science is the conceptual framework used to organize data and ideas. Essential changes in scientific understanding are embodied in changes in conceptual frameworks. These frameworks are usually formalized in terms of explicit theory that describes three things:

The interlocking system of laws that constitute the formal terms of theory; identification of observables in terms of indicators by which they will be indexed; and the relationship among different observables, between theoretical constructs and observables, and of constructs to one another.

This conceptual framework was called a nomological net (Cronbach & Meehl, 1955) and can be visualized with the metaphor of a fish net, with the nodes of the net being theoretical constructs (nomologicals) and the strands connecting them the functional laws that relate one construct to another. To have science, rather than philosophy or literature, at least some of the laws must explicitly be related to observables. Observations must be quantified at least to the extent of identifying the conditions under which an event is present and those under which it is absent.

The system of laws constituting a theory can be in terms of fixed probability statements that hold always and everywhere, or they might be statistical, embodying varying likelihoods that depend on contingencies, such as those produced by the total context within which events occur. Evolutionary theory, for example, involves a complex web of interacting factors, and most statements are of the *if . . . then*, variety—sometimes with a lot of *ifs* and a lot of *thens*. To know more about a theoretical construct it is necessary to elaborate the nomological net, which can be done by adding a new construct that serves as a primitive term in the structure. This addition advances the theory as long as the new construct is supported by reliable observations. The net is also improved if adding a new term makes it possible to eliminate others, thereby reducing the total number of nomologicals; this results in greater parsimony, as revealed by explanatory elegance and efficiency.

Reliable measurements are the heart and soul of science. The same observer should record the same event when it is observed on a subsequent occasion (intraobserver reliability), and different observers should record the same event when the same object is observed at the same time (interobserver reliability). It is difficult to ensure that measurements are indicators of what they are supposed to measure—that they are valid. If I want to measure intelligence, the concept "intelligence" must be defined explicitly, and the operations to measure it should exhaust the construct as defined. To establish validity it usually is necessary to rely on more than one way of measuring a construct, including such items as vocabulary, analogies, verbal problems, numerical problems, reaction time, spatial problems, and a variety of performance measures. One also must show how different lines of evidence converge to give a similar answer, a process known as establishing construct validity (Cronbach & Meehl, 1955). Various indicators should combine to provide a more reliable and valid estimation of intelligence than any one of them, and if strong discrepancies exist, the reasons for them should be investigated, because the underlying construct might not have been conceptualized adequately.

In experimentation, it is important to allow the variable of interest to interact within a representative background of variables with which it competes, cooperates, and interacts, to understand its force in the natural ecology. Whereas the true experiment, in which all variables but the one of interest are eliminated or held constant, can help establish the possible importance of a variable, it must be studied in a representative context to understand its real importance. It also is important to measure constructs that are critical to a theory using different methods and apparati, to establish the generality of conclusions independent from the specific ways it has been studied—to establish construct validity.

Contexts of Discovery and Justification

Several distinct tasks must be performed if an adequate and useful theory is to be developed. First, a theory must be invented. Based on current understanding of reality, it considers how the world should be viewed, using hunches and guesses to create an idea about how all these things come together to produce the reality of concern. This initial stage is common to all storytelling, be it religious, philosophical, literary, or pseudoscientific. Eminent philosopher of science Sir Karl Popper (1959) referred to this as the context of discovery, a term coined by Hans Reichenbach, that involves a series of events that are not specific to science. Some (e.g., Francione, 1995; Regan, 1983; Rollin, 1989; Singer, 1990a) asserted that this initial subjectivity undermines the epistemological basis of science, a position I believe is not only wrong, but could well reduce science to the consideration of empty minutiae.

Popper (1963, p. 50) wrote, "Thus science must begin with myths, and with the criticism of myths; neither with the collection of observations, nor with the invention of experiments, but with the critical discussion of myths, and of magical techniques and practices." He drew a sharp line between the context of discovery and what he called the context of justification. The latter requires that observations be made to bring evidence to bear on theoretical expectations. That is, observations are gathered to justify a theory or, better, to falsify it (more on falsification in a moment). I maintain that Popper created too marked a difference between the contexts.

It is helpful to make some rough distinctions between discovery and justification in science, and I believe the following propositions are specific enough to do this.

1. To make it reasonable to engage in science, one must believe that the universe contains *lawful regularities*. These can take the form of general universals that are always true, other things being equal, or consist of probabilistic statements whose truth depends on the actions of other variables as well as the inherent variability of nature. If time and energy are to be devoted to understand regularities, any form of strict indeterminism must be rejected and at least a weak form of induction accepted, even if only at the level of a belief that "facts" represents more immediately accessible sensory experiences shared by different observers, and that these facts reflect something of an external reality.

2. *Empiricism* is one way to discover these regularities. There must be the conviction that it is possible to make observations, and that these observations are related to whatever conceptualizations are developed.

a. Empiricism is based on *measurement*, which requires at the lowest level that identification can be made whenever an event is present or absent. Such a primitive identification can be important at this point for both science and nonscience. It is here that logic and mathematics enter the picture. The methods of subjective philosophers and those of scientists do not differ up to this point. Philosophers rely on evidence of the senses and on internal consistency of the reality concocted based on these senses, just as do scientists, whereas mathematicians work within the confines of pure logic. Measurement at the level of identification is as important for philosophers as much as for scientists.

b. Scientists must propose an additional measurement scheme, even if it continues to be as crude as simple identification (presence or absence of an event). To proceed, scientists must provide an *operational translation* of conceptual variables that is explicit enough to allow the occurrence of some observable event to be taken as an instance of some latent conceptual entity. This requirement does not imply that constructs depend on an operational *definition;* it simply insists that translation rules between events and concepts are necessary for measurement.

3. Measurement consists of the *public assignment* of numerical values to events, the simplest being 1 for presence and 0 for absence. Transformation rules from observation to scalar values must be public in the sense that they can be communicated to qualified observers, qualified in the sense of being capable of performing and understanding the measurements. At a crude level, philosophers reach the level of logic and mathematics, but they do not necessarily move to the level of public observation and operational translation; they often rest their case on logic and employ refined strategies of argumentation.

4. For scientists, public assignment of values must meet the two reliability standards mentioned above.

a. *Intraobserver reliability:* The same qualified observer must assign the same weight to the same event on different occasions of its occurrence.

b. *Interobserver reliability:* Different qualified observers must assign the same weight to the same event. When these two requirements are met, empirical generalizations logically can be derived from premises based on a shared observational base.

5. A consistent *internal logic* should be applied to relate theoretical terms to one another, observables to observables, and observables to theoretical terms. At this point the central task is to develop the nomological networks of Cronbach and Meehl (1955), and latent variables (theoretical terms) should be created that embody the relationship of latent variables to observationals, and between different manifest variables (also being immediate observationals).

6. Admissible theoretical terms and their relationships one to another should be evaluated in terms of *alternatives* that are capable of being *falsified.* The concept of *verisimilitude* is important; it refers to the relative truth-likeness of the theoretical structure, a quality that should increase as study proceeds.

These are some of the essential steps that must be taken to pursue the nature of reality in the manner of science. Attention and care must be devoted to establish adequate conceptual frameworks, but it should not be forgotten, as H. I. Brown (1977) emphasized, that it is continuing research, rather than established results, that constitutes the life blood of science. The only permanent aspect of science is research, which is a continuing attempt to interpret nature in terms of an a priori theoretical framework. This framework plays a fundamental role in determining what problems should be solved and what are to count as solutions. Fundamental theories play a crucial role in determining what is to be observed, and the significance and meaning of observational data can change markedly whenever a scientific revolution takes place.

Although research is the life blood of science, the critical events are theoretical changes driven by research, with sense impressions the starting point and concepts the end point. Even the most basic observations are preceded by a particular interest, question, or problem, in short, by something theoretical. The idea of pure inductive theory, free from any theoretical constructs, can be rejected; all facts are tainted with some kind of subjectivist bias.

I have discussed the distinction between discovery and justification to underscore the need for strategies and methods that have high heuristic value, thereby enhancing the likelihood that important factors and relationships will be discovered. Two problems must be avoided. One is introduced by always using the same procedure to study a phenomenon, which leads to a risk that what is found is not general, but specific to the one test procedure. The other is the use of traditional statistical methods of analysis that merely ask whether an obtained effect is large enough to reject the idea the effect is due to chance, to reject the null hypothesis, and then using the mere fact that other than a chance effect is involved to justify a belief in the favored hypothesis.

Procedures that enhance theoretical discovery should be emphasized continually throughout the research process: Identifying and investigating the workings of important variables will likely lead to understanding of phenomena; a serious difficulty is encountered if research does not include variables that are important but that have not been identified carefully enough to study. The two conceptual contexts of discovery and justification should be kept in mind during all stages of science, and methods of justification should not impede the heuristics of discovery.

Discovery is contributed to by anyone who considers a problem (philosophers, novelists, poets, priests, or scientists), and some activities pursued in the name of discovery have a reasoned logic. Only when measurement begins and justification is involved does the work specifically identified as science begin. No matter how sophisticated the quantitative or technological aspects of research procedures, the importance of the discovery process must never be forgotten, and the importance of heuristic aspects of scientific theories must be stressed continually.

The Importance of Competing Hypotheses One way to enhance the likelihood of discovering strengths and limitations of a theory, as well as to lead to discovery of new information that adds to the theoretical framework, is to pose empirical tests of hypotheses in terms of plausible alternatives that compete as explanations. By developing alternatives it is possible to avoid many limitations on the breadth of generalizations made when using only a single guiding hypothesis. Discovery is of paramount importance in developing science and the importance of justification should not be overemphasized. Although justification is important, the problems related to it are relatively simple compared with those for discovery.

The value of considering alternative competing hypotheses extends beyond investigation of research problems within a single discipline, such as behavior or physiology. The most significant advances in science are often realized by considering findings within the boundaries of one discipline in combination with those from other disciplines. Ghiselin (1971) identified the advantage that was gained in the biological sphere when both Darwin and Wallace read the economist Malthus and were led independently to formulate the theory of natural selection; here established normal theory in one discipline (economics) led to revolutionary theory in another (biology).

To move toward the realist's goal of developing theories that "carve nature closer to the joints," it might be well to consider findings from disciplines at different levels of analysis (e.g., social, behavioral, physiological, and neurophysiological). Information gathered at these different levels regarding the same issues (e.g., communication) should be examined as carefully as alternative hypotheses at the same level to detect violations of accepted facts at other levels. This does not imply that any level will be reduced to another, but only that principles and processes operating at one level might provide insights regarding those at another, and boundary conditions and constraints can be set on any one level by principles and processes operating at others.

Falsifiability Popper (1959) maintained that all observation statements have a degree of subjectivity because an arbitrary (but necessary) decision has been made regarding what to observe, how to observe it, and how to represent observations quantitatively. Any primitive observation, fact, experiment, or experience contains implicit theoretical assumptions because all are based on selection of innumerable events that are occurring at any one time. The only way to justify a basic observation is by recourse to a lower-level inductive inference, and this process leads to an infinite regress. Somewhere, a theoretical premise has to be accepted as basic, and this produces reliance on "more immediate experience," a parsimonious system of basic premises, but a system that still is based on a network of hypotheses. Because there is no such thing as pure induction, absolute verification is not possible—it is impossible to verify theories empirically. What must be done is to test theories against experience, which implies *falsifiability* rather that verifiability.

For a statement to be useful scientifically it must be possible to refute the statement by experience. The statement "It will or will not rain here tomorrow" is not empirical (Popper, 1959); it cannot be refuted—it is vacuous because it "predicts" all possible outcomes, which really means it predicts nothing at all. The statement "It will rain here tomorrow" is empirical because it can be refuted by taking a look tomorrow; the statement "It will rain three inches here tomorrow" is of greater empirical interest and value because it asserts more by making a more risky prediction. The empirical method is characterized by its manner of exposing the system to be tested to falsification: The system is examined by making severe tests based on risky predictions. In this way one system emerges as the fittest through exposing all systems to the fiercest struggle for survival. A theory, then, is rejected by a better theory rather than by negative results.

Facts are not amassed to construct a model of reality, but to test theories, first by a logical examination of conclusions—a test of internal consistency. The logical form of a theory can be investigated to be sure that it is more than a mere tautology, as in the statement, "It will or will not rain here tomorrow." One theory can be compared with others by asking if it explains more and better on the same level of reality; if it contains more nomologicals that are more tightly tied together. It is important to determine whether the theory contradicts accepted "knowns" at other levels; theories about behavior should not violate what is known about operating characteristics of physiological systems. It also is important that the theory predict things currently not known, and that some of these predictions be correct, or the theory's *heuristic value*.

The empirical method is characterized by its manner of exposing the system to be tested to falsification (Popper, 1959). As noted, these should be severe tests in the sense that they involve fewer primitive terms, apply to a broader range of phenomena, and predict phenomena that have not been so far observed. It is also preferable that tests do more than predict a difference that will appear between groups treated one way or another; in other words, tests should predict the magnitudes of expected differences, or the *effect sizes* (Meehl, 1986). Popper (1963, p. 229) wrote: "Truth is not the only aim of science. We want more than mere truth: what we look for is interesting truths—truth which is hard to come by."

Imre Lakatos (1970), a student of Popper, characterized Popper's "recipe" as "Boldness in conjectures on the one hand and austerity in refutations on the other. . . . Intellectual honesty does not consist in trying to . . . establish one's position by proving (or 'probabilifying') it—intellectual honesty consists rather in specifying precisely the conditions under which one is willing to give up one's position" (p. 97). Lakatos proposed what he called sophisticated methodological falsificationism that considers a theory acceptable only if it has corroborated excess empirical content over its predecessor (or rival); that is, it leads to the discovery of novel facts. He agreed with Popper that a theory can be considered falsified if and only if another theory has been proposed that has more empirical content (meaning that it predicts facts that were improbable or even forbidden by the first theory), it explains the success of the previous theory, and some of the excess empirical content is corroborated.

Lakatos pointed out that in reality we never test a single theory. Rather, a maze of interlocking theories makes up a research program. When a theory is proposed there will not be a simple negation of it. Because of the interlocking theories, as Lakatos phrased it, "nature may shout 'inconsistent,'" making it necessary to search through the maze and decide where error resides. What could be called a *theoretical hard core* is of direct interest, but it has a *protective belt* of auxiliary theories surrounding it. Auxiliary theories involve measurement and statistical and psychological theories that underlie testing methods, testing instruments, research design (e.g., whether each subject is tested in only one of the conditions, or whether all subjects are tested in all conditions), range of subject types, and validity of the testing instruments to measure what they are supposed to measure.

A host of methodological, conceptual, and procedural problems make it impossible to decide whether negative results cast doubt on the core theory, whether they are produced by inadequate statistical theories used to translate between observations and theory, or on auxiliary theories involved in constructing the measuring instrument, the testing situation, or categorization of the people tested. If data falsify the predicted outcome it is not possible to know what it is that is falsified: Is the core theory incorrect, are one or more of the auxiliary hypotheses incorrect, or were the experimental conditions not appropriate? The core theory is shielded from negative data by the protective belt provided by auxiliary hypotheses, making it difficult to know whether it is the core theory itself that is at fault, or one or more of the auxiliary hypotheses. Little progress can be made toward developing a progressive science unless it is recognized that a complex web of issues is involved in evaluating any core theory.

It is possible to protect a core theory from disconfirmation by ad hoc adjustments of some aspects of the auxiliary hypotheses to accommodate observed anomalies. This may be legitimate, but if such ad hoc adjustments have to be made over and again, it might mean the enterprise has become what Lakatos called a degenerating scientific program. Less and less is understood and explained as more and more research is done, because each new finding makes it necessary to add another primitive term to some aspect of one of the theories, resulting in loss of parsimony and an undesirable gain in ad hocness.

Because of these complex methodological realities encountered when bringing empirical data to bear on theories, another student of Popper challenged Popper's ideas. Feyerabend (1975) considered himself an epistemological anarchist and insisted that no methodological rules have to be adopted. "Manmade" factors, in the form of underlying predispositions or assumptions made by the scientist, assume such a dominant role it is not possible to conduct an objective study. Investigators accept some pet theory at the outset of a research effort, this theory is elaborated, and alternatives are not seriously considered. Because some success and explanatory power are found in even a partially correct theory, empirical support will be claimed for whatever is interesting and intriguing about the preferred theory, leading to even less tolerance for alternatives. It becomes less likely that incompatible facts will be discovered, or even looked for. Adverse facts will be explained by slight accommodations of, and tinkering with, the favored theory; popular science books will spread the theory; it will be applied to distant fields; and no research money will be granted to evaluate rebel theories. Feyerabend considered this to result in the construction of what appears to be tremendous empirical support; the construction of this edifice would enhance the likelihood that the theory would enjoy an undeserved long life.

These conclusions led Feyerabend (1975, pp. 47–48) to state, "The separation between the history of a science, its philosophy and the science itself dissolves into thin air and so does the separation between science and non-science." Finally, "Hence, we are not dealing with an alternative [discovery and justification] either, we are dealing with a single uniform domain of procedures all of which are equally important for the growth of science. This disposes of the distinction" (p. 167).

Feyerabend also deplored the use of methodological rules, proposing that a pluralistic methodology should be adopted—one that uses ". . . aesthetic judgments, judgments of taste, metaphysical prejudices, religious desires, in short, *what remains are our subjective wishes*" (p. 285). As indicated earlier, there is no reason why taste and judgment should not be a respected part of the scientific enterprise—in fact they are critical components of it. However, it is useful to make a demarcation between nonscientific aspects that enrich the enterprise and scientific aspects that concern the adequacy of data and their permissible generalization to theoretical statements. I believe much of what Feyerabend wanted to achieve through a pluralistic methodology is embedded in the proposals of Lakatos. Procedures used to establish construct validity, as developed by Cronbach and Meehl (1955), formally include pluralism as an essential aspect of theory development and evaluation. Feyerabend's polemic provides a helpful reminder of the arrogance that is often found among scientists, and that has led the establishment to insist that one dominant method be used to evaluate everything; for example, a preference for single-variable experimental designs of the Newtonian type, rather than correlational studies in which all variables are measured as they occur in the natural population under specified conditions (Brunswik, 1956). Many researchers, especially those in the behavioral sciences, have developed powerful methods of multivariate design and analysis to exploit the strengths of pluralism to develop powerful explanatory systems. With these methods one can investigate the merits of competing alternative models by evaluating the explanatory adequacy of each alternative to account for the obtained pattern of results (Bentler, 1980; Joreskog & Sorbom, 1984.

Progress and Verisimilitude

Progress in science should be viewed in terms of theoretical pluralism rather than theoretical monism. Kuhn (1962) developed an often-cited monistic conception of a research paradigm that contains accepted examples of actual scientific practice, including law, theory, application, and instrumentation that provide the coherent traditions of scientific research. This paradigm represents concrete models of scientific practice that are passed on to students of a science, and constitute general agreement regarding fundamentals. While clearly some paradigmatic theories tend to be accepted uncritically, which students are required to master during their training, there is an alternative way to view science. Rather than viewing it in terms of a reigning paradigm that must be overthrown by revolution to accomplish change, as did Kuhn, it may be more effective to conceive of a battleground of research programs. A dominant core theory might prevail, but it is always being challenged, anomalous facts have been recognized, and, as Lakatos stated, these anomalies are acknowledged and placed in an ad hoc quarantine—but not forgotten. When enough anomalies are recognized, a competing research program will likely evolve, and it will be successful over rivals when it accounts for the anomalous findings and displays greater heuristic power. It does this by accounting better for those facts that have been discovered, and anticipating novel facts expanding the realm covered by the theory. The new theory might contain aspects of the old, but it adds new features. A better way to conceive of scientific change is in terms of evolution rather than revolution. The positive heuristic in such a construal is enhanced by pluralism and discovery.

Darwin (1871) stated the case nicely in the last chapter of *The descent of man:* "False facts are highly injurious to the progress of science, for they often endure: but false views, if supported by some evidence, do little harm, for every one takes a salutary pleasure in proving their falseness; and when this is done one path towards error is closed and the road to truth is often at the same time opened" (p. 909).

Some of those opposed to animal research attacked science in general and raised specific objections regarding the permissibility of using animals as subjects. An example can be found in the informative book by the legal scholar Gary Francione (1995), codirector of the Rutgers Animal Rights Law Center. He stated, ". . . science as a body of knowledge should not be viewed as presenting 'truth' in some abstract sense, or as constituting an epistemologically superior form of knowledge. This recognition is slowly eroding the pedestal upon which science has presided for many years" (p. 175). His model is a caricature of the modern philosophy of science discussed in this chapter, and his attacks are directed at a straw man. He characterized science as an enterprise that seeks only to describe the physical world in terms of empirical observation, to make testable claims, and to produce knowledge through institutional imperatives that effectively lead to intellectual neutrality among scientists. He is correct to this point, but he assumed that if subjective influences exist, all of the science is flawed and untrustworthy. He wrote, "More and more, science is viewed as a political enterprise that does not possess the imprimatur of 'objectivity'" (p. 177). He also made the strange statement, ". . . induction in science assumes a certain uniformity in nature, but such uniformity must either be established empirically, which is circular, or established formally, which means that the principle of uniformity does not refer to anything in the world" (p. 175). If this statement is taken seriously, no science is worth considering and certainly should not have any legitimate epistemological standing.

The basic subjective assumptions on which all of science (and logic and mathematics) is based would leave only a tottering house of cards. I argued above that science is based on acceptance of the idea there are lawful regularities in the universe, and one way to discover their nature is through empirical measurement. If these basic assumptions are rejected, it would be a waste of time to pursue scientific investigations, and speculation, argument, and activism should proceed without science as an impediment.

Francione enumerated some of the points I have made in this chapter (p. 177): "The close relationship between fact and theory suggests that facts cannot even be formulated in the absence of theory and that theory, then, cannot be refuted unequivocally by means of theory-based facts. No fact may qualify automatically as the falsification of a theory. Furthermore, observation itself is subject to interpretation. An investigator may '*not know what he is seeing* . . . until his observations cohere and are intelligible as against the general background of his already accepted and established knowledge'" [the material in single quotation marks is quoted from Hanson (1969)].

As discussed, no fact reveals the "truth," and no purported fact can falsify a theory. A theory is made up of a network of basic and auxiliary hypotheses. A fact can disconfirm some aspects of a theory, which means those aspects should be changed and a remodeled theory subjected to yet another severe test to push it to its limits. If the theory withstands the new test, more and even riskier tests (riskier in terms of extending the theory to explain phenomena not understood at present) should be made, and progress should occur with varying degrees of success, but, it is hoped, toward greater verisimilitude. One problem with Francione's view is that he insists on construing matters as true or false; if something is not completely objective, it is totally subjective, an example of two-valued logic to which we all fall victim too often.

Strong subjective biases influence science, such as what, how, and where reality is to be observed. However, guidelines fall into place whenever the process of justification (observation or experimentation) and the public business of science begin. The objectivity of science lies in the public methods and explicit chain of logic used, and these are open to examination by all interested and competent parties, competent in the sense of possessing the requisite information to evaluate issues pertaining to the adequacy of research design, statistical methods, and instrumentation.

Francione (p. 174) objected to reductionism ". . . that requires one to reduce an object to its constituent parts in order to understand it," and he would have us believe this is an inherent part of science. To be sure, it can be a useful part of science, but it is just as important to understand the rules by which elements are organized, with qualities emerging when more and more elements are involved due to complex interactions among them. These matters are especially critical when a functional view is taken to decide why and when elements and interactions combine, especially if a conceptual framework is to be developed that is adequate to understand reality from a variety of perspectives and levels. Little of these aspects smack of the reductionism of which Francione wrote.

Francione's view of the nature of science led him to suggest that one should reject reductionism, and that it would be more profitable to investigate alternative approaches to health care such as holistic and homeopathic medicine. Undoubtedly, many homeopathic treatments based on the wisdom of earlier times and of other cultures may embody sound principles of physiology and psychology, and many could be accepted in preference to technologically driven procedures favored by clinicians in modern industrialized society. The adequacy of holistic methods remains to be investigated, and their effectiveness should be demonstrated through evaluation research bearing on clinical outcomes. If such studies are done and their results are positive, many surgical and chemical procedures might well be discarded. But until they are done I for one am not willing to forego treatments based on accepted medical information when I am in dire straits. I am reminded of the Emily Dickinson poem, written in 1860 and published in 1891 (Johnson, 1961): "'Faith' is a fine invention/When Gentlemen can *see*/But *Microscopes* are prudent/In an Emergency."

Even if it is decided that more natural remedies should be used, most would want their effectiveness studied by the best methods of modern evaluation research—double-blind controls, carefully matched samples of patients, random assignment to groups, adequate sample sizes, prospective design, and appropriate statistical methods to evaluate results and assess the importance of confounding variables. Whether animals are required in performing such research is a separate question that is considered in chapters 9, 10, and 11. Science as an enterprise, although flawed by human frailty, is the best way to obtain certain kinds of answers to well-framed questions. Many of Francione's quarrels concern the problem of making proper generalizations based on evidence at hand rather than formal aspects of research.

Because all observations, facts, and data are imbued with some quality of human subjectivity, it is almost certain that any unifying theory will not be true in all aspects. Background assumptions are always made when performing even the simplest observations: Certain events are chosen for observation, and important aspects of underlying reality might not be included. It may be necessary to change and refine the theoretical network being developed to explain phenomena of interest. This does not mean science is in an inevitable subjective crisis, moving from one half-truth to another. If objective reality is assumed, and the laws that regulate this reality have some stability, as more becomes known and more observations and experiments are conducted, many expectations and explanations will be rejected and the investigative focus directed elsewhere. If these new directions enrich the nomological network through the addition of new nomologicals accompanied by understanding how primitive elements interact to produce outcomes, the explanatory network should improve steadily. The test of whether one model of reality is more adequate than others is whether it leads to better understanding and explanation of outcomes, and this is decided in terms of whether it is possible to predict future outcomes and encompass past results using the new model. When a theory makes better and better predictions and conclusions, although it might not be absolutely true, it has greater truth-likeness, the quality of verisimilitude.

In many areas of biological science it is certain that understanding of organic functioning has steadily improved due to better understanding of primitive elements involved in complex processes. This better understanding leads to a clearer conception of how basic elements interact to produce the structures that support organic functions, accompanied by increased identification of the influences that should be examined to conceptualize underlying realities more clearly and understand the relationship of different levels of reality that determine organic functions.

Universe of Generalization

An important consideration regarding permissible generalizations based on a research study is embedded in the preceding discussion. If studies are theory driven, they will apply to a broader universe of events than those that have been examined, even if the application is little more than an empirical generalization. To ensure that research results can be generalized beyond specific questions, the nature of the universes of events and individuals to which results can be applied must be specified in advance to ensure that specifics of the research are representative of that universe (see Petrinovich, 1979, 1989).

Cronbach, Gleser, Nanda, and Rajaratnam (1972) developed a multivariate view of reliability that sharpens the concept of the universe of generalization for a given observation. They wrote, "The decision maker is almost never interested in the response given to the particular stimulus objects or questions, to the particular tester, at the particular moment of testing. . . . The universe of interest to the decision maker is defined when he tells us what observations would be equally acceptable for his purpose. . . ." (p. 15). An observation can be representative of a number of different universes of generalization; it might provide adequate support for some generalizations and be inadequate for others. Everything a research scientist does is intended to be generalized to something. The only possible exception I can conceive of is if the aim is to know only about this individual, at this time, and in that place, and I believe this is seldom of interest in science.

A theory is always a general statement about a specific set of occurrences. This set of occurrences can be conceived to be universal, to hold widely, to apply only to certain individuals at certain times and places, or to apply only to this individual in this place. A theory always applies to a universe of occurrences, and the question of sampling representativeness always rears its ugly head whenever a theory is about anything. The permissible extent of a theoretical generalization is never known until limitations produced by the particular experimental conditions, task variables, and subjects used in a particular study have been explored.

Misconceptions Regarding Research

Many doubts, reservations, and objections to using animals in research are based on misunderstandings and misconstruals of points developed in this chapter. I discuss a few that are commonly expressed, and reserve discussion of concrete objections regarding the planning, conduct, and evaluation of specific kinds of research to later chapters.

Singer (1990a, p. 40) complained: "Among the tens of millions of experiments performed, only a few can possibly be regarded as contributing to important medical research," and (p. 49), ". . . much research is trivial, obvious, or meaningless," and (p. 50), ". . . many, many experiments still being conducted . . . offer no prospect of yielding really momentous or vital new knowledge." In another context Singer remarked: "There has never been and never could be a single experiment that saved thousands of lives" (p. 81). All these statements miss the point, because no research program dealing with complex processes ever depends on a single experiment; progress toward understanding comes about because better and better questions are asked and more and more irrelevant factors are ruled out. With hindsight it is relatively simple to scorn studies that, even though well conducted, were way off the mark in terms of what we know now, experiments that, given our current knowledge, would not be done. When we examine the history of science we can see that some of the most interesting discoveries that led to immense theoretical breakthroughs in understanding were met with initial outrage by the intellectual community, often being rejected when submitted for publication. Sometimes early studies in an earthshaking series that led to critical advances had to be done with little financial or intellectual support and only minimal facilities, until the intellectual establishment was forced to deal with the accruing anomalies introduced by the research. When the implications of these new findings were explored they sometimes provided a foundation on which refined theoretical structures were built.

It is not possible to decide whether or not a novel research direction is a profitable one until a step or two has been taken in that direction. It may well be possible to reject an approach after data have been collected, analyzed, and interpreted. By refusing to make risky tests of current theory, however, progress would be slower because investigators keep looking in the same place for the same things. These might be the wrong places to look, and the things being sought might be the wrong things. It would be an instance of the familiar story of the drunk on his hands and knees searching under a lamppost: When asked what he was looking for he said, "The car keys. I dropped them in the alley, but I'm looking in the street because the light is better."

One problem with Singer's statements is that the progress of science should be viewed as the development of an interlocking series of theoretical elements—a conceptual framework that constitutes a research program. Given this perspective, it is clear that no single experiment is likely to falsify a theory. A theory is discarded when a better alternative is developed that explains more of what is known and predicts new facts that are not known. Even if some results are not understandable in terms of an available theoretical framework, the results do not lead people to give up the search and start anew. During the progressive phase of research, anomalies should be ignored to focus on the positive heuristics, and the program should be followed until anomalies become so numerous they lead to a suspicion that a degenerative phase has been reached. When this occurs, it is time to search for a rival program, and if the research field is an active one, several available alternatives probably can be tailored to start the cycle moving in a more productive direction.

None of this subjectivity diminishes the power of science as long as it is moving toward better and better understanding of more and more. Better understanding is indexed by the degree to which new models are more able to account for the unknown variance in data than are alternatives. If answers to questions were known, it would not be necessary to do research at all, in science or philosophy. At the very least, we should take Darwin's reminder to heart that, with failure, at least one path toward error is closed and the road to truth is often opened at the same time.

Bernard Rollin and the Philosophy of Science   Bernard Rollin wrote three books that consider issues regarding the treatment of animals: *The unheeded cry* (1989), *Animal rights and human morality* (1992), and *Farm animal welfare* (1995). Here, I consider his arguments regarding philosophy of science and principles of scientific methodology, because they provide an informed criticism of science, and they suffer because they are based on an outmoded and slanted view. I single out these three books not because they are bad, but because they represent an informed view, consider many important issues that have been discussed in this chapter, and make their points in a comprehensive and clear manner. I maintain, however, that his characterization of science, especially of the biological and behavioral sciences, is inadequate and inaccurate. I confine myself to matters regarding philosophy and methodology of science and consider specifics regarding experimental findings later.

Rollin (1989, p. 9) begins by noting; ". . . every invasive use of animals in scientific research involves a tacit moral judgment: namely, that the data gained in such research are of greater importance than the pain or suffering or death or fear engendered in the animals in the course of gathering such data." This statement evaluates science from a utilitarian perspective—what practical good will be provided by the new knowledge—a view that often prevails. However, other considerations, such as advances in basic understanding of the universe, can be said to be as important as the market value of information.

He accuses scientists (1989, p. 29) of obscuing, ". . . the deep moral issues by burying them under an avalanche of empirical data," which he believes results from an over reliance on "reductionist minutiae." Rather than relying on controlled experimentation in laboratory settings, he believes the study of behavior (p. 39) ". . . must necessarily be 'uncontrolled' and anecdotal." Trust should be placed in disinterested reports of people who do not stand to gain by the information they disseminate and who have no professional theoretical bias. He considers these sources of information to be preferable to those who stand to gain from their findings, or who approach their findings (as do both scientists and animal rights activists, by the way) with strong theoretical prejudices. The training of research graduate students in construed (p. 40) to produce narrowly trained individuals who serve ". . . as cheap labor for whatever research happens to be funded." He continues, "Scientists are pressed into doing research in recognized, safe, narrow, non-risky, non-boat-rocking mainstream accepted areas" and "Innovative or revolutionary research . . . is discouraged or selectively ruled out." In support of these arguments he appeals to "an increasing number of scandals involving 'fudged' data, falsified data, sloppy data, and so on," suggesting that ". . . obviously, the reported cases are only the tip of the iceberg."

This bill of indictment led him to conclude that ". . . scientists are humans, just like everyone else, even in their scientific moments, contrary to what positivistic ideology and the commonsense of science would have us believe" (p. 41). Again, he suggested that reliance should be placed on disinterested observations of neutral observers with no vested interest in results, rather than on the "generally unchecked results" of scientists with careers at stake. Observations made by these "disinterested" observers would be corroborated by those of other observers "with whom they have had no truck." Given these views regarding the necessity for research involving animals to be done by disinterested observers, his suggestions regarding farm animal welfare are puzzling. In *Farm animal welfare* he made many excellent suggestions regarding the kinds of research that should be done by agricultural researchers, ranchers, and animals slaughterers. He expressed the belief that the good will and humane characteristics of those people involved in and supported by the meat industry can be counted on. (His suggestions regarding farm animal welfare are be discussed in chapter 14.) I wonder why commercial agribusiness observers can be trusted, and scientists uniformly are to be distrusted? His positive view of beef producers in particular is in stark contrast to his negative characterization of scientific researchers. He concluded his discussions stating that, when seeking to understand animal behavior, studies should be done under natural conditions (at least initially), and that a trained observer is not required to do them. It can be agreed that whenever scientific instrumentation is involved trained personnel are required, but it is not apparent why this fact necessarily invalidates the outcomes.

A few comments are in order. Of course, scientists are human, and as such have biases and interests that can influence the results of their work. That very reason is why the minutiae involved in research design are insisted upon; why control groups must be used; why observers and experimenters should not know what treatment subjects have received, as far as that is possible; why background influences should be measured so they can be ruled out by statistical control whenever it is not possible to control them experimentally; and why peer review of research is insisted upon before funding is granted, while it is conducted, and before it is published. It is never possible to eliminate all subjective bias, to detect all fraud by unscrupulous individuals, or to realize at the outset that the course being pursued is a hopeless one. The scientific community insists on a high degree of objectivity, and unusual results found in the course of investigations have to be cross-validated. Unusual results that have profound implications tend to be replicated in several laboratories on publication—witness the profound advances in understanding the human genome that have occurred in the past few years (see Petrinovich, 1996, for a review of this research). Findings by human genetic researchers have been earthshaking, there have been numerous replications of unexpected findings, and many of these findings have led to improvements in therapeutic procedures. The results of these careful scientific moves promise to yield significant advances in understanding the basic cell mechanisms involved in the development of cancer and immunodeficiency syndrome, and detection of inborn genetic defects.

Although considerable scientific progress has been enjoyed, problems remain due to the fact that scientists are human. I documented the dangers to free inquiry posed by allowing individuals, corporations, and universities to patent basic genetic findings in order to reap enormous economic benefits (Petrinovich, 1996). Undesirable aspects of human selfishness are not peculiar to science. Fraud, greed, and dishonesty tend to be present in many human endeavors, be it religion, education, philosophy, commerce, the military, the arts, or sports. Such undesirable tendencies seem to reflect an aspect of human nature that surfaces in enterprises that have economic and social implications. One advantage of science is the insistence that formal steps of justification be communicated in a public manner, making it easier to detect malfeasance there science than many other activities. At least at the level of data acquisition, safeguards are in place to enhance objectivity that are not available for many other endeavors.

It is not obvious that those in the antianimal research community would make objective observations any more than those in the proresearch community. History supports the view that it was reliance on pure anecdotalism by naturalists that drove the discipline of animal behavior onto the shoals of subjectivity, eventually setting the stage for the onslaught of American Behaviorism in the period between 1930 and 1960 (see Petrinovich, 1973). Contrary to Rollin's (1989) characterization, it was the qualitative (but at the same time, objective) natural history observations of early ethologists that led the study of animal behavior away from overreliance on the laboratory and made it possible to substitute meaningful, quantifiable observations for subjective anecdotalism and objective trivialization.

Rollin (1989, p. 61) noted: ". . . many extra-logical, extra-rational cultural factors enter into and shape philosophical and scientific changes," and (p. 63), ". . . science succumbs to the same 'foibles' as philosophy . . . scientific theories are adhered to despite the presence of holes and contradictions, and even in the face of empirical falsifications." He is correct when he remarks that scientific positions, as philosophical positions, change with value changes. He is remiss when he does not remember that justificatory procedures in science provide an important corrective to the unbridled subjectivity that is the essence of many other valid ways of knowing the universe. I hope the preceding discussion of the pluralistic nature of research methodology that can be employed to develop adequate conceptual frameworks strengthens the belief that scientists attempting to construct general theories are aware of the pitfalls and difficulties involved in establishing constructs to explain behavior, and that Rollin's simplistic characterization of science is rejected.

As I have held throughout this chapter, Rollin's (1992, 1995) position that science views itself to be value free is misleading. Most sophisticated scientists, acquainted with contemporary ideas in philosophy of science, would not subscribe to this belief. As developed earlier, the context of discovery is of paramount importance, as is the choice of problems and methods, and the generalizations drawn. This context is as vulnerable to the perils of subjectivism regarding values as is true for philosophy or literature. Science is/should be/can be value free in terms of those activities falling within the context of justification. Within this context it enjoys an epistemological advantage, and I believe the progress realized in a variety of fields, such as archaeology, astronomy, genetics, biochemistry, biophysics, anthropology, psychology, and sociology, is due to the way knowledge is pursued, applying the procedural safeguards that are the essence of science.

Rollin (1992, p. 61) asserted: "Scientific ideology must be shown up for what it is: bad philosophy. . . . what will count as fact, as a legitimate object of investigation, or as data relevant to a given question, rests squarely on valuational presuppositions." I agree, and believe that those issues are recognized by most biological and behavioral scientists. What should be done is to ensure that the logic of argumentation is sound, that the operational translation of variables is defensible and public, and that generalizations logically follow from results. Difficulties plaguing science are due to the fact that it must move back and forth between stages of theorizing and measuring. Because science has assumed this added burden of measurement does not mean it is bad philosophy it must do things in addition to philosophy, and it is possible, but not easy, to do them adequately.

A second piece of bad philosophy in Rollin's (1992, p. 62) view is represented by his incorrect notion that scientists accept the ". . . common sense of science's shibboleth that ethics is subjective and not rationally adjudicable." I reviewed extensively the scientific research done to understand ethical and moral views (Petrinovich, 1995), and proposed that research has illuminated factual issues relevant to morality. Research on moral intuitions and on the structure of ethical beliefs has been based on extensive discussions of basic principles developed by moral philosophers. Studies have attempted to move to the level of obtaining empirical data within the context of justification, to add relevant information to the argument.

To counterbalance the negative views of science offered by Rollin, Singer, and Francione, it is of interest to consider the more positive appraisal of Woodward and Goodstein (1996). Most scientists are motivated by the desire to discover important truths and to help others do so as well. Regardless of public communication of results and a degree of cooperative effort, scientists prefer that they, rather than their competitors, make discoveries in order to receive recognition, career advances, and resources that reward success. The first to make a discovery gets nearly all the credit, and the discovery might even be named for that individual.

Competition increases the likelihood that investigators will pursue a range of lines of inquiry, because that enhances the probability of discovery by adding to the nomological net. Whereas competitiveness is good, in terms of leading to an active and progressive science, it also can lead unscrupulous individuals to scientific misconduct and fraudulent claims.

Competitive aspects of the structure of science guarantee certain safeguards. Important and unexpected findings always stimulate rivals to attempt to falsify those findings. Thus it is dangerous to perpetrate fraud because of such checks and balances. Critics are quick to pounce on misinterpretation and overinterpretation of data. Failure to report contrary data is soon corrected by the research of others, who not only replicate the critical study, but make tests of alternative hypotheses that will expose its inadequacies.

Woodward and Goodstein noted that Nobel prizes are received for constructing theories that predict new effects, providing the theories are subsequently verified. Another way to receive credit is to refute a well-established theory. This conceptual give and take provides most of the energy that keeps science progressing.

One of the most important ethical tools is peer review, which determines whether journals will publish submitted papers and whether agencies will grant financial support to research projects. Although peer review cannot detect instances of intentional misrepresentation, it is good at separating good science from nonsense. Woodward and Goodstein warned that conventional reviews may delay a truly visionary or revolutionary idea, but suggested that may be the price paid for conducting science in an orderly way. Their conclusion is that distinctly scientific forms of misconduct require the expert judgment of a panel of scientists who can understand and assess the particulars of the research. This is because such a panel have the background and training that enables them to detect, understand, and deal with data fabrication, adequate research design, appropriateness of instruments, acceptable norms for presenting data, and appreciation of the importance of experimental data within the total structure of the science.

I find it neither fair nor accurate to condemn those who pursue science as ignorant, self-serving, and evil in intent. Many scientists are sophisticated regarding problems involved in pursuing science, and attempt to develop conceptual models based on measurements made within an explicit operational framework. Rather than maligning these practitioners, I believe the issue would be better joined if attention were devoted to questions of how to deal with conflicting values that typify pro- and antianimal research advocates. There should be forthright discussion regarding certain questions. Is it reasonable to hold that animals have rights, and if so, what does that imply? When competing interests exist between individuals and species, how can one decide among them? Can one establish rational scalar values to allocate scarce resources, and is rationing of valuable goods defensible in a just society? Can utilitarianism be defended as a reasonable system to organize decisions in a just society? Is speciesism an undesirable prejudice on a par with sexism and racism?

In the remainder of this book I focus on these specific questions in the belief that this is a more profitable enterprise than attributing bad intentions, moral weakness, undesirable sentimentality, or selfish motives to those on one side or the other. Disagreement is not necessarily undesirable when basic issues in morality are involved. However, refusal to tolerate different opinions regarding morality is a frequently occurring evil that can lead, and has led, to great cruelties and injustices, especially when some members of society have power to enforce their arbitrary moral standards on all members. After reviewing basic information regarding the developing capabilities of the human fetus, neonate, and infant, I proceed to philosophical arguments regarding animals, and then consider practices that have occasioned strong disagreement.

5

Development of Sensing and Acting

When considering evolved similarities between humans and nonhumans and the mechanisms that bond young to their social community, much of the preceding discussion focused on emotional factors producing social bonding. Because neonates require extensive care, bonding mechanisms exist for almost all species of birds and mammals. These mechanisms enhance the likelihood healthy young will emit behaviors that evoke acceptance and nurturance, especially by the primary caregiver, usually the mother.

Another important topic involves the nature and development of the abilities that have been called *cognitive*, a term used rather indiscriminately to accommodate processes that intervene between stimulus input and response output. Considerable discussion of cognitive processes has taken place among observers concerned with continuities and discontinuities in the characteristics of different species. Many studies investigated the development of cognitive capacities of a large number of species, especially the human infant. Capacities studied include basic aspects of sensitivity to external stimuli, perceptual processing of those stimuli, basic associative abilities of organisms of different ages, extent of complex problem-solving abilities, development of various communication and language systems, and evidence that an organism has a theory of mind.

The development and functioning of language systems and characteristics of the mind are of special interest, because some maintain that the complexities of human language and aspects of the mind have emergent properties not comparable with simpler systems of other animal species. Others propose that some animals, for example, chimpanzees and dolphins, possess language systems that, albeit simpler, are qualitatively similar to that of humans. If there are strong similarities between humans and nonhumans, some demand that members of nonhuman species be accorded the same moral standing as human infants, mentally impaired adults, and senile humans no longer able to function cognitively. If a distinction is drawn between cognitively impaired humans and animals that display a similar level of functioning, some consider this an instance of an arbitrary, unacceptable, and undesirable *speciesism*, a position that is contested in chapter 8.

On the other hand, if critical dissimilarities exist between humans and nonhumans, it can be posited that humans belong to a qualitatively different category of being. Dissimilarities in functional abilities are cited to support beliefs that it is morally permissible to treat humans and nonhumans based on different rules. Even if dissimilarities are accepted, questions remain regarding specification of the kinds of permissible differential treatment, and for what reasons. The significance of similarities and differences between species is addressed in chapters 10 and 11, where the morality of animal research is considered.

In this chapter the literature bearing on the development of sensory and motor capacities of the human fetus and neonate is reviewed to gain an understanding of the initial path adult humans travel before they attain the status of sophisticated symbol manipulators. This provides a point of reference to compare the cognitive attainment of humans with those of other animals, especially nonhuman primates. In chapter 6, the development of human perception, cognition, and language and the nature of mind are addressed and compared with abilities of other species.

Some of this chapter will read like a review article with citation after citation; it should, because in part it is. This strategy reflects my background as a research scientist, and was chosen to provide an overview of the facts on which I base subsequent conceptual arguments. Much of the detailed information in this chapter can be skimmed, beginning on page 125. Conclusions the data support are stated on pages 127–128, and 135. The material concerning facial recognition and imitation should be read in its entirety, along with the conclusions on page 141.

Half-empty or Half-full?   Supposed continuities and discontinuities between nonhumans and humans have been cited to support and decry using animals in research. It is important to understand the nature of continuities and discontinuities, and to decide what their relevance is to the permissibility of animal research. Those who approve and disapprove believe in strong continuities among animals of all species. Both camps appeal to Darwinian conclusions regarding how natural selection can account for continuities. Both accept the idea that historical factors have produced similar solutions to enhance successful differential reproduction, given the particular ecological and social circumstances faced by organisms of different kinds.

Supporters of animal research identified continuities ranging across genetic, cellular, neurochemical, neurophysiological, and behavioral levels, and cited the value of studying basic mechanisms under controlled circumstances for a number of reasons, among them, to enhance the understanding of the workings of the universe, and to alleviate nonhuman and human suffering. These arguments often stress the importance of understanding each species, as well as of pursuing a reductionist strategy to study and understand the simple elements of which complex organismic systems are composed.

The same facts regarding continuities have been used by opponents of animal research to contend that, because animals have the capacity to enjoy pleasure and to suffer pain much as humans, they have the right not to be subjected to experimental procedures damaging to their well-being. These objections are variously phrased in terms of animal welfare, interests, desires, or rights. For example, Regan (1983, p. 120) wrote: ". . . the same categories of thought (interests, benefits, harms, etc.) that illuminate the most general features of human welfare are equally applicable to animal welfare."

Both supporters and opponents point to the other side of the coin and use discontinuities to uphold their positions. Supporters emphasize crucial discontinuities that make humans special. Often these are cognitive, and involve the idea that only humans have an autobiographical sense and understand concepts regarding their future welfare, of causation, and of intentionality. Their complex language is an emergent phenomenon that sets them off from all other species. This language system permits a profound understanding of the transient nature of individuals, while also supporting appreciation of the enduring nature of the human community, and emphasizing the nature of the human mind. Because of profound differences in modes of adaptation, those insisting on a reductionist strategy consider it necessary to conduct research with animal species that differ in many respects, to understand the workings of basic mechanisms of adaptation in the face of different demands, even if the ultimate interest is only to understand the human condition.

Opponents of animal research use discontinuities to hold that, in the face of profound dissimilarities in physiological functions and the essential emergent qualities involved in human psychological functioning, it is not reasonable to expect research results obtained in animals to illuminate the human condition. For example, Singer (1990a, p. 35) wrote: "If there are differences even among closely related species of monkeys, generalization from monkeys to humans must be far more questionable," and (p. 52), "So the researcher's central dilemma exists in an especially acute form in psychology: either the animal is not like us, in which case there is no reason for performing the experiment; or else the animal is like us, in which case we ought not to perform on the animal an experiment that would be considered outrageous if performed on one of us." In other words, to understand humans it is necessary to study humans directly, and it is suspect to cause animals to suffer, given differences between them and humans, differences that erect an insurmountable barrier to reaching the desired goal of understanding human functioning and alleviating human suffering.

Often, the facts on which different opinions are based differ only minimally. Rather, the arguments resemble debates between those who would describe a cup's contents in terms of it being half empty or halffull. As with the physical analogy, the reality does not change, but the implications of that reality can, depending on a number of subjective decisions. These decisions concern such things as the purpose of the research and the permissibility of using animals for those purposes, and are based on a set of underlying moral beliefs and interpretations.

Questions regarding cognitive function often are phrased in terms of how much difference there must be for something to be classified as different in kind, rather than different only in quality. Francione (1995) asserted that differences between humans and other animals are, for the most part, those of degree and not of kind. Regan (1983) believes that, in terms of our "animality," it would be surprising if human welfare differed in kind from animal welfare. Another physical analogy can be used to question assumptions regarding the relationship between quantity of units and quality of function. If a computer has a small amount of memory, it can perform certain kinds of functions. If that memory is increased, it can solve larger problems of the same kind more quickly—obviously the addition of more memory units produces a quantitative enhancement. However, with the addition of a very large number of memory units, it becomes possible for the computer to solve problems of a totally different kind. The addition of more and more hardware units of the same kind makes it possible to develop programs to accomplish functions that were not possible before. Thus, new software can be evolved, and the supercomputer can be considered to be a different kind in terms of the problems it can solve and the concerns it can address. Indeed, it is a different functional entity because it possesses more basic units.

Probably no overall agreement can be reached regarding the permissibility or impermissibility of all kinds of research using animals. It might be helpful, however, to develop general principles that can be applied in most cases, and attempt to obtain agreement among reasonable people. When disagreements arise they can be evaluated on a case-by-case basis. In this way, advocates of different positions might be able to understand the bases of their opponent's disagreements and express the bases on which their own position rests; it might even be possible to arrive at acceptable compromise positions. Failing agreement, the bases of disagreement will at least be explicit, and political action can be directed to sway decisions that bear on basic differences for dispute, rather than moving immediately to a "might makes right" ethic that leaves losers dissatisfied and lessens the likelihood that reasoned debate will resume.

The value of such rational methods of conflict solution were discussed at length in *Living and dying well* (Petrinovich, 1996), where methods were described to resolve a number of social conflicts to the satisfaction of all parties. These methods have been extremely useful when people of good intent were faced with the problem of justly allocating scarce resources, especially such things as limited health care resources.

Fetal and Neonatal Development

To understand the foundations of human nature it is helpful to consider the development of the human fetus and neonate from a functional, developmental view. Although human neonates enter the world in a vulnerable state, and require careful nurturance for several years to survive, they cannot be characterized as simply empty slates awaiting the breast of succorance to sustain their present, and the hand of experience to write their future. They appear with well-tuned sensory capacities that direct them toward certain classes of stimulations, and are outfitted with a set of motoric tendencies to respond in certain ways. These sensory capacities and response potentials have a strong affectional base, tend to elicit nurturant responses from adult caregivers, and enhance the likelihood the infants will develop the critical cognitive and behavioral abilities required to develop into reproductively successful moral agents. These early developments enhance the likelihood that continuing neurophysiological, sensory, and motoric development will proceed efficiently, and set the stage for the emergence of perceptual, cognitive, and linguistic characteristics of all normal members of the community.

I will not review the enormous literature that bears on these developmental factors, but touch on only a few salient examples. Good, comprehensive reviews are contained in books by Bower (1982), Johnson and Morton (1991), Locke (1993), Mehler and Dupoux (1994), and Hauser (1996), all of which are well-organized and readable accounts of the primary literature.

The human fetus undergoes considerable neural, sensory, and motor development in utero, and these developmental processes set the stage for progress along paths that will lead to effective mature functioning. The aspects I discuss are critical stages in the development of human nature, are relevant to the moral arguments developed in chapter 3, and can help us understand essential differences between humans and other animals.

I present a few important details regarding prenatal development, especially those in sensory, motor, and nervous systems. I then provide a snapshot of the organism at birth to give a glimpse of ways in which the fetus and neonate evoke emotional responses that result in nurturant attachment from members of the human community. These emotional bonds support the neonate's entry as a person with moral standing (personhood) and provide the foundation to support the elaboration of cognitive abilities.

Neural Development

The fetus is capable quite early of making limited limb movements, and is sensitive to auditory, tactile, and chemical stimulation. Patterns of these motoric and receptive capacities indicate considerable development of sensory receptors and nervous system throughout gestation. While in utero the human brain grows from almost nothing; a neural groove (the forerunner of the central nervous system, CNS) develops at the end of the third week after conception (gestational age, GA), and major subdivisions of the CNS are appearing by the second month GA. The brain is about 50 grams at midgestation, about 200 grams by thirty weeks GA, and about 350 to 400 grams at birth. Most neurons that exist are produced during gestation, although the brain continues to develop in size, weighing about 1000 grams at one year and about 1350 grams at twenty years (Lecours, 1982; Nowakowski, 1987).

Although humans are born with almost the entire number of neurons they will ever have, brain mass at birth is only about 25% that of the adult brain, reaching 45% by six to seven months and 93% to 95% by the end of the fourth year (Shatz, 1992). This increase in weight is not due to the addition of new nerve cells, but to an increase in length of elements connecting neurons to one another (axons and dendrites), an increase in density of these connections (synaptic density), and development of myelin (a white insulating tissue) and glial cells of various kinds that provide structural support, participate in metabolic processes, and defend against inflammation and infection (Shepherd, 1988).

Growth of the brain and changes in density of connections occur regardless of overall quality of environmental stimulation, suggesting the system is well buffered from environmental variations, and that normal sensory and social experiences are sufficient to provide the requisite minimal stimulation necessary for neural development. Brain development consumes 87% of the basal metabolic rate of neonates, a figure that drops to 64% at two years, and declines to 23% for adults. This suggests that rapid neurological changes occur for a considerable period of time following birth, and they consume a large proportion of available metabolic resources.

Huttenlocher (1990) reviewed developing anatomy of the central nervous system in the human fetus, infant, and child, concluding that gross cortical development differed greatly for different areas in time and rate as well as in pattern of development of different cellular layers of the cortex. The cortical volume of primary visual cortex expands rapidly during fetal life and the first four postnatal months, reaching maximum volume by four months of age and with a slight contraction during late childhood. This early development of neurons in the visual cortex could mean that further increase in brain weight throughout childhood is due to growth of connections in cortical association areas, especially the frontal cortex. The total number of neurons in human visual cortex remains constant from twenty-eight weeks GA until about seventy years of age. About 10% of the maximum number of synapses in visual cortex are present at birth, with the maximum reached at eight months of age. In contrast to the case for neurons, there is a significant loss of synapses in the cerebral cortex during postnatal development; synapses in the visual cortex decrease to 50% to 60% of the maximum by eleven years of age.

Huttenlocher interpreted these patterns to indicate that synaptogenesis in the visual cortex develops more quickly for sensory (afferent) inputs than for motor (efferent) systems. It appears that new synapses are constantly forming and old connections disappearing, with little change in total number of synapses. As noted earlier, only about 10% of the maximum number of synaptic connections is present at birth, with a rapid burst in synaptogenesis at four months of age (correlated with a sudden increase in visual alertness), and a switch from primarily retinal or subcortical (thalamic lateral geniculate) function to cortical function that involves the development of additional visual functions, such as binocular interaction.

The development of visual function is considerably plastic for at least four years, and this plasticity is related to a large number of unspecified or labile synaptic contacts. It appears the primary visual cortex has an earlier developmental schedule than most other cortical regions.

This pattern of cortical development for humans is different from that for most other animal species. Research done by the Rakic group (Rakic, 1995; Rakic, Bourgeois, Eckenhoff, Zecevic, & Goldman-Rakic, 1986) revealed that overproduction of synapses does not differ for diverse regions of cortex of the rhesus monkey as it does for humans, with the overall synaptic density for the monkey almost at adult levels at birth. Nowakowski (1987) found no proliferation of neurons in the adult nonhuman primate brain, meaning that all neurons of the adult CNS are produced during early development. This contrasts to the extensive development in humans, for whom dendritic branching continues for many years.

The extensive programmed cell death in monkeys and mice does not seem to occur in humans (Huttenlocher, 1990), which means that it might be more important in less complex neural systems. In the cerebral cortex, synapse elimination rather than cell death is more important as the complexity of the system increases. In more complex systems, such as the large human cerebral cortex, the genome would be insufficiently large to allow for specification of all synaptic connections, even though approximately 30% of the entire genome is expressed in the brain (Nowakowski, 1987). Nowakowski endorsed a view similar to that proposed here: The issue should not be phrased in terms of whether nature or nurture is the major contributor; the crucial questions regarding neural development concern the nature of changes, and where and when they occur.

The preceding discussion considered fetal and infant development in terms of global quantitative changes of different regions of the CNS. A great deal is also known about qualitative aspects of the development of sensory and motor systems in the fetus. Patterns can be understood in terms of the organism changing from an aquatic life in utero to a terrestrial one after birth, and many fetal development patterns enhance an infant's ability to cope with the demands of the neonatal world.

According to Smotherman and Robinson (1995), behavioral developments reflect the infant's close adaptation to the sequence of environments it encounters during early life. These developments expedite emergence of new behavioral capacities that, in turn, provide the foundation for behaviors that are important functionally. The fetal environment was characterized by Als (1995) as one that provides the fetus with a securely inherited, evolutionarily promised environment sufficient to support development during a period when the brain is growing more rapidly than at any other time in the life span. The problem for preterm infants is that they suddenly must develop in variable extrauterine settings during this critical time, rather than continuing in the relatively supportive and homogeneous uterine environment.

The interplay between sensory information and experience in utero lays the groundwork for species-appropriate patterns (what Als referred to as evolutionarily "good-enough"), whereas extrautero patterning presents unexpected challenges ("violated" situations) that can lead to malfunction or distortion of brain development and function. Premature activation of frontal cortex pathways may inhibit later differentiations, and this could interfere with appropriate development, especially of cross-modal connection systems important for complex mental processing and regulation of attention. The frontal lobes have developed structurally to a unique extent in humans, and one of their functions is to inhibit impulsive reflexive reactions in order to support expression of voluntary control mechanisms. Als (1995, p. 462) suggested: "In the good-enough full-term situation, it [the fetus] appears to be nurtured in the social-emotional communicative matrix of good-enough parenting in good-enough social groups. In violated situations, it requires special attention for preventive and ameliorative care." Although the uterine environment is relatively stable and predictable, fetal behavior is plastic and responsive, reflecting its ability to adapt continually to changing environmental conditions in utero (Smotherman & Robinson, 1995).

Sensory Systems

In utero, the fetus is bathed by a complex array of chemicals, many of which would be the same for most developing individuals. Some of these pervasive chemicals, however, provide qualitatively variable stimulation for different individuals. Among the most constant and prevalent stimuli are those associated with tastes and odors, and they are ingested and respired by the developing fetus. Mechanical stimuli are also present in the form of vibratory and vestibular influences produced by the mother's movements and her heartbeat, as well as auditory stimulation provided by her heartbeat. Another important source of extrauterine sound stimuli is vocal, especially the mother's voice—sounds that are transmitted in a filtered form through the liquid medium. In the review below I focus primarily on the human fetus and neonate, because the purpose is to support the theory that the organism has a set of genetic predispositions, probably evolving to facilitate its entry into the community as soon as possible after birth.

Chemosensory

Fetal Abundant sensory stimuli are available in utero, but does the fetus have the necessary structures to sense them? The main olfactory system is organized most intensively during the first trimester of gestation (Schaal, Orgeur, & Rognon, 1995), at which time a sheet of receptors capable of sensory performance is present. The laryngeal, pharyngeal, and epiglossal taste buds, main olfactory epithelia, and vomeronasal and trigeminal systems, all involved in chemical reception, are present.

The sensory apparati of several modalities are well developed morphologically in the fetus, with chemosensory modalities arising shortly after that of somesthetic and vestibular modalities, but preceding auditory and visual modalities (Schaal et al., 1995). This morphological development (and as we will see, functional onset) occurs before birth. Rats, for example, are born less advanced in attaining some senses than are humans; their cutaneous and vestibular systems develop prenatally, but auditory and visual areas develop postnatally. The same order is found for different modalities for both rats and humans (Ronca & Alberts, 1995).

Organization of the precocious human chemosensory system is completed during the last month of fetal life (Schaal et al., 1995), and the system is functional. Odor tests given as early as the first hour after normal term birth indicate that neonates can detect increasing concentrations of odorants, although they are not as sensitive to low concentrations as are adults (Schaal et al., 1955). Preterm neonates (28–32 weeks GA) were almost as sensitive to a mint odor as full-term ones (40 weeks GA), which means the chemosensory system is functional well before normal birth. When full-term neonates were tested at twelve hours of age (before their first feed), they responded positively to odors that adults find pleasant (both fruity and milky odors) and negatively to unpleasant ones (fishy or rotten). This effect probably is mediated subcortically because it was observed in an anencephalic baby that lacks a cerebral cortex. It is likely that the pattern of responses is based on genetically established sensitivity to odor categories, because neonates would have had no experience of some of the odors with which they were tested.

Prenatal chemosensory events are detected by the fetus. If the mother eats foods strongly flavored with cumin or curry the flavorings are detectable in the amniotic fluid, and would therefore be available to the fetus. The breathing rate of fetuses between thirty-two to thirty-six weeks GA accelerated when mothers drank two cups of coffee (regular that or decaffeinated), which indicates not only that the fetus is influenced by the prenatal chemosensory environment, but that this particular effect is due to some other influence than caffeine.

Neonatal Makin and Porter (1989) suggested a possible adaptive significance for chemosensory preferences. They exposed two-week-old bottle-fed babies to two gauze pads; one contained the odor of an unfamiliar lactating mother's breast, and the other either the odor of the same woman's armpit or breast odor of a nonparturient woman. Babies preferred the odor of the lactating mother's breast. They had never been breastfed or had any direct exposure to milk, so preference could not be due to postnatal familiarization or associative learning.

Porter, Makin, Davis, and Christensen (1991) tested the preference of two week-old bottle-fed babies for the odor of an unfamiliar lactating mother's breast compared with that of the infant's own formula. The babies preferred the lactating mother's breast odor, even though they had only been exposed to the odor of the formula. Schaal et al. (1995) interpreted these findings to mean that the fetal chemoreceptor system may be genetically predisposed to detect particular odor cues critical for neonatal survival. In the natural course of events the baby would be breastfed, and this predisposition would be facilitated by the "strongly reinforcing power" of initial interactions with the mother. This pattern of genetic predispositions can be influenced prenatally and strengthened by postnatal events. It appears to represent biases that ensure the infant will respond in ways critical for survival, and it should be expected to occur in other modalities.

Audition

Fetal Many studies have assessed fetal auditory sensitivity and function because the auditory system is well developed quite early, fetal response to sounds can be detected in utero, and controlled sound stimuli can be presented to the fetus. The prethalamic acoustic pathways begin to myelinate at five months GA and are completed at the fourth postnatal month. The postthalamic pathways begin to myelinate at birth, with the process completed by three years of age (Lecours, 1982). A review of the research concerning human fetal auditory perception led Lecanuet, Granier-Deferre, and Busnel (1995) to conclude that early prenatal experience to sounds contributes to the maintenance, tuning, and specification of the auditory abilities necessary for neonates to process sounds that will be important postnatally.

Using ultrasound techniques to record fetal responses, Crade and Lovett (1988) found that human fetal auditory responses begin at twenty-four weeks GA. Fifer and Moon (1995) noted that morphological, anatomical, and electrophysiological studies indicate the fetus is capable of responding to sound as early as twenty-five to twenty-six weeks GA.

When auditory stimulation is delivered through a loudspeaker placed one meter away from the mother's abdomen to fetuses between twenty-three and forty weeks GA, motor and cardiac responses begin to appear at twenty eight weeks. Wide-band sounds elicit greater accelerative changes in heart rate, and a greater increase in motor responses than do pure-tone or narrow-band sounds of the same amplitude. The level of response increases as the pitch of narrow-band noise increases.

At twenty six to thirty four weeks GA the fetus shows a reliable heart rate response to speech stimuli, and at thirty-six to forty weeks GA it responds to maternal speech. This means it has sensitivity to speech sounds, and special sensitivity to the mother's voice.

At thirty-six to forty weeks GA the heart rate of French fetuses gradually ceased responding (habituated) to a pair of French syllables spoken by a female voice, and the response recovered (dishabituated) when the order in which syllables were spoken was reversed, indicating the fetus discriminated between the stimulus patterns. A short French sentence spoken by either a low-pitched male voice or a high-pitched female voice was presented to fetuses at thirty-seven to forty weeks GA and repeated until the heart rate was stable at presentation of the voice. A change from one voice to the other produced deceleration of heart rate, and this change was greater than if they experienced only silence. Again, the pattern indicates that the fetus is sensitive to voice and can discriminate between two voices.

Neonatal Prenatal auditory experiences affect the infant profoundly as early as a few hours after birth, making it unlikely the effects are due to postnatal experience. To facilitate entrance into the community, to establish emotional attachment to its mother, and to ensure its survival when it is most vulnerable, it is useful for the neonate to be able to discriminate the mother's voice and respond to it. DeCasper and Fifer (1980) found that neonates who were less than seventy two hours old preferred their mother's voice. Fifer and Moon (1995) summarized a series of studies indicating that neonates less than seventy two hours old would learn to suck a pacifier when a syllable (pat-pat-pat) was paired with the mother's voice rather than suck in response to another syllable (pst-pst-pst) that was paired with silence or with another woman's voice. This means that neonates can discriminate between sounds, can learn to associate a syllable with the mother's voice, and prefer the sound of the mother's voice.

Forty-eight-hour neonates preferred the mother's voice filtered in a manner that mimicked the sound as it would have been heard *in utero* over the sound of the mother's unfiltered voice (Moon & Fifer, 1990). If born in a monolingual environment, the infants preferred the sound of a female voice speaking the sounds of the language (either Spanish or English) they had heard in utero (Moon, Cooper, & Fifer, 1993).

Vision

Fetal Although visual receptors are not subjected to external visual stimulation in utero, pronounced visual capacities and preferences appear at birth. At birth abrupt changes occur in the types of inputs that besiege the CNS: Visual inputs assume a paramount role in behavioral development throughout infancy and adulthood, whereas the role of postural responses decreases. The role of auditory influences changes from those that play a role in emotional adjustment to those that allow the infant to acquire speech and language (Lecours, 1982). As discussed earlier, the visual pathways and the primary visual cortex undergo considerable development during the fetal period and are capable of primitive function at the moment of birth.

The optic radiation of the thalamus (the major subcortical way station to the cortex) begins to myelinate at the eighth month GA and is completed during the fifth postnatal month (Lecours, 1982). Trevarthen (1982) considered the eye, as an optical instrument, to be stamped with adaptive structure far in advance of when it is able to function. There are ". . . elaborate prefunctional activities that foreshadow the use of gesture and speech in communication because communication is vital to psychological development after birth" (p. 9). He also noted that the subsequent development of brain systems ". . . is constrained by intrinsic relations and not just inserted in a compliant random nerve network by patterns of stimuli reinforced by simple homeostatic principles" (p. 8).

Neonatal Johnson (1990) discussed major features of cortical maturation related to development of vision in early infancy. There are four neural pathways.

1. A pathway from the retina to the superior colliculus is involved in generation of eye movements toward easily discriminated stimuli. The peripheral retina is quite mature at birth, whereas the central macular region is immature. The superior colliculus already has the layered structure typical of the adult by twenty four weeks GA, and this pathway begins to myelinate at about seven months GA. The thalamic way-station from the eye (lateral geniculate) to primary visual cortex doubles in total volume between birth and six months.

2. There is a broad-band cortical pathway from primary visual cortex to superior colliculus, and another from primary visual cortex to middle temporal cortex, and subsequently to superior colliculus. Dendritic spines in the primary visual cortex become more numerous in the weeks after birth, reaching a peak at four to five months before declining to adult levels at two years.

3. A frontal eye field pathway mediates detailed and complex analyses of visual information. This field probably is not functional at one month after birth, begins to develop at three months, and continues until the infant is six months old.

4. An inhibitory pathway from substantia nigra to superior colliculus is involved in control of visual attention, which may begin to function at one month.

At birth, subcortical visual evoked potentials are present, but only a few of the components related to the visual cortex can be detected. Electrophysiological evidence supports the idea that cortical functioning develops rapidly throughout the first few months, with major changes occurring in the second postnatal month.

The neonate can track moving objects at birth, but the tracking is jerky, the movements are of fixed sized, and there is no anticipation of target movement. The neonate more readily orients toward stimuli presented in the temporal than in the nasal visual field, and with stationary patterns it attends to the frame of a figure rather than to internal elements. However, if internal elements move, the neonate attends to them, as would be the case when the mother's eyes and mouth move as the neonate views her face. Laplante, Orr, Neville, Vorkapich, and Sasso (1996) found that newborns (mean age 65.6 hours, range 42–127 hours) could detect changes in stimulus rotation.

Johnson proposed that early neonatal vision is based on subcortical structures such as the superior colliculus. From birth to one month the visual field decreases and expands again by two months. Two-month-old infants become more sensitive to targets in the nasal than in the temporal visual field, as do adults. Smooth eye tracking of targets begins at about six weeks and is quite smooth at two months, with more attention paid to internal features of patterns. These functional changes seem to be due to maturation of primary visual cortex. By two and one half months the infant understands causal relationships between two moving objects, by three to six months visual tracking becomes anticipatory and perceptual constancies appear. These changes probably are due to the maturation of the middle layers of visual cortex and develop at the same time as do binocular functions, such as optokinetic nystagmus and stereopsis.

A newborn infant is able to see quite crudely, being myopic and astigmatic. Any object farther than 20 centimeters away is a blur, and in terms of Snellen values the two-week-old's visual acuity is about 20/600, which improves to about 20/50 by one year of age (see Held, 1982). Wertheimer (1961) reported that a neonate tested two minutes after birth responded to sound by looking in the direction of the source, indicating integration between auditory and visual systems at birth.

Most adults have a slightly reduced acuity to oblique edges as targets compared with vertical or horizontal ones. This oblique effect has been found for infants as young as six weeks, leading Leehey, Moskowitz-Cook, Brill, and Held (1975) to conclude this effect reflects an innate bias in the visual system, rather than being due to greater experience with the vertical and horizontal edges that predominate in an urban environment, as has been suggested.

The evidence reviewed above shows the neonate was well primed in its supportive homogeneous uterine environment and is able to respond in adaptive ways to the variable extrauterine environment. These response tendencies can all be considered to enhance the likelihood the neonate will respond to and receive attention of a primary caregiver. The next question concerns what the infant is able to do about it when important visual and auditory stimuli are encountered.

Actions

Fetal Not only does the fetus have sensory systems that function effectively at birth, but the groundwork has been laid that will enable it to act on the world. In a review of milestones in the development of fetal movement patterns, James, Pillai, and Smoleniec (1995) noted that normal fetal movements in the first half of gestation begin by the end of the first trimester; they are fluid and done with little variability. This pattern contrasts with the jerky and repetitive movements of anencephalic fetuses for whom no distinct patterns can be recognized, suggesting that important cortical developments take place even at this early age. The first movements observed in the fetus, at about fourteen weeks GA, are in response to stimulation around its mouth (Maratos, 1982).

In later periods of gestation, movements become increasingly sophisticated and integrated, and the diurnal pattern of behavior is beginning to develop by twenty to twenty two weeks GA. At twenty four to thirty two weeks GA movement is characterized by periods of quiescence lasting 6 minutes or more. These quiescent periods are associated with development of inhibitory neural pathways, probably involving the cerebral cortex given that quiescence is not observed in anencephalics (James et al., 1995).

Lecours (1982) noted that morphological asymmetries have been observed in frontal and temporal lobes as early as the twenty-ninth week GA. Fibers crossing the midline between the hemispheres are present at about ten weeks GA, with major crossing fibers of the corpus callosum developing rapidly from the end of the sixteenth week GA to birth, a developmental burst that continues to the end of the second year of postnatal life.

The fetus not only engages in general activity patterns, but some important specializations begin to appear as early as twelve weeks GA. Stromswold (1995) reviewed evidence indicating the fetal brain begins to lateralize during gestation. The right temporal plane appears at thirty weeks GA, and the left plane first appears seven to ten days later. Neonates show strong laterality biases as revealed by head position preferences (Hepper, 1995). Most spontaneously turn the head to the right, and if the head is held in a midline position they turn it to the right. Ultrasound observations indicate that about 90% of fetuses suck the right thumb, the percentage of right-handed adults in a normal population. This thumb preference is present from as early as fifteen weeks GA, and correlates with head-turning preference and with the preferred hand used to grasp at fifteen to eighteen months. This means the developmental origins of laterality are evident early in gestation, and Hepper (1995, p. 408) suggested ". . . sucking the right thumb differentially stimulates the left and right brain hemispheres and this begins the development of hemispheric specialization and the subsequent laterality of function."

Neonatal Neonates show rhythmic side-to-side movements of the head in response to a gentle stroke on the cheek or corner of the mouth (Prechtl, 1982). These movements are replaced by directed and graded head-turning movements toward the stimulating source, followed by reaching toward the source with the mouth and grasping it with the lips. This motor pattern involves rhythmic mouth, tongue, and jaw movements, and an intricate coordination with swallowing and breathing that facilitate food taking at birth. These sucking movements are accompanied by a flexor synergism of arms and fingers and extension of the legs.

Infants as young as four days have a right-ear advantage for syllables and a left-ear advantage for music like noises (Mehler & Christophe, 1995). At birth, any speech stimuli activate the left hemisphere, whereas later in life only the native language enjoys that privileged status. Even at two days of age infants show a preference for short utterances spoken in the native language compared with those in an unfamiliar language. Mehler and Christophe suggested that this preference results from their having paid attention to prosodic properties of speech in utero, which allows them to classify inputs according to whether they are drawn from a familiar versus unfamiliar language.

"Smiling" movements involving both sides of the face were observed in both premature and full-term infants during periods of rapid-eye-movement sleep (Prechtl, 1982). Smiles appear spontaneously before they become linked to appropriate releasing visual stimuli (e.g., faces of caretakers). These spontaneous smiling patterns are reliably recognized by observers and are responded to positively by caretakers, even though it is unlikely the neonate is expressing anything intentionally, it merely is engaging in an innate movement pattern that benefits its ultimate survival likelihood.

Bower (1982) discussed the importance of the smile in the social development of infants. The first smiles may be seen in the first few hours after birth but observers judge them to be incomplete, because they do not include crinkling of the eyes as do real smiles. During the third week of life real smiles appear, and parents often want to spend more time with the infant once this occurs. The infant's smile at this time is elicited by the human voice, particularly a female voice. By the fifth week the most effective stimuli eliciting smiling are visual, the appearance of a face and particularly the eyes. The first real smile in response to another person's smile occurs at about ten to twelve weeks of age (Astington, 1993), about the same age the infant recognizes the mother's face from a group of face photographs (Dannemiller & Stephens, 1988). The next milestone is about nine months later, when smiles are directed preferentially toward the person who is responsible for daily care.

Crying is another early expression, and only humans cry with tears (Hauser, 1996). Early in life tearful crying elicits an almost immediate parental response. Later it is used to manipulate the parent, and Hauser suggested it is one of the first manipulative behaviors of the infant, exploiting the fact that adults are designed to respond to those who cry.

Facial Recognition and Imitation

The capacity to produce and perceive stimuli identifying individuals as members of a particular category, especially as conspecifics, is a ubiquitous feature of all animals, with the face being the most critical source of information (Hauser, 1996). Hauser reviewed studies indicating how the primate brain was designed to detect not only faces but particular features of a face, and characterized the nerve cells that are highly responsive to facelike stimuli as "face-sensitive" rather than "face-specific." The general pattern of interspecific differences in primate facial structure and expression can be understood by examining the communicative actions characteristic of members of each species within the context of its socioecology.

Although human neonates have very poor acuity they, like other primates are especially predisposed to attend to facial stimuli. Babies only a few minutes old (median 9 minutes) preferentially attended to a schematic face more than to one that had scrambled features or a blank face shape (Goren, Sarty, & Wu, 1975; Johnson, Dziurawiec, Ellis, & Morton, 1991). Babies less than one hour old prefer a slowly moving schematic face with appropriate features to a blank face or to one with the same features scrambled, even if they had never seen a face before (see Johnson & Morton, 1991). Walton and Bower (1993) presented newborns, age eight to seventy eight hours (mean 34.8 hours), with four different faces, followed by a composite of the four faces and then a composite of faces they had not seen. The time of the first look at the composite picture was greater than at the noncomposite, which means they recognized the difference between them. Because the mother's face usually would be the most frequently presented, it would make the greatest contribution to the face prototype an infant will form and should be preferred for that reason.

Meltzoff and his collaborators reported that very young infants can imitate adult facial expressions. He and Moore (1983) tested a group of neonates (mean age) 32 hours, the youngest 42 minutes, and found they imitated mouth opening and tongue protrusion. Six-week-old infants imitated the same two facial gestures made by either a stranger or the mother, indicating that no special relationship or attachment was necessary for the infant to imitate successfully (Meltzoff & Moore, 1992).

Neonates who had no experience with anyone before testing during the first hour postpartum imitated a person pursing the lips and widening the mouth (Reissland, 1988). When twelve 21-day old infants were exposed to adults to performing different body actions (lip protrusion, mouth opening, tongue protrusion, sequential finger movements) they imitated each action (Meltzoff & Moore, 1977). In another study, displays of mouth opening and tongue protrusion were presented to 30-day-old infants sucking a pacifier while watching the displays (Meltzoff & Moore, 1989). The infants imitated each display appropriately, even while they were sucking on the pacifier. This control procedure rules out the hypothesis that the infants' imitation depended on some form of motor resonance while viewing the display—they were actively sucking while watching.

To determine whether infants could master delayed imitation, Meltzoff and Moore (1994) assigned six-week-old infants to one of three experimental conditions. In one the experimenter demonstrated mouth opening, in another tongue protrusion at midline, and in the third tongue protrusion to the side. The infants were tested on three successive days, which provided a test for imitation immediately after the demonstration, as well as a delayed test twenty four hours later before the second and third demonstrations. Facial imitation occurred in both immediate and delayed tests. This means the infants had memory for the specific facial action displayed by the experimenter twenty four hours before, indicating the ability to remember characteristics of an individual seen twenty four hours before.

Meltzoff (1995) reported that 14 to 16-month-old infants could imitate actions, even novel ones they had not seen before, after retention intervals of two and four months, although they had not been allowed to engage in immediate imitation when the act was displayed. He suggested that imitation after these lengthy delays means it probably plays a significant role in human development, and supported this suggestion by conducting field studies showing imitation plays a role beyond the laboratory.

These studies of facial imitation were replicated in twelve independent laboratories in more than twenty four experiments (Meltzoff, 1996), and they reveal that, at birth the human infant has some basic imitative ability that does not require extensive interactive experience, experience with mirrors, or a history of reward. Facial imitation is an automatic response made to stimuli that have the configuration of a face, especially a moving one.

Hauser (1996) noted that there is no evidence monkeys can imitate one another, and only weak evidence apes can imitate at all. He characterized humans as "imitators par excellence," and Meltzoff dubbed humans "*Homo imitans.*" Imitation may be part of basic human biological endowment: Infants are comparing proprioceptive information from their own unseen facial movements to visual information from adult displays. They appear to be imitative generalists (Meltzoff, 1996), because they can imitate a range of novel and arbitrary acts, imitation is its own reward, and it is a bidirectional activity between infants and parents. He considered imitation to be a species-typical trait manifest in newborns so that they "act like" other humans.

Meltzoff emphasized that developmental studies found rich nonverbal "dialogues" often occurring while a mother and infant are facing one another, as well as during early feeding episodes. One function of imitation is to establish social identity. Infants use it to reidentify particular people after a break in perceptual contact. When different individuals appeared and then reappeared, the infant was able to perform the appropriate action associated with each individual. Bower (1982) concluded that through imitation the infant affirms its identity at a primitive level—it knows it is one of us. He considered imitation to be one of the earliest social interactions between humans.

Thus we have abundant evidence that neonates are able to recognize facial stimuli at the moment of birth, and this ability is not the result of learning. Slater (1993, p. 132) reviewed this literature and concluded that neonates prefer to look at patterned rather than unpatterned stimuli, at moving rather than static ones, at three-dimensional rather than two-dimensional ones, and at high-contrast rather than low-contrast stimuli. He wrote: "These visual preferences are often so powerful that *all* newborns tested with a particular pairing will look more at the preferred stimulus. These preferred stimulus characteristics are found in the face and combine to ensure that the face will be one of the most attention-getting and attention-holding stimuli encountered by the infant."

Hauser (1996) considered studies of facial recognition to indicate that humans are born with an innate predisposition to respond to the simple features characteristic of faces and find them perceptually salient, even though these simple feature might not be ones that adults would accept as a face. The features not only attract the infant's attention, they also guide its visual tracking system. One of the most salient features that compels an infant's attention is the eyes, and Hauser suggested this could mean feature detectors pull eyes out of the visual array of the face. He concluded, "A brain that has such simple featural demands is well designed, however, because the most important thing for an infant to know is whether someone is looking at her, and most importantly [sic], looking after her" (p. 361).

Conclusions

This review indicates that neonates have strong innate preferences for odors associated with mother's milk, even though they have never been nursed. Prenatal experience predisposes them to recognize and prefer the sound of the mother's voice, as well as the sound of the language that they heard prenatally. Neonates are tuned to be especially sensitive to, and to discriminate between, stimuli that are associated with caregivers, especially facial stimuli.

Now that some functional capacities have been traced through their fetal and neonatal stages, the development of more complex aspects of sensation, perception, and cognition are addressed in the next chapter. The discussion is extended to consider language development, and the characteristics of a theory of mind capable of expressing and recognizing intentionality.

6

Cognition and Mind: Humans and Nonhumans

In this chapter I characterize the perceptual and cognitive development of human infants. Relatively little attention is given to the voluminous literature bearing on nonhuman development, because that literature is not germane to the basic position being developed here. Human neonates appear in a state that qualifies them as human moral patients, particularly responsive to the sights and sounds of those in their community. These emotional and communicative behaviors are universally shared by humans. Although members of other species respond and nurture neonates and young of their own kind, humans quickly acquire a set of communicative and cognitive capacities leading them to develop a theory of mind (ToM) that supports a sense of cause, intentionality, and morality.

Human Infant Cognitive Development

An immense body of research and theory covers the human infant and the cognitive abilities that are used to infer the existence of mind. Early developmental research was stimulated by the studies and conceptions of Piaget, and a rich literature addresses the infant's intellectual capacities. A few critical high points in the development of an infant's basic perceptual abilities through the first year of life are summarized. They are important because they represent the first steps toward a theory of mind and higher-order intentionality necessary to qualify as a moral agent. Discussion concentrates on changes in visual perception, because these have been studied intensively and play a crucial role in infants' early emotional and intellectual development. Major psychological growth occurs between two and one half and five months of age, and includes understanding of simple physical principles, appreciation of the existence and constancy of discrete objects, and understanding that an object persists when it is not in sight.

Other developments occur between five and eight months of age, including the ability to understand continuity of movement, a tendency to reach to the future position of a moving object, appreciation of simple physical causation, and ability to follow an adult's eye gaze, which demonstrate the beginning stages of ToM. Between eight and twelve months infants can inhibit reaching for visible objects in a manner that reveals they exercise choice and control, crucial attributes to understanding intentionality. Gopnik and Meltzoff (1997) analyzed infant perception, cognition, and action, and identified early critical stages occurring at six and nine months of age.

The basic foundation on which human cognition develops is established by this time, with later developmental benchmarks occurring in the second to fourth years of life, which are discussed briefly when the development of speech, language, and cognition are considered. Material regarding speech and language is examined to consider what a complete ToM might include, what developmental steps might be involved in attaining it, and how understanding principles of causation might represent a critical step in the establishment of morality. Finally, a few cognitive attainments of nonhuman primates are described to contrast them with those that typify normal human development.

As noted in chapter 5, at birth the brain has only 25% of the mass of the adult brain, and increases in mass are due primarily to the development of connections, insulation, and metabolic processes. Large numbers of studies focused on functional changes in visual and cognitive functions during the first year of life. Rather than describe the particulars, only the conclusions are presented, with references to the primary and secondary sources that describe the experiments.

Most studies of very young, preverbal infants tested habituation and dishabituation to repeated presentation of visual displays, the behavioral measure being the time an infant looks at the visual display. The same display is repeatedly presented until the time the infant spends looking at it has decreased to a constant level on each presentation (habituation).

Then the display is changed and looking time is recorded. If the new display is consistent with the one to which the infant has been habituated (or is a transformation that is physically possible), little increase in looking time occurs (little dishabituation), whereas if it is inconsistent with the original (or is an impossible physical event), looking time increases (dishabituation). When looking time becomes short, it indicates that the infant has come to expect the characteristics of the visual display and spends little time looking at such a boring event. However, when that expectation is violated by a new display, the infant expresses surprise, as indicated by looking at the new event for a longer time. Infants similarly express surprise when an event violates their understanding of physical principles; for example, if an object would have had to pass through a solid barrier to be where it now appears.

Developmental regularities imply the existence of genetic predispositions that control the maturation of physiological structures and concomitant psychological abilities. By the time infants are two and one-half months of age they understand some aspects of physics, such as object permanence, continuity of motion, and that objects will be displaced when hit by a moving object (Spelke, Vishton, & von Hofsten, 1995; Baillargeon, 1995). By three months they recognize animate movements of the human body (Bertenthal, Proffitt, & Cutting, 1984) and the unity of objects, and understand physical cohesion and shape constancy (Caron, Caron, & Carlson, 1979; Milewski, 1979). Four-month-olds understand that objects move continuously, perceive figure-ground organization (Spelke et al., 1995), and remember objects after 10 to 15 seconds (Diamond, 1991). The visual system undergoes rapid changes during this period, and these changes are exploited to develop more veridical processing methods.

By five months infants understand that objects exist when out of sight, have a rudimentary understanding of the number of objects present (Wynn, 1992; Geary, 1995), and reach for the future position of an object that is no longer visible, although there is dissociation between seeing an object and being able to reach it, an ability that begins to develop at about eight and one-half months of age (Diamond, 1991). Diamond believes this lack of inhibitory control occurs because area 6 of the prefrontal cortex, which inhibits reflexive behavior, has not yet matured. These are important data because they reveal a general pattern that will continue to emerge with age: Infants are able to perceive and understand characteristics of a visual display before they are able to act on that knowledge.

Between eight and twelve months they become more and more able to inhibit dominant responses, and by twelve months have a primitive model of physics, have begun to develop cognitive capacities that will make it possible to understand causality, and appreciate that others have intentions that might be related to their own. Until they are about eight months old infants commit what is called the A, not B error; if they have found an object at one place (A) and the object is then hidden at another place (B), they search at A, even though they have watched the object being hidden at B only moments before. According to Diamond, two abilities are required by the A, not B task: One is memory, and the other is ability to inhibit the tendency to repeat the rewarded reach at A.

Leslie (1994) suggested that a theory of body mechanism (ToBy) begins to develop at around three to four months, and that what he called the theory of mind mechanism $system_1$ (ToMM$_1$) begins to develop at about six to eight months. One of the first signs of this system is following eye gaze. At six months infants demonstrate what is called joint attention: They turn, and visually search the side of the room the mother is looking at, but do not localize the target; by nine months they look to the correct side and locate the target if it is moving; by twelve months they locate even stationary targets the mother is looking at, becoming more and more accurate as they grow older (Butterworth, 1995).

At this stage infants are able to appreciate and store knowledge about goal-directed actions. As discussed in the next section, Leslie believes that the theory of mind mechanism $system_2$ (ToMM$_2$) begins to develop during the second year of life, emerging between eighteen and twenty-four months. During this period, infants are able to construe the behavior of other agents, making them able to infer attitudes of those others.

As noted in chapter 5, profound changes in the nervous system occur during this time that continue until infants are twenty-one months old: These include increases in the elongation of dendrites and number of neurons in the visual cortex; the optic radiation of the thalamus is completely myelinated at five months, the lateral geniculate nucleus of the thalamus has doubled in volume (to 45% of the adult volume) by six months, the fibers from the superior colliculus have begun to myelinate at seven months, and a maximum number of synapses are present in visual cortex by eight months. These neurological developments enable the infant to perceive the world, revise their theories about that world, and act on it in increasingly appropriate ways.

By nine and one-half months infants can separate line of sight from line of reach (Diamond, 1991), and between eight and twelve months they first become able to inhibit the dominant response tendency to reach automatically to where they see an object, even though the reach is blocked by a transparent solid wall. Diamond (1991) reported that lesions of the dorsolateral prefrontal cortex in the monkey disrupted this performance, resulting in exactly the same sorts of errors as those made by seven and one-half to nine-month-old humans. She concluded: "The ability to inhibit making the predominant response frees us to exercise choice and control over what we do. That is, it makes possible the emergence of intentionality" (p. 105).

Infants age nine and one half months realize that the presence or absence of a protuberance in a cover signals the presence or absence of an object beneath the cover (Baillargeon, 1995). They are not able, however, to infer anything regarding the relative size of the object until they are twelve and one half months old. Thus, by the time infants are twelve months old, they have built up a primitive model of physics, psychology, and number (Carey & Spelke, 1994). The authors concluded that a single system of knowledge is involved in object perception and physical reasoning in infancy, and that the domain-specific system is the same as for the domains of psychology and number.

Spelke et al. (1995) suggested that perception and reasoning emerge early in infancy and are closely related to one another, but are distinct from capacities to act on objects. Perceptual and cognitive mechanisms are attuned to the most reliable environmental constraints that provide the firmest foundation for learning, and knowledge about principles of cohesion, continuity, and contact remains central to human perception and reasoning throughout life; Sperber (1994) concurs. Hauser (persual communication) added that the human brain probably capitalized on the consistencies that existed in the EEA.

Gopnik and Wellman (1994) hold that, rather than having successive modules that come on line, knowledge has a starting state providing an innate mapping of inputs onto representations, and these starting conceptions are revised and reorganized as a result of countervailing evidence. All of these concept suggest that the human infant is a highly efficient and precocious information processor as soon as the neurological apparatus becomes available to support such processing, and these abilities to perceive and act on the world develop with the universal regularity typical of evolved mechanisms.

Development of Speech and Language

One of the most striking and ubiquitous cognitive characteristics of all normal humans is acquisition of spoken language. Speech develops spontaneously with mere exposure to sounds of language and does not require systematic teaching. There is a strong regularity in the time and rate of articulatory development of speech sounds and acquisition of syntactical and grammatical forms. Infants who are not able to hear learn to communicate through the medium of signing, and signing systems show developmental timing and regularity similar to those for speech.

I discussed the development of human speech and the beginnings of language in *Human evolution, reproduction, and morality* (Petrinovich, 1995, pp. 74–91) and concluded that they initially serve the function of attachment and emotional bonding, processes that lay the foundation for communication through speech. Language development (whether spoken or signed) is an adapted and evolved process involving innate computational mechanisms that define grammatical categories of such things as noun, verb, and auxiliary. Stromswold (1995) considered the remarkable uniformity of language acquisition to imply that categorical membership, rather than meaning, determines syntactic behavior. She believes infants are born with the ability to learn the categorical membership of words, that is, which words are nouns and which verbs. They rapidly display knowledge that objects are expressed by nouns, physical actions by verbs, and attributes by adjectives. This innate knowledge allows them to infer the category words belong to without having to go through an extensive process of learning about individual words in order to form generalizations.

Speech Reception

Studies of infants indicate that words are categorized phonemically and are organized into grammatical categories, rather than stored individually. Words are placed in phrase units that constitute the basic levels of linguistic analysis, and these cognitive processes of categorization are shared with adults, enabling children to learn variable parts of language in such a way that their developing grammar is synchronized with the grammar of their community.

When language development is conceived in this way, it is possible to understand how huge chunks of grammar become available to the child all at once (Pinker, 1994). If language development is thought of as a chunking process, it is unnecessary to acquire dozens or hundreds of rules; it is necessary only to set a few mental "switches." Natural selection would be the driving force that favored those in each generation whose speech hearers could best decode, as well as hearers who could best decode the speakers. Those favored individuals would be most likely to communicate, survive, reproduce, and successfully rear young. Hauser (1996) proposed that over the course of evolution by natural selection, dramatic alterations in the morphology of structures involved in human speech production were favored, but with few alterations in the mechanisms that underlie speech perception. This suggests the two systems might have a different evolutionary basis, each operating according to different principles and through independent mechanisms.

In chapter 5, several salient processes that appear during fetal development were identified that initiate the neonate into the human social and language community at birth. Among these processes is a prenatally developed preference for the mother's voice. In fact, the infant prefers the mother's voice when it is filtered so that it resembles her voice as it would have been transmitted through the aquatic prenatal medium, rather than her terrestrial voice. Not only is the infant able to discriminate and demonstrate a preference for the mother's voice (and human voices compared with noise or silence), but it discriminates and prefers intonation patterns of the language community with which it was surrounded prenatally.

The neonate is a complex pretuned developmental bundle, primed to proceed along paths that will lead to the comprehension and production of spoken language. Mothers smooth these developmental paths by speaking to infants in a distinctive pattern called "motherese" (Fernald, 1992), which is used in infant-directed vocalizations in all cultures that have been examined. Infants are more receptive to vocalizations spoken in motherese, and the characteristic intonation patterns also are used when teaching new words to infants later in life. Deaf six-month-old humans also respond and attend to signed motherese (Masataka, 1996). This style of signing is characterized by a significantly slower tempo, the same sign is repeated often, and movements associated with each sign are exaggerated.

Infants imitate vocally before the onset of meaningful speech, and infant babbling sounds differ across cultures. Although they are able initially to discriminate speech contrasts of any human language community, this generalized ability is lost by about ten to twelve months of age, and infants come to group speech sounds as do the adults of their language community (Werker, 1989).

Many of these developmental principles are applicable to the development of signed language by deaf infants (Newport, 1991). As for many other evolved adaptations, the facility to develop language does not persist throughout the lifetime of the organism; there are privileged times when the organism is highly plastic, but this plasticity disappears quickly. It is possible to learn a second language as an adult, but the process is slow, and intonation patterns of a second language learned in adulthood are seldom mastered as fully as the native language. It is likely that different mechanisms are involved in learning first and second languages.

Neville (1995) recorded event-related brain potentials (ERPs) when attention was directed to visual stimuli, and when language was being processed by normal adults, congenitally deaf adults, and normal children. Different subsystems were active during visual and linguistic processing, and they displayed different degrees of activity-dependent modification. Congenital deafness led to major alterations in visual system development; deaf adults were faster than hearing adults at detecting motions of peripheral targets, and peripheral attention-related ERPs were several times larger than those for hearing adults.

Individuals who became deaf after the age of four years did not show the increased ERPs or the enhanced peripheral attention that accompanied adult auditory deprivation. This suggests critical periods for development of these abilities between birth and four years of age. For normal adults, ERPs to auditory stimulation in the temporal (primary auditory) region of the brain were large, but in the occipital (primary visual) region they were small. For six month-olds ERPs were equally large for both regions, indicating less specificity and more redundancy of connections in the young. These findings accord with reports by several investigators (e.g., Spelke et al., 1995) that considerable intermodal integration exists during this period.

Neville examined the pattern of ERPs during linguistic processing. She found that when individuals were doing semantic processing (e.g., the meaning of nouns, verbs, and adjectives that make reference to specific objects and events) or grammatical processing (e.g., structural or relational information using articles, conjunctions, and auxiliaries), different neural mechanisms were active. It probably is biologically meaningful to consider these two grammatical systems to be separate subsystems within the language substrate.

Several investigators studied biological processes involved in speech perception. Eimas (1982) considered the mechanism responsible for perception of speech to be a species-specific adaptation that evolved for the sole purpose of processing speech. Categorical perception allows infants to categorize inherent variation in the speech signal along those acoustic continua that are critical when making phonetic distinctions of human languages, as well as when organizing segmental units into syllables. He considered the perceptual processes of infants to be constrained and shaped by genetic factors, and to be well matched to the demands of linguistic processing and acquisition of language.

At ages three and four months infants could integrate two sounds, one presented to each ear, and they could form a coherent speech percept if it was possible to create one from the two sounds (Eimas & Miller, 1992). Infants integrated information from the two sources to form a unified phonetic percept, as do adults. These results support the idea that percepts of auditory events are organized entities, and their representations are due to innate processes that begin in the womb during the later stages of pregnancy.

Infants as young as one month group speech sounds into segments that constitute the syllabic structure of language (Eimas, Siqueland, Jusczyk, & Vigorito, 1971). Categorical perception is characteristic of many aspects of infant sensitivity, including colors, object perception, and a number of nonspeech dimensions (Jusczyk, 1982). Examinations of these perceptual groupings led Jusczyk to suggest that specialized mechanisms found for speech perception might be part of a general psychophysical mechanism used by infants to analyze the welter of stimuli encountered in the world. Adults group facial expressions into naturally occurring categories (Etcoff & Magee, 1992), and it might be expected that infants will be found to do so as well. Kuhl (1992) maintained that infants enter the world with innate knowledge about natural psychophysical boundaries that enable them to break up the continuous sound stream into functionally meaningful categories. Her research suggests this process is well in progress by the age of six months.

Three-month-olds are capable of intermodal learning only if auditory and visual stimuli are presented in a synchronous manner, indicating that by this age there are inherent constraints on the kinds of audiovisual relations infants can learn (Bahrick, 1988). Infants age eighteen to twenty weeks recognize a face articulating a sound perceived visually, and prefer looking at it rather than one in which sight and sound were not synchronous (Kuhl & Meltzoff, 1988). When ten to 16-week-old's were presented with a video of a person speaking with the audio track out of synchrony, they preferred the synchronous sound (Kuhl, Williams, & Meltzoff, 1991). They even looked away from as asynchronous presentation (Dodd, 1979).

Not only are infants more receptive to those aspects of sounds that make up the language they will come to use, but they are preadapted to engage in "conversations." Condon and Sander (1974) recorded movements of infants as young as two days old to speech sounds and described an organized pattern between adult speech and a neonate's body movements. An orderly tendency to take turns develops from this initial responsiveness. This interactional synchrony is specifically human, is elicited only by speech, but does not depend on the particular language spoken (Bower, 1982). These characteristics do not typify the behavior of any other primate. Accompanying this initial stage of synchrony is the ability to imitate, with facial gestures being particularly salient. Imitation may function to elicit and maintain social interactions between an infant and other humans, and initially may be more important than the developing behaviors of smiling and vocalizing (Maratos, 1982).

When the mother vocalizes, the neonate fixates on the talking face, which causes the mother to engage in vocalizations characterized by a higher fundamental frequency and an exaggerated frequency variation. This pattern of exaggerated intonation might give infants clues to parse adult utterances, a process that helps them acquire the speech structure of their language. The fact that infants learn the art of vocal turn taking very early provides them with a frame within which vocal dialogue can develop. Taking turns is part of a social contingency mechanism involving a social behavior emitted by the infant (vocalization while gazing at an adult) and a social behavior emitted by the adult (vocalization that occurs while gazing at a child) (Dunham & Dunham, 1995). The eye-detection system that would initiate this pattern is considered to be an adaptive mechanism that developed early in the evolutionary history of humans to detect "eyes directed at me," and this mechanism specifies the object on which the agent's next action is targeted (Baron-Cohen, 1995b). A number of studies showed that infants normally follow the gaze of other individuals at an early age, which could enable them to develop the concept of joint reference. All of these developments usher them into the social community and enhance the likelihood that caregivers will bond with them.

Speech Production

Crying is the first vocalization at birth, probably due to acute distress involved in switching to a completely different oxygenation system (Locke, 1993). Sixteen-hour-old neonates can discriminate between their own vocalizations recorded a few hours earlier from recorded vocalizations of other newborns (Martin & Clark, 1982). If the neonate was quiescent when the sound was presented, it would begin to cry at the sound of voices of other neonates, but if it was crying it would stop at the sound of its own cry.

These first cries appear to be involuntary, driven by subcortical structures and becoming voluntary as cortical structures mature. Hauser (1996) proposed that strong selection pressures may shape the nature of the infant's cry, as well as the parent's perceptual sensitivity to in. Infant cries are individually distinctive and appear to be designed for long-range propagation—as anyone who has been a parent can attest. Adaptations involved in actions and reactions to crying regulate parent-offspring relationships.

Human infants begin to make nondistress vocalizations early, but infant monkeys and apes do not engage in any such vocal play, in fact, no other mammal does anything similar to babbling. Locke (1993) summarized the research identifying stages of early vocal behavior of human infants using the following scheme. The first stage is phonation (0–1 month) in which nondistress sounds are associated with an open vocal tract. Next is a "goo" stage (2–3 months) in which crude syllables with round velar stops, /g/, are produced repetitively with an irregular distribution. This is followed by an expansion stage (4–6 months) in which the vocal behavior diversifies and there are more vowellike sounds, as well as bilabial trills ("raspberries"), squealing, and grunting. Well-formed syllables are emitted during a reduplicated babbling stage (7–10 months) that starts suddenly, is different from what occurred before, and is remarkably similar to speech. Next is variegated babbling (11–12 months) during which monosyllabic strings, such as /daba/ are emitted. Locke (1993, p. 176) considers the six month-old to be ". . . an old hand at vocal communication and 'conversation'." Although the content does not sound much like articulate speech, babies have begun to partition the voice into syllable-size elements during babbling.

The abrupt onset of babbling between six and ten months occurs in all languages that have been studied. A strong universal tendency regulates the earliest babbled sounds; /m/ is babbled in 97% of languages, whereas /r/ occurs in only 5%. Babbling provides vocal self-stimulation, which provides useful sensory and motor feedback advancing the processes involved in acquisition of speech. Although the deaf babble, they emit a smaller number of syllables and at a later age. Universal babbling reveals few cross-cultural differences that can be differentiated perceptually or acoustically. Early babbling patterns are the same for deaf and brain-damaged infants, suggesting that they represent biological universals that are well buffered from disruptions during development.

Locke suggested that the onset of babbling marks the onset of left hemisphere control of speechlike activity, indicating the beginning of neural preconditions for the development of spoken language. He reviewed the literature on the development of precisely timed motor behavior of babbling and development of repetitive activity of the right hand, and concluded that, in the second six months of postnatal development, the left hemisphere assumes control of speechlike activity. Babbling represents the functional convergence of motor control and sensory feedback systems.

Early developments in the nervous system, sensory capacities, and motor abilities unfold in orderly and uniform patterns, and adapt the human infant to its community's communication structure. The infant not only has the capacity to elicit responses from caregivers, it also is able to respond appropriately to signals from caregivers. These early communicative behaviors serve two functions; they establish emotional contact with the social universe, and lay the foundation enabling the infant to communicate with that universe. Early developmental stages that support speech reception and production usher the infant into the linguistic world, and set it up to play the endless verbal games that characterize human existence.

Theory of Mind

Not only do humans have adaptations that enable them to relate to and communicate with others, they develop the ability to understand the intentions of others; to appreciate that others also have intentions, and that these intentions might be different from (or the same as) their own. This ability is referred to as a theory of mind (ToM), and it seems to undergo a process of regular development for all normal humans, and in fact is another inherent part of human nature.

Extensive theorizing regarding the nature of ToM was begun by philosophers and psychologists who recognized implications of the data described here, and brought them to bear to understand such enduring problems as the nature of intentionality. Dennett (1991) spoke of the "intentional stance," by which he means that when a rational agent exhibits intentionality, or "aboutness," the agent's actions can be explained (or predicted) on the basis of the content of these mental states. The term intentionality comes from the Latin, *intendere arcum in*, which means "to aim a bow and arrow at" (Dennett, 1991). The arrow has become a mere "logical" arrow, aimed abstractly at a thing in the world. Certain mental states, such as beliefs and desires, can be about either mental or nonmental states. Dennett (1978) discussed a second-order intentional system, one to which we ascribe not only simple beliefs, desires, and intentions, but beliefs, desires, and intentions about beliefs, desires, and intentions.

Dennett (1978) considers nonhuman animals to have first-order intentions, but probably no second-order ones. " . . . [We] will grant . . . that Fido *wants* his supper, and *believes* that his master will give him his supper if he begs in front of his master, but we need not ascribe to Fido the further *belief* that his begging induces a *belief* in his master that he, Fido, wants his supper." (p. 274).

A first-order intentionalist is a behaviorist—perhaps a clever one—but it does not have a ToM module designed to generate second-order beliefs (beliefs about the beliefs and mental states of others). Chimps are natural psychologists in the sense that they might have second-order intentional systems (Dennett, 1995). Even if this possibility is granted, they lack a crucial feature shared by all human natural psychologists: They never get to compare notes in order to engage in disputes over attributions, but have to generate knowledge all on their own. "Naked animal brains are no match for the heavily armed and outfitted brains we carry in our heads" (p. 391).

Baron-Cohen (1995a) noted that the phrase "theory of mind" has come to serve as shorthand for the capacity to attribute mental states to oneself and to others, and to interpret behavior in terms of mental states. There has been strong interest in the workings of the mind, and this interest resulted in several models for and theories about ToM (see Carruthers & Smith, 1996). Research programs and theories were developed by individuals in a number of disciplines, including philosophy, primatology, cognitive science, and developmental psychology, and the separate and collaborative cross-disciplinary efforts resulted in output that displays a strong hybrid vigor.

Infants have to relate to the adults with whom they will be interacting, and must understand which of the behaviors they see are important. They need to develop communication skills and a sense of self, be able to understand and communicate their intentions, and understand that others have intentions. These early steps support, and are accompanied by, growing ToBy, which involves understanding mechanical actions, and ToM, which has two components: The first concerns actional properties and goal-directedness; the second allows the infant to infer something about intentions of others.

One of the earliest complex attributes that appears in human infants is ability to imitate actions; it appears at birth and becomes increasingly sophisticated over time. Meltzoff (1990) found that fourteen-month-olds looked significantly longer at, smiled more at, and directed more behavior to an adult who imitated the infants' actions than they did to a control adult who played with a toy but either did not imitate at all or did not imitate the infant's specific movements. Meltzoff (1996) interpreted this to mean that infants recognize not only that another person moves when they do, but that the other moves in the same manner. This imitation could be a first step toward appreciating a world of interacting people, which leads the infant to realize it is a part of that world and its patterns of action and reaction.

The next step is to develop an idea that it is a distinct, differentiated individual. Bower (1982) suggested the infant formulates both a concept of self and a concept of others through social development. The ability to imitate seems to be manifest in all human cultures, and represents early ability and willingness to interact with any person.

The infant must now move toward understanding that it has mental states and that others have similar states. Human adults do not consider other people as mindless entities, but beings who have mental states, such as beliefs, expectancies, and desires (Meltzoff, 1996). Infants do not blindly imitate actions they observe an adult make, but infer what the goal of the action is. Their imitative behavior indicates they understand the intention of the actor, and not just the specific actions performed. There is little evidence for this kind of imitation in other primates.

Infants do not assume all objects have intentionality. When similar movements in space are traced by an animate and an inanimate device, only the animate behaviors are imbued with intentionality. The capacity to understand intentions of another person could mean that infants have a ToM, and I contend that aspects of a complete ToM represent characteristics that develop only in young humans. The complete ToM, together with an understanding of rules and causation, is the hallmark of moral agency.

I made passing reference to the tripartite domain-specific schema of ToM that Leslie (1994) developed to characterize cognitive development: Mechanical (ToBy), actional (ToMM$_1$), and attitudinal (ToMM$_2$). He considers these processes to be three separate aspects that define the quality he calls agency. ToBy is evident by three or four months of age, and is a mechanics module that involves understanding ". . . .of cohesive, solid, three-dimensional objects embedded in a system of mechanical relations, such as pushing, blocking, and support" (p.124). He phrases these developments in terms of modularity because he believes such a mechanism would ensure rapid and uniform knowledge acquisition in domains having adaptive significance for members of the species, with benefits accruing from componential organization at more central levels of perception. Leslie suggests this mechanism would confer the ability to participate and benefit from the cultural transmission of knowledge.

This conception is different from Piaget's (1954) view of the infant's developing knowledge of the physical world. He believed infants were not able to construe the physical world as a rigid three-dimensional space containing stable physical objects whose behavior is regulated by causality until the end of their second year.

Leslie regards ToMM systems to be concerned with intentional properties. ToMM$_1$, which develops between six and twelve months, refers to an agent's ability to represent actional properties, which includes interactions between agents, as well as goal-directedness. ToMM$_2$ develops during the second year and supports the infant's ability to infer something about the attitudes and intentions of others—what Baron-Cohen (1995a) calls mind reading. Mind reading does not mean we have special telepathy, only that we have the capacity to imagine or represent states of mind that we or others might have, and use this knowledge to predict behavior. We cannot help mind reading because it is a consequence of our biology, just as is our capacity for language.

Baron-Cohen (1995b) advocated the name "folk-psychology" to remind us that we are simply considering our everyday way of understanding people. Carruthers and Smith (1996) believe that folk psychology (the mind reader) is embodied in an innate, genetically endowed ToM module in the normally developing child. This initial basic theory is based on the assumption of an innate starting point for the attention biases and similarity spaces that give a kick-start to the acquisition of a theory of mind which also requires a learning process similar to that suggested by Gopnik and Meltzoff.

Baron-Cohen and Swettenham (1996) proposed that another basic mechanism, the shared attention mechanism (SAM), would be added to (or included in) Leslie's tripartite scheme (it could either be a specialized component of $ToMM_1$ or an independent one). It identifies that you and another organism are both attending to the same thing. Development of SAM is universal and independent of culture; children the world over show gaze monitoring and protodeclarative pointing. It evolves to guide behavior whenever the goal of an action is uncertain (Baron-Cohen, 1995b) In the face of such uncertainty, the first place to look for information to disambiguate the goal is a person's eyes. Baron-Cohen presented evidence that if SAM is impaired in a normally sighted person, ToMM will inevitably be impaired. He showed that children with autism suffer from mind-blindness due to damage either to SAM or ToMM, and characterized the psychological and neurobiological factors of the social brain, suggesting which might be involved in autism. He assumed that, in the blind, SAM functions by touch and hearing, allowing these individuals successfully to avoid problems of mind-blindness.

Gopnik and Meltzoff (1997) criticized the use of modularity to characterize the cognitive development of children. Instead, they proposed what they called the "theory theory." Whereas sensory modules may be innately structured to provide input for cognitive processing, the important structures are central ones that are revised and restructured as the child accumulates evidence about the world. Input modules direct attention, perhaps on the basis of innate calculations of a modularized perceptual system, and this input allows the infant to accumulate information on which to make empirical generalizations about such things as the relations between actions and events. When enough information is amassed and anomalies to theoretical expectations occur, the infant is led to revise its theory of reality. Gopnik and Meltzoff believed this to be a sensible proposal given that "Infants and children have infinite leisure, . . . they are free to explore the cognitive problems relevant to them almost all the time. They also have a community of adults who . . . are designed to act in ways that further the children's cognitive progress" (p. 25).

The infant begins at birth with an initial theorylike structure that is modified, revised, and restructured in response as evidence accumulates through experience in solving problems. The infant's early theories are simple and constrained to such concerns as there being a world of three-dimensional, amodal objects. They are elaborated to support understanding of the movements of objects by six months of age, and by nine months infants not only search the environment, but display surprise, reaching, and visual tracking, activities that indicate an abstraction of some of the underlying structure of both physical and psychological causality. At this age infants begin to produce communicative intentional behaviors that obey the rules of spatial contact, and attempt to influence people by producing gestures and vocalizations.

Later, linguistic input has striking effects on conceptual development, with children who hear language relevant to a particular conceptual problem being more likely to solve that problem than those who do not. Gopnik and Meltzoff believe that evidence regarding the effectiveness of differential experience supports the theory theory over modularity theories. Another line of evidence in that direction is the fact that cognitive developments in different domains are independent of one another. Although understanding of object appearances, actions, and kinds appears on average at about the same age, these stages are relatively independent of each other in the order and rate of development for individuals.

Causation and Morality

Premack and Premack (1994, 1995) related the child's development of simple ideas regarding causation—those involved in Leslie's ToBy—to bear on the formation of principles of morality. They considered the attribution of intention to be central to morality and also a fundamental component of ToM. Most animal species react appropriately to movements of physical objects, but only humans seek to explain the significance of these movements. The Premacks interpret this to mean that other species have no ToM at all, and the domain-specific theories that have evolved in humans represent a fundamental emergence.

These investigators (1994) determined that one of the most important ideas involved in the development of morality is attribution of cause: A two one-half-month-old distinguishes objects that move only when acted upon by another self-propelled object. When shown an object that starts and stops its own motion, the infant considers the object to be animate and intentional, and this occurs as early as three years of age. Three essential features required to attribute goal seeking to an intentional object are that its actions must be directed to a constant end, it must repeat the action, and its repeated acts must not be repeated exactly.

A set of abstract physical thought experiments was used to illustrate how positive and negative values could be attributed to objects. The net value of an act is determined by relationships between the actions of intentional objects. If an object, B, acts to hinder another's, A's, attempts at an action, negative intention could be attributed to B—a harmful attribution. If C acts to help B hinder A's action, C's act could also be seen as harmful in intent. If two bouncing objects are shown and one of them becomes trapped in a virtual hole, an infant might interpret the action of a second object that restores the motion of the first as positive helping. A second kind of helping occurs when one object assists another to move from an existing to a preferred state. An example would be if one ball that bounces higher and faster than another, lifts the ball bouncing with lesser height and speed, and the second thereby bounces higher.

The Premacks also assessed the importance of possession; an object could be considered possessed if it is connected to another and the two move together. An example of such a state of possession was provided by Kummer and Cords (1991) who found that an object attached to a macaque monkey and moved with it was treated by other monkeys as owned by the monkey to whom it was attached, making it impermissible for others to attempt to take possession of it. The Premacks believe that monkeys need a physical basis to interpret possession, whereas human infants probably do not. Thus possession is an important primitive because it has the power to bring into the moral domain objects that ordinarily lie outside it, stating (1994, p. 156): "Once value is assigned to actions, reciprocation follows, and in many respects it is reciprocation that is the crux of morality."

Another important physical factor influencing morality is the group, relationships among intentional objects. An infant could consider intentional objects of equal size and strength that move together to be members of a group, and such uncoerced comovement takes precedence over physical similarity. The concept of group entails powerful consequences: Members should reciprocate acts perpetrated by other members; members should act alike; and members should act positively toward one another.

Viewing intentionality in this manner supports the idea that "ought" is an innate concept (1994, p. 158); "If an antecedent is satisfied, the individual expects that a consequent will follow. This can be given the quality of ought or 'should' by reading, not that the 'consequent *will* follow,' but rather that it '*should*' or '*ought* to follow.'"

They summarized their theory regarding the basic form of moral belief in terms of six primitives: (1) Morality is a property of intentional objects; (2) the action of one intentional object on another is judged positively or negatively; (3) reciprocation of the value of an action is expected; (4) possession extends the moral domain to nonintentional objects, and although nonintentional objects are not assigned valence, those directed at possessed nonintentional objects are; (5) the concept of power is presupposed by both possession and group; and (6) when intentional objects of equal power move together they are perceived as a group, and knowledge of internal properties of the group develops earlier than knowledge of external group properties.

From this list of primitives they proposed a general form of moral belief using three terms: (1) Beliefs regarding relations between intentional objects; (2) coding these relations in terms of right and wrong—the former enjoined and the latter forbidden; and (3) distinguishing the group to which the participants belong from all other groups, and only relations among members of this group count. Although the primitives have an innate basis in physical causality, human moral beliefs result from a conjunction of innate and learned factors. The primitives supply a frame into which the content of moral beliefs is poured, and these beliefs reflect the power struggles of culture. These ideas are still programmatic and require empirical support (which I understand is forthcoming), but they eliminate some of the mystery regarding how humans might progress from simple notions of interaction and causality to develop and elaborate and intuitive moral sense.

Summary and Conclusions

This review of data and theory supports the conclusion that the human fetus is a bundle of genetic predispositions thriving in the benign intrauterine environment. These predispositions lead to behavioral predispositions that enhance the likelihood it will be accepted and survive in the more unpredictable extra-uterine environment that will challenge it from the moment of birth. In addition to the many constant intrauterine stimuli encountered, variable stimuli influence the course of development. The most salient of these are chemosensory, but important motor, auditory, and vestibular stimuli not only promote physiological development, but also tune the fetus to attend to environmental events it will encounter. Sperber (1994) suggested the presence of a general attention device, the function of which is to bring representations into a temporary buffer to be processed by specialized modules. In his view, attention fits "snugly" into a modular picture of thought.

Prenatal auditory experiences have an especially important role to pretune the fetus to speech sounds it will encounter. The universal importance of this auditory adaptation lends credence to theories that language is a critical aspect of human nature, so critical that genetic space is allotted for preadaptations to support its development. The power of these influences is demonstrated by the neonate's immediate preference for the mother's voice and the sound of the language heard in utero.

Prenatal development of the predisposition to detect and respond to facial stimuli is even more striking, because visual receptors are not exposed to external prenatal stimulation to channel development. The immediate ability to recognize faces provides a compelling argument that such recognition is subjected to selection pressures, and it also represents a universal aspect of human nature. Neonates are not only able to recognize faces, but are able to imitate facial expressions and recognize adults from their facial expressions. This ability to imitate is almost unique to humans; in fact, evidence for its existence in any other species is weak. The ability to imitate may represent an important step in forming a sense of self-identity.

Humans have a language ability with an almost limitless repertoire and an immense breadth of reference, whereas in other animals language forms a closed set with specific, invariant meanings (Wilson, 1975). The human infant is primed to communicate to comprehend and produce language whether spoken or signed. Early stages of vocalization and babbling unfold in a uniform manner for infants who are exposed to any language community, with the particulars of the specific language constraining the developing perceptual and production systems as language progresses.

The ToM concept is important because it involves attributes that probably are specific to humans. Some animals are able to appreciate the mechanical causality involved in simple actions (ToBy), a stage attained by humans by the time they are three or four months old. However, it is unlikely animals of any species other than some nonhuman primates possess a ToM that involves Leslie's $ToMM_1$, which arises between six and twelve months in humans, involving an understanding of goal-directedness. $ToMM_2$, which is seen during the second year, involves ability to mindread attitudes and intentions of others, and probably is a human emergent. These intentional capacities are built on a social base that supports recognition of other people and an early emerging concept of self, with goal concepts developing very early in life.

Understanding physical causality and the ability to infer that objects, especially animate ones, have intentionality is considered important to the formation of a sense of morality. The specifics of moral intuitions are elaborated within cultural contexts, but all embody several physical constraints recognized by all intentional agents: Beliefs regarding relations between intentional objects are coded right or wrong, and beliefs regarding the relations among members of the group to which one belongs are important in early valuations. Characteristics of ToM, combined with the nonreferential and complex syntax of human language that unfolds with exposure to any language community, make it possible to establish, understand, abide by, and enforce the rules that characterize the moral code.

Nonhuman Primate Cognition

I close this chapter by examining the characteristics of nonhuman primate cognition and posit tremendous differences between humans and nonhumans, making it reasonable to propose a set of emergent qualities that comprise basic human nature. Cognitive abilities are not pertinent to arguments regarding the personhood that depends on a biologically mandated social contract. Rather, they come into play to determine the status of moral agency that depends on the ability to understand causation, intentionality, and systems of rules that confer duties and responsibilities that moral agents must respect.

Animals do not possess the requisite capacities to be held to such responsibilities. The only possible exception that has been suggested to these restrictions regards the cognitive abilities of the great apes, especially chimpanzees. Most would not maintain that humans should prosecute or punish nonhuman primates for transgressions against the laws of human, or even primate, society. In chapter 8 I propose that differences in the conception of duties and responsibilities appropriate for animals and humans represent an underlying speciesist reality embedded in every moral agent's thinking regarding humans and other animals. The cognitive ability of animals becomes a moot point in terms of the basic moral position advanced here. A brief examination of cognitive abilities of primates is useful to gain perspective regarding differences in this area that exist between humans and other primates.

Hauser (1996) presented a detailed and balanced view of the communicative functions of animals and humans that emphasized evolutionary, ecological, and cognitive principles, and I recommend his book to those interested in such matters. The intent of the discussion of human development in this chapter is to characterize the human infant's neurological, sensory, and motor development as related to early perceptual and cognitive capacities. I have written here and elsewhere (Petrinovich, 1995, chapter 9) that birth marks a significant stage at which the neonate must be accorded moral standing as a human, and that this stage is determined not only by distinct biological and psychological characteristics peculiar to humans, but by patterns of emotional and communicative behaviors of the neonate interacting with caregivers. The next critical development leading to the status of moral agency involves development of ToM, which is specific to and between humans.

The development of human speech, the beginnings of language, and the evolution of both have been discussed here and elsewhere (Petrinovich, 1995, chapter 4), and the relevance of these characteristics to the evolved human social condition have been outlined (Petrinovich, 1995, chapter 5). The cognitive characteristics of the human species permit the development and appreciation of a full-blown, linguistically directed cognitive world, with ability to manipulate abstract relational concepts with almost unlimited flexibility.

I examine the case of the chimpanzee, which is considered to be the closest phylogenetic relative to *Homo sapiens*, to understand the chasm between humans and other species in terms of cognition, culture, language, and intentionality. An important methodological point is that many tests of chimp behavior involved animals that had undergone enculturation in the human world and were chosen because of their humanlike qualities (Gomez, 1996; Tomasello, Kruger, & Ratner, 1993). Many of these tests could result in underestimation of primate cognitive abilities, just as testing humans with nonsense syllables provides a poor estimate regarding verbal abilities. Gomez distinguished between chimps who are raised in the wild, those having friendly and frequent contact with humans in a zoo, and those who have been extensively and individually hand-reared by humans, often with intensive training procedures. He cautioned that, although hand-rearing could bring out chimp-specific behaviors that either would not have emerged or might eventually have appeared in time, it could also produce human-specific expressions of attention that make it easier for them to pass tests in which they have to react to humans.

Tomasello (1994, 1995) observed that mother-reared chimps hardly ever imitate novel actions, whereas those raised like human children and exposed to a language-like system of communication learned imitatively, much as do two-year-old humans. He concluded that a humanlike sociocultural environment is essential to the development of humanlike social-cognitive and imitative learning skills. Over researchers (Rumbaugh, Savage-Rumbaugh, & Sevcik, 1994) believe language skills appeared spontaneously in bonobos because they were reared from birth in a language-saturated environment where communication was emphasized. Experience with certain features of the human environment is required for chimps to engage the capacity to imitate, especially to imitate a different (human) species (Hauser, 1996). I agree with Hauser, who concluded that a great deal has been learned from attempts to teach chimps novel and artificial communication systems, but these studies do not contribute much to our understanding of communication systems that evolved in response to naturally occurring problems in the species-typical environment.

Chimpanzees have received intensive training to learn a language system that has some of the characteristics of human syntax (Gardner, Gardner, & Van Cantfort, 1989; Premack, 1986; Rumbaugh, 1977; Savage-Rumbaugh, 1986; Terrace, 1979). These programs demonstrated that chimps can master extremely complex tasks, and they certainly qualify as "clever behaviorists." Some observers determined, however, that not even a degenerate version of human language has been developed in an ape (Wallman, 1992). This conclusion was based on the belief that none other than humans have been able to acquire and use grammar, a system of nested abstract rules for the production and interpretation of utterances dictating the permissible relationships among elements of a set. Chimps require years of intensive shaping and thousands of training trials to acquire considerably fewer than 300 vocabulary items.

As noted above, chimps do not take turns in conversation, as do human children, although they do use symbol systems as a tool to do "chimpanzee cognitive psychology" (Pinker, 1974). They can master very complex tasks, but humanlike language does not seem to be one of them. Pinker (1995, pp. 138–139) neatly summarized the situation: "Chimpanzees require massive regimented teaching sequences contrived by humans to acquire quite rudimentary abilities, mostly limited to a small number of signs, strung together in repetitive, quasi-random sequences, used with the intent of requesting food or tickling. . . . This contrasts sharply with human children, who pick up thousands of words spontaneously, combine them in structured sequences where every word has a determinate role, respect the word order of the adult language, and use sentences for a variety of purposes."

Another methodological point is that much of the evidence offered to attest to the nature of chimp minds is based on anecdotes. Such evidence can be extremely valuable, but it should be supplemented by systematic observations or experimental manipulations either in the field or laboratory to avoid problems due to sampling bias, and to guard against the possibility an observed behavior has been picked out of context. Such biases could lead to misinterpretation of the meaning of behavior within the overall behavioral context, or lead one to regard extremely rare behaviors as representative of species-typical behavior.

It is necessary to be just as careful when selecting behavior for study in the laboratory. Patterns of behavior must be understood in the natural environment before theories are constructed to explain behavioral processes. Careful ethological studies of animals in representative environments should precede any manipulative study of molar behavioral processes (Petrinovich, 1973, 1976). After such systematic observations have been made, they can be included as variables for systematic study in either the field or laboratory, and represented with the frequency, distribution, and covariance occurring in nature. Presenting interacting variables in this manner makes it possible to understand their prevalence and strength; it is not possible to understand the strength of interaction if they are presented without preserving frequency, distribution, and covariance.

There is no question but that anecdotal and observational evidence has greatly enhanced our understanding of behavior patterns of chimps. F.B.M. de Waal (1982, 1989, 1996) presented a multitude of instructive examples that emphasize the importance of cooperation and altruism in chimp societies, suggesting they even develop a sense of justice and fairness. Such observations can be useful to generate ideas, but the ideas must be tested against alternative explanations and examined with more systematic observations and experiments (van Hoof, 1994).

In addition to these methodological concerns, strong political overtones exist. *The great ape project* (Cavalieri & Singer, 1993) is a manifesto demanding that these animals (humans, chimpanzees, gorillas, and orangutans) be admitted to the moral community as equals and are entitled to the right to life, protection of individual liberty, and protection from torture. The project was predicated on the fact that nonhuman primates are unable to fight for themselves. Contributors to the book characterize themselves as determined people willing to overcome the selfishness of their own group (humans) to advance another group's cause. One problem with the basic premise is difficulty understanding how nonhumans are equal if they are unable to press their case, they lack the communicative abilities and cognitive qualities, such as intentionality and the ability to mind read, that human moral agents possess.

Some of the argument was based on anecdotes from individuals with a declared bias, and these biases make the factual bases at least suspect. For example, Patterson and Gordon (1993) attempted to explain away reports that gorillas failed to pass a mirror self-recognition test, stating that the animals were inhibited by the presence of unfamiliar observers who made them so self-conscious they could not exhibit behaviors indicating self-recognition. Patterson claimed her gorilla, Koko, could pass the mirror test, but only when she tested it. It is difficult to establish objectivity or to assess reliability when only one observer, admittedly committed to a certain outcome, is able to conduct testing successfully, with all other observers automatically ruled out. Another problem is that little of Patterson's research was published in peer-reviewed scientific journals, making it difficult to judge the adequacy of her findings in terms of commonly accepted scientific norms.

Deborah Blum (1994), in her excellent journalistic representation (appropriately entitled *The monkey wars*) discussed the views of Roger Fouts, one of the leading advocates of chimpanzee welfare and a proponent of their advanced cognitive capacities. Fouts bitterly attacked the scientific establishment representated by the National Institutes of Health (NIH) and National Science Foundation (NSF) on the grounds that scientists who are members of peer-review panels object to his proanimal political stance and for this reason refuse to support his style of research. He asserted that this lack of support injured his scientific reputation and consigned him to a secondary status in the scientific establishment. His position is well represented by Blum, and her book should be considered if one wants a balanced discussion of the different views and perspectives of pro- and antinonhuman primate research communities.

Methodological and political issues aside, what can be concluded regarding the nature of chimps' cognitive abilities, the level of their ToM, and their level of intentionality? Hauser (1996) concluded (as I have here) that human infants are born with the ingredients for ToM because they show evidence they are sensitive to an object's goal and its directedness, are aware that self-propelled objects are driven by internal mechanisms, and understand that direction of gaze and attention provide important hints regarding what other individuals think or feel. Research bearing on primate cognition provides only weak evidence that apes have ToM, and indicates that Old World monkeys do not. Hauser (personal communications 1997) pointed out, however, that the number of experiments conducted on ToM in nonhuman animals is small, making it premature to decide absolutely about the presence or absence of that capacity.

No convincing experimental evidence supports the hypothesis of cultural transmission among chimpanzees, and if any true cultural transmission is present at all, it is at best inefficient Wrangham et al., (1994). There is not a single case of habitual tool use in the wild by bonobos, as exists for chimpanzees (McGrew, 1994). Not all free-ranging chimps use tools, but such behavior is likely to be typical of chimpanzees, although they have no comprehensive, habitual repertoire of that nature. Controlled experiments failed to support claims regarding full-blown imitation of tool use in any nonhuman primate (de Waal, 1994).

Chimps attend only to general functional relations between tool and food, and to end results obtained by the demonstrator (Tomasello, 1994). In contrast, human children use the same techniques and methods that are demonstrated, so they are truly engaged in imitation, and chimps only in emulation. Emulation is a type of social learning in which subjects reproduce an observed end result without copying the behavioral methods used by the demonstrator, whereas in imitation learning the focus is on the demonstrator's methods.

van Hoof (1994), Tomasello (1994), and Hauser (1996) agree, and what often has been considered imitation is the result of local or stimulus enhancements, which means that chimps are drawn to the locality and object being used by other chimps, and then learn the procedures for themselves. van Hoof (1994) discussed the one report that found chimps able to teach by actively molding the behavior of the young, noting that if it is replicable, chimps would be the only nonhuman species able to do so. However, lack of evidence for teaching by animals of species other than humans may be due to the low quality of current data, and more research should be performed to obtain more thorough understanding before any definite conclusion is reached (Caro & Hauser, 1992).

Comparing cognitive abilities of human infants and chimpanzees, Povinelli (1994, 1996) stated that between eighteen and twenty-four months of age a striking turning point occurs in human development during which several abilities emerge, many of which were described in the section discussing ToM. Chimps are able to follow gazes by five years of age, but it is not clear they have a mentalistic appreciation of the meaning of attention shown by others—they may not subjectively understand attention.

Povinelli found that chimps could respond appropriately if a human had knowledge of an event versus when the human was ignorant. The significance of this research was questioned by Hauser (1996), who suggested that it is not comparable to the state of affairs for humans. The chimps in Povinelli's experiments required several hundred trials to distinguish between knowledgeable and ignorant humans, whereas this ability appears rapidly and spontaneously in humans at the proper developmental age.

Baron-Cohen (1995a) studied the ToM of young humans afflicted with autism, which seems to be a lifelong disorder. He characterized the key symptoms as abnormal development of social and communication abilities that become apparent during the first few years of life. The play of these children lacks flexibility, imagination, and pretense. Autistic children have components of mind that allow them to interpret stimuli in terms of their wants and desires; they can use the word "want" in spontaneous speech, for example. They also can detect when a person is looking at them. However, they are not able to build the triadic representation necessary to specify and verify that the self and another agent are attending to the same object or event (a principal function of SAM, as discussed above). Lacking the ability to understand joint attention, they cannot establish a shared interest between self and another person. Because they do not have an intact SAM, virtually all aspects of ToMM are impaired. Baron-Cohen believes SAM is required to trigger ToMM. Autistic persons fail the false belief test (make the A, not B error) and do not understand the nature of beliefs involving psychological causes of behavior. In general, their understanding of beliefs remains at a level below that of normal three- to four-year-olds. Through a brain model he developed, Baron-Cohen attempted to show that autism is produced by a break at some point in a proposed neural system involving the orbitofrontal cortex, superior temporal sulcus, and amygdala.

Baron-Cohen (1995a, chapter 7) summarized comparable data for nonhuman primates. Macaque monkeys show more emotional disturbance when shown a picture of a conspecific displaying full face with eye contact than to one with a face turned away. This means they probably have an eye-detection mechanism, just as do autistic children. Baboons, macaques, and a number of other Old World monkeys and apes use and react to eye contact, and engage in mutual gazing. Chimps look in the same direction as another chimp, which might indicate they are able to make the attentional contact necessary for basic communication. However, it is unlikely that SAM is available to them because their gaze-monitoring seems more reflexive than for humans (Povinelli & Eddy, 1996). Given that SAM is not present, the chimp would be unable to develop ToMM, as discussed above. I conclude that nonhuman primates are not mind readers.

Hauser (1996, p. 652) concluded, "An organism without a theory of mind . . . will be frozen in action-reaction state, with no understanding of why others feel the way they do or why they might have different beliefs or desires. They simply don't know how to care, though they behave as if they do." If one accepts this conclusion, and I do, these beings are moral patients and should not be accorded the status of a moral agent.

Now that basic evolutionary, philosophical, developmental, and cognitive principles have been examined, it is time to consider issues regarding the permissible use of animals by humans. In the next two chapters I discuss basic philosophical views held by two of the leading animal welfare advocates and ways in which they are applied. In chapters 9, 10, 11, and 12, I turn to moral problems involved in using animals in biological and behavioral research.

II

Animal Issues

7

Animal Rights

In this chapter the question of animal rights as presented by Regan (1983) is discussed, followed in chapter 8 by a consideration of the utilitarian animal liberation views of Peter Singer (1975, 1990a). Views of other philosophers regarding the treatment of animals by humans are addressed in relation to those of these two leading exponents of the animal welfare movement. In chapter 4, issues in research methods and the philosophy of science were presented in the hope of engaging in a meaningful discussion of the value of scientific research in animals, and these comments are referred to again in chapters 9, 10 and 11.

The Conflict

There have been impassioned arguments, actions, and reactions regarding the moral status of animals. Various theories have been advanced by moral philosophers, some insisting that animals have rights, and some strongly against that possibility. Some say that these issues should not be posed in terms of rights, but should emphasize utilitarian respect for relative interests. These dialogues sparked active debate within the scientific community among those who want to consider issues in terms of animal rights or liberation, those who prefer to speak of animal interests and welfare, and those who believe that the needs of humans always take priority over those of nonhumans; and then there are those who would rather not even think about it.

One wing of animal liberation activism strongly disapproves of any use of animals whatever as means to human ends. Others go only so far as to content that factory farms where meat, eggs, milk, and by-products such as leather are produced should be abolished. Still others believe all consumption of animal products is morally impermissible, no matter how animals are raised. There have been spirited arguments that all research using animals should be stopped at once, and that animals should not be used in circuses, be ridden, worked, or kept in zoos. Animal welfare advocates agree less regarding the permissibility of keeping animals as pets or companions, or to assist blind and handicapped persons.

All this has led to direct political action by both proponents and opponents of animal welfare. (I tend to use the generic term animal welfare to refer to all animal advocates whether they be rightists or utilitarians.) Proponents have engaged in acts of civil disobedience, destroyed research facilities, and threatened researchers. Laws and regulations have been introduced to support various positions regarding the permissibility of using animals in research and to teach students. Numerous political actions involved much lobbying, shouting, and pamphleteering by people on both sides. Every citizen has the responsibility to consider these issues and take a position, whether it is one of considered action or inaction, and examine the bases for conclusions with care, as I do here.

The first position considered is that of Tom Regan, who believes animals have rights that confer a moral standing that makes it impermissible to use non-human-animals in any way that infringes these rights. The second position is that of Peter Singer (considered in chapter 8), who arrives at the same end point in terms of policy recommendations, but by a different philosophical route. To him, relevant concerns involve the interests an animal has to live a satisfactory life, interests that maximize pleasure and minimize pain and suffering. Singer developed a detailed theory against the evils of speciesism, which he considers to be the moral equivalent of racism and sexism, a position I challenge.

Animal Rights

The most complete and extensive position in support of animal rights was described by Regan in *The case of animal rights,* published in 1983. This book contains a clear presentation of how moral issues should be evaluated, and I discussed it in an earlier book (Petrinovich, 1995). Here, I summarize the major points of Regan's theory to capture their richness and thoughtfulness, even though I disagree with most of what he says. I comment on points with which I have difficulty, suggest why I believe rights views generally fall short, and propose that an evolutionarily grounded utilitarianism is preferable. The chapter concludes with a discussion of the legal status of animals. All page references to Regan in this chapter are to his 1983 book unless otherwise indicated.

Animal Awareness

The first step in Regan's theory is that animals possess awareness to the extent that they can experience pleasure, feel pain, and suffer. He maintains convincingly that such awareness exists for animals of many species, and that it exists independent of whether they have language abilities, a position disputed (none too successfully) by Frey (1980, 1983). When referring to animals, Regan usually means mammals (p. 172), but sometimes he specifies terrestial mammals (p. 240). At the end of the book he includes all mammals less than one year of age that have the physical characteristics qualifying them as being a subject-of-a-life, a status that entails more than being alive and conscious (p. 391). The subject-of-a-life criterion requires that individuals have beliefs, desires, perceptions, memories, a sense of the future, an emotional life (together with feelings of pleasure and pain), preference and welfare interests, ability to initiate action in pursuit of desires and goals, and a psychophysical identity over time.

It is important to Regan that individual animals be considered to have inherent value, even though they do not meet the subject-of-a-life criterion (p. 245). Elsewhere, he relaxes the definition of animals to include chickens and turkeys, which do not seem to satisfy the criterion (p. 349). He proposes this inclusion to demonstrate "how difficult it is to draw the line," and that it is impermissible under any circumstances to treat farm animals as renewable resources. Writing six years later (1989), he still found it difficult to decide where one should draw the line between those who are and who are not subjects-of-a-life.

His notions regarding awareness are supported by appeals to the evolutionary continuity of mental experience (see Hauser, 1996), and to numerous studies and observations of animals done both in the natural environment and laboratory. Ethological studies (ethology can be defined broadly as the study of animals in their natural habitats) established that animals (especially birds and mammals) behave in ways that signify a degree of intentionality and purposefulness, and it is reasonable to characterize some of their behaviors using cognitive terms such as beliefs, expectancies, and desires. I discuss these points further when I consider Singer's animal liberation position, which is based on these same assumptions regarding animal awareness.

Preference Autonomy and Interests

According to Regan, individuals should be considered autonomous if they have preferences and the ability to initiate actions to satisfy them (pp. 84–85). Preference autonomy leads to preference interests, dispositions to want and seek certain states of being and to avoid others. Animals benefit to the extent that they live in an environment that provides opportunities to satisfy preferences related to needs, and they also have a welfare interest to be in an environment where these interests can be pursued and satisfied (p. 90). It is important to establish that animals have intrinsically worthwhile positive interests that are comparable with those of humans, and that entitle them to enjoy a similar degree of satisfaction.

Regan (1980) stated that an animal's interest in avoiding pain is just as important to it as it is to a human infant. How relative strengths are to be estimated when interests in such things as avoiding pain are in competition remains a muddy concept throughout much of his work. The assumption that animals have an interests to avoid pain is reasonable. The sense of pain undoubtedly developed evolutionarily to enable animals to sense and avoid danger, and a defective pain system lessens an individual organism's likelihood of survival.

Moral Agents and Moral Patients

The distinction between moral agents and moral patients is central to much of Regan's thinking, and I discussed that distinction at length in chapter 6 of *Human evolution, reproduction, and morality,* and briefly in chapter 3 of this book. Moral agents are those who meet all subject-of-a-life criteria; they make up the moral community, are of direct moral concern, and have direct duties toward all individuals who are part of the community (p. 152). In contrast, moral patients lack prerequisites that would allow them to be held morally accountable for what they do, and for this reason they cannot do right or wrong. Moral agents can do right or wrong and must respect the rights of moral patients (p. 154).

Midgley (1983) suggested no one can have a right who cannot understand and claim it. Some maintain, as do I, that moral agents have indirect duties to moral patients as a consequence of being moral agents. Others contend that if duties of any kind are due in respect of a nonhuman animal or a human who is not a moral agent, that being has corresponding rights. On the other hand, Rodd (1990) suggested that "rights" should be considered to be a technical term to describe valid claims resulting from verbal agreements between moral agents. I defended such a position in chapter 3, but broadened its base to include biological tendencies that evolved to enhance the strength of the social contract between family members and the community.

Regan proposed that moral agents can be harmed by being killed or caused to suffer thus; there is a duty not to harm individual moral agents. He extends this duty to regulate the permissible treatment of moral patients by moral agents. He concluded (pp. 189–192) that his views meet the critical requirements to support ideal moral judgments, as outlined in chapter 4 of his book and chapter 1 of *Human evolution, reproduction, and morality*. I disagree with the key element of his position that all animals have equal inherent value.

Justice and Inherent Value
One condition of an ideal moral judgment is that it is impartial to comply with the formal principle of justice, based on the requirement that all individual animals are given their due so that similar individuals are treated similarly (p. 232). Regan (1979) raised a central point when considering infants who have not yet developed high level cognitive capacities, as well as irreversibly comatose humans. Human infants are comparable cognitively with many animals, all of whom have an interest to avoid pain, and none of whom understands concepts of right and wrong. Both Regan and Singer say it would be inconsistent to accord moral standing to one class of beings that would be denied to the other

whenever the two classes have similar capacities. I believe that this different treatment does not involve an inconsistency if it is accepted that the status of personhood signaling humanity can provide an adequate ground to support the differentiation. Both the human infant and animal are moral patients, but the former is a member of the human social community. Midgley (1983) noted that the basic trust people display to those around them cannot depend on language because it is found in young infants (discussed at length in chapters 5 and 6), people display it toward their elders, to each other, and to people who do not share the same language or have acquired no language at all. All of these individuals are properly considered members of the human species and can be accorded agency.

The case of the irreversibly comatose person is different. Here we have a former person who now has no interests and may suffer no pain, but is accorded legal rights and considered to be a special moral patient. I maintain that this special moral status is based on the fact that members of the community accept conventions that regulate societal interests. This acceptance leads to a necessity to honor commitments, even though an individual is no longer rational or sentient. The contract is important because those currently in the society want their own wishes and property bequeaths respected at their demise, and the living have a deep emotional attachment to dying relatives and a lasting respect for the no longer sentient person that the dead and dying symbolize. This contract creates a difference between comatose human moral patients and animal moral patients, even though the latter might have sensibilities that exceed those of the former. This view of the comatose human moral patient does not invoke rights as the operative moral principle; human moral agents have indirect duties and responsibilities toward all moral patients. When animals are accepted as pets, a special set of contractual responsibilities is assumed toward them by their owners or companions, and that accords them a special moral status.

Regan believes formal justice requires equality for all individuals, that this equality is based on the fact that different individuals have an inherent value, and that all moral agents are equal in inherent value. The argument regarding equal inherent value of moral agents runs as follows: Individual agents have a distinctive value independent of their pleasures, preferences, or abilities. He uses the analogy of a cup, wherein inherent value is contained by the cup itself, not as a receptacle for what goes into it. He wants to avoid problems that would arise if some individuals are considered to have such different values that their moral standing would be higher, and that higher standing is used to justify favoring those who have such virtues and excellence over those who do not. Favoring virtues in this way leads to a possible justification for slavery, racism, sexism, and elitism, in his view.

He rejects the idea that moral agents have inherent value in varying degrees: "All moral agents are equal in inherent value if moral agents have moral value" (p. 237). It can be posited that if individuals are considered to have certain essential values that cannot be abrogated—freedom from harm, freedom of respect and dignity—it is possible to allow for real differences in the value of different individuals, and that these differences are not relevant to an agent's basic moral standing. I consider individuals to have different value, but there is a basic level of freedoms below which none should be allowed to fall.

Regan regards equal inherent value not to be something that can be lost through an individual's actions; it does not wax and wane, and it is independent of the interests of others. Regarding humans who are not irreversibly comatose (1979), all have inherent value, but it does not follow that all have an *equal* inherent value beyond those that guarantee the essential freedoms cited above. He does not want to consider "severely mental enfeebled" individuals to have unequal inherent value, even though they cannot lead a life with the range of values that characterize normal adult humans. Such a concession ultimately would be troublesome to Regan's basic position, and could open the flood gates to permit comparisons between animals of the same and different species in terms of the potential richness of their lives, a point he does not want to concede.

He concedes the possibility that some animals might possess rights not possessed by others, some might not possess any rights whatever, and some might possess certain rights not possessed by some humans. When considering marginal human cases, decisions to be made must depend on having the capacity to suffer. This way of characterizing rights adds up to a vague and equivocal position. Although he states animals should have the same inherent value as marginal humans, he equivocates regarding what particular inherent values (hence, rights) are possessed by humans who have different qualities.

Regan reaches a puzzling conclusion when considering a lifeboat dilemma in which either a severely mentally enfeebled child or a normal adult could be saved. Perhaps it would not be unreasonable, other things being equal, to save the adult, because that individual has greater inherent value than the unfortunate child, and he bases this greater value on the adult's richer potential life (p.137). He continues with the mysterious statement that the manner in which such cases ought to be decided does not have to be resolved: ". . . the view that not all humans are equal in inherent value does not entail that those with greater inherent value can treat those with less in any way they please (e.g., as slaves)." These difficult matters should be set to one side, but this creates a problem because this conclusion could be construed to support an elitist position; when choices are to be made one should favor the elite and educated producers in society because they have potentially richer lives, which would accord them greater inherent value. If the proposal in this form is used to compare nonhuman animals and humans, animals would lose out against almost any normal human, as does happen when Regan considers the lifeboat dilemma involving a decision of whether to drown one of four human occupants or one dog. I consider his discussion of equal inherent value to be murky and inconsistent, and address his resolution of fantasy dilemmas in a special section below.

Midgley (1983) expressed similar concerns when examining problems involved in estimating relative value. One example was of an animal considered to have one-tenth the emotional capacity of a human being. She questioned whether the animal's value should be discounted by one-tenth of full value, and if it could even suffer another discount because it does not enjoy the emotional bonding value that humans enjoy with one another. She asked rhetorically whether this makes the animal worth one-tenth of a human, one-hundredth, or maybe one-twentieth. And what if an alien species appears that is ten times as intelligent as humans—do they move to full par and we to one-tenth of their value? She suggested that attempts at detailed arithmetical claims are useless, cannot possibly be made consistent, and usually are morally shocking. I suggest the overriding factor is the special interest parents feel for their own children and kin, which stresses the paramount importance of the species bond, a bond that is discussed at length when the concept of speciesism is examined in chapter 8.

Regan's position that moral agents should have equal inherent value is crucial because it forms the grounds on which the possession of rights are to be based. He holds that a necessary and sufficient condition to have basic moral rights is to have inherent value (1979). He characterizes inherent value by listing its "most noteworthy" features: (1) If any being has inherent value, this value is logically independent of any other being's interest or respect of that value; (2) having inherent value makes it improper to treat an individual as though the value was only a means; and (3) if an individual has inherent value, there is an obligation to treat that individual with respect. These foundational qualities are the stipulated basis for the concept of rights.

If it is conceded that moral patients have *some* inherent value, he believes it must be conceded that the inherent value of moral patients is equal to that possessed by moral agents. He pursues this argument because it is improper, in his view, to consider individuals as only receptacles of different amounts of inherent value, as this leads to an indefensible (and "unsavory") utilitarianism. Inherent value is not reducible to something that goes into receptacles, but is an absolute characteristic that either exists or not. His statement of this position is (p. 238): "To suppose otherwise leads us again to assume that moral agents are merely receptacles of valuable experiences and so may be treated in ways that optimizes these values without the victim being treated unjustly." Those with moral standing then, are equal in inherent value; all have it whatever their race, sex, or species; and any harm done must be justified because it produces the best consequences for each individual affected by the outcome (p. 239).

As noted above, he does not adhere to these principles consistently when dealing with difficult moral situations or fantasy dilemmas, and this inability, in my judgment, is due to a basic inadequacy in his position. For example, he might correctly consider his son's and his neighbor's son's interests to receive a medical education as equal, yet help only his son (1980). This, he states, does not necessarily treat the neighbor's son and his own son's equal interests differently, nor does he believe he has done anything morally reprehensible. I am puzzled by the first claim, but concur with the latter. He justifies these conclusions by referring to duties to his son, duties he does not have to the children of others. I fail to grasp his assertion, however, that different treatment of individuals who have equal interests does not violate the principle of equality of interests. I suggest this is another instance of the powerful influence of kinship bonds on human decision making, and he is sidestepping that fact. Whenever kinship bonds are involved, an equal interest no longer is equal, because the impact of this evolved aspect of human nature exerts a powerful influence abridging the neutral principle of equal treatment. The importance and priority of this evolved factor should be acknowledged and embedded in the basic structure of any moral system. Failing to do so leads him to serious difficulties that subvert the basic rights principle he upholds.

There is also a justice principle, insisting that respect be given to all individuals who have inherent value. Because those who have any inherent value have equal inherent value, all, moral agents and patients alike, must be treated equally, and the aggregate effects of the amount of inherent value in the population is irrelevant. As mentioned, Regan is not always consistent in his application of this principle of equal inherent value. He permits too many exceptions (what he calls special considerations) to make it acceptable as a basic principle to guide applied ethical decisions.

Narveson (1987, p. 36) chided Regan for carrying around a "fairly deep satchel of intuitions" that are called special considerations. Narveson observed that love relations are relations of deep self-interest, leading one to prefer those one has chosen as friend, lover, spouse, with whom one has special relationships. These self-interests are moral relationships generated by rational agents to promote their own well-considered long-run interests. I add that they are the deep, evolved nature of all humans and they power the moral engine. They are not mere special considerations that must be appealed to whenever a decision violates moral intuitions.

Regan (pp. 189–193) believes he has satisfied the necessary standards to arrive at a moral judgment: Conceptual clarity, adequacy of scope, precision and consistency, impartiality, verifiable factual information, and intuitive acceptability. Questions can be raised regarding whether he satisfies the criteria of clarity and rationality with his notion that all animals have equal inherent value. He allows too many exceptions, especially whenever kinship is involved in otherwise equal situations, and whenever one individual is favored because of a potential for a richer life. His theory also fails to meet the criterion of impartiality; when resolving some hypothetical dilemmas he introduces special considerations solely to challenge the permissibility of conducting research on animals for the benefit of humans.

Rights

Arguments regarding justice and inherent value involve the question of whether moral patients have rights. Regan's crucial point is (p. 279): "Because moral patients have inherent value and have neither more nor less inherent value than that possessed by moral agents, they have the same right to respectful treatment possessed by moral agents *and* they possess this right equally—that is, moral agents and moral patients have an equal right to respectful treatment." It is a direct duty of moral agents to respect rights of moral patients, and this respect is not to be construed in terms of "kindness" to animals, or as the result of "sentimentality" in respect to human infants and elderly humans. The treatment of moral patients—human and nonhuman—should be in terms of respect for their inherent value.

All individuals of any inherent value are entitled to equal respect for their rights, although Regan equivocates from time to time regarding how equal "equal" is—at times some are more equal than others. His rights view considers four principles: The minimize harm principle; minimize overriding principle; worse-off principle; and the principle of liberty. He also brings special considerations into play when difficulties are encountered regarding the intuitive acceptability of decisions that follow from his statements.

Minimize Harm Principle   In a situation in which all options will produce harm to innocent individuals, the option resulting in the least total sum of harm should be chosen. Regan rejects this principle using his familiar idea that individuals should not be treated as receptacles of value. He favors a respect principle, maintaining that all individuals are to be treated in a manner honoring their postulated equal inherent value. It is not permissible to cause gross harm to one individual to prevent minor harm to a large number of individuals, because this would not respect the former individual's inherent value, even though the aggregate harm might be less when considered over all individuals. This notion opposes the classic utilitarian position.

Minimize Overriding Principle (Miniride)   Regan would use this in place of the minimize harm principle (p. 305): "Special considerations aside, when we must choose between overriding the rights of many who are innocent or the rights of few who are innocent, and when each affected individual will be harmed in a prima facie comparable way, then we ought to choose to override the rights of the few in preference to overriding the rights of the many."

If the choices available are to inflict a comparable harm to A alone, to harm B, C, and D, or to harm all four, it is necessary to compare the harm done when each individual is compared with each of the others in turn. When this comparison is made Regan considers it better to override the rights of A because the comparison of A with each of the others never results in any differentially greater harm, and the equal inherent value of each protects the rights of the many (B, C, and D) by overriding the rights of the few (A). He does not believe this decision is driven by aggregate value, but is the outcome of the series of individual comparisons. If the harm to A is the same as that to each of the others, I fail to see how he can choose who to harm without bringing in some idea of aggregation. He extends this position (p. 307), asking whether it is permissible to sacrifice one innocent person in order to save fifty, and decides it is permissible to kill the one because the decision shows equal respect for the inherent values of all individuals involved, although he maintains that their equal rights are being counted equally. Either I am missing something, or a utilitarian-style aggregation is sneaking in under disguise.

Worse-off Principle   The worse-off principle is relevant when harms done to different individuals are not comparable. Once again Regan says the proper test is a comparison of each individual with every other one. He frames it as follows (p. 308): "Special considerations aside, when we must decide to override the rights of the many or the rights of the few who are innocent, and when the harm faced by the few would make them worse-off than any of the many would be if any other option were chosen, then we ought to override the rights of the many."

If the harm that A faces greatly exceeds the harm done to the many (such as death or permanent incapacity of A compared with only suffering of B, C, and D), A should not be harmed. The relative harm done to A would be greater when tested against that to each of the other individuals. When harms are not comparable, the critical factor determining whose right overrides considers the harm done to A compared with that done to each of the other individuals, rather than the sum of A's harm compared with the sum of harm to the others. This implies that it would be permissible for each of the many to be blinded by disease rather than to cause the death of one individual who could be killed to make a vaccine to save the others. This conclusion fits the pattern of intuitions revealed in our study of human moral intuitions (Petrinovich & O'Neill, 1996). Regan use this principle to avoid utilitarian calculations that base decisions on aggregate outcomes. I speak to this issue in chapter 8 when I discuss Singer's utilitarian position and Regan's disagreement with it.

Special Considerations   When developing each operative principle Regan refers to special considerations that suspend the normal application of the miniride and worse-off principles (p. 317). One special consideration (p. 324) is due to voluntary agreements regarding duties and responsibilities involved in a social contract, emphasizing that these are entered into voluntarily. Another involves lessened responsibility toward those who voluntarily engage in hazardous endeavors. Yet another occurs when there is historical background, with those involved in their present predicament because their basic rights were violated in the past. He also suggests a special consideration due to the moral bond between friends and family members. These bonds are special not because of an explicit and agreed-upon social contract, but because they represent crucial societal relations between loved ones built on mutual trust, interdependence, and performance of mutually beneficial acts.

He believes (p. 317) one should suspend application of the miniride and worse-off principles to spare significant harm to friends, even though it makes a stranger worse off. However, if harm to a stranger is great (e.g., death) but harm to a friend is minor, the special consideration of friendship should be set aside and the normal application of the worse-off principle honored (p. 316). He denies this is a case of a "theory's grasping at straws to save itself" (p. 316) in this instance, and considers it preposterous to suppose an individual's familial obligations exist for the benefit of other members of society; kin and friends stand in a special relationship. There is no consistency regarding when a special consideration should and should not be invoked, and it is necessary (and difficult) to decide what degree of harm is significant enough to weigh the balance in favor of a stranger rather than friend or kin.

Narveson (1987) expressed uneasiness regarding the ad hoc character of these special considerations, because some moral relationship always could be generated by any agents who wanted to promote their own well-considered, self-seeking interests. The awkwardness of special considerations and the manner in which they are invoked appear at times to involve utilitarian calculations (by whatever name), and to favor kin and friends when difficult decisions involving them are to be made. Accepting evolutionary factors as basic (rather than special) considerations is more satisfactory and leads to a more consistent and rational basis for moral theory.

For Regan (p. 317), the miniride and worse-off principles should not be suspended when circumstances involve a slave trader who must consider harming a fellow slave trader rather than one of the slaves. Such a suspension is not appropriate because the fact that the institution of slavery is "unjust to the core" invalidates the contract between slave traders. The problem with this is that "valid moral duties" must be determined on a case-by-case basis, which gives as much weight to special considerations as to any general moral principles that presumably guide moral decisions. The evolutionary principles discussed in chapters 1 and 2 are universal ones that can be applied in all circumstances where kin and friends are involved, especially if there is a possibility of reciprocation by the latter.

Liberty Principle Rights views recognize the right of the individual, subject to special considerations, to do what is necessary to avoid being made worse off relative to other innocent individuals, even if the actions involve harm to those other individuals. To avoid the problem that anyone could claim rights and use them as a license to engage in what would amount to moral anarchy, Regan proposes the liberty principle (p. 331): "Provided that all those involved are treated with respect, and assuming that no special considerations obtain, any innocent individual has the right to act to avoid being made worse-off even if doing so harms other innocents." This principle is necessary to give individuals the right to pursue their own welfare while acting within moral constraints that apply to all moral agents.

Criticisms of the Rights View

Regan applied these moral principles to several problems to illustrate how they could be used to make decisions in the course of everyday life as well as to resolve hypothetical dilemmas. A major question is whether he is able to meet the requirements he established for making ideal moral judgments: Are his principles compatible with accepted facts, are they consistently applied, do they have adequate scope, and do the conclusions stand the test of our intuitions?

Little agreement exists concerning the qualities an organism must have in order to have rights. Several qualities have been suggested and debated, among them needs, interests, desires, beliefs, and powers to reason. Another problem concerns the relative importance of different rights when they come into conflict, and it becomes necessary to decide which right will prevail at the expense of another. Regan holds that rights should remain as stipulated primitives, and as such they become fundamental and axiomatic; Leahy (1991) considered this to be taking refuge in a theology of inherent value. If the axiom on which a right is based is not accepted, we are adrift in a sea of disagreement regarding the stipulation, and no closer to fundamental agreement.

I suggest matters should be considered from an evolutionary perspective, grounding basic moral principles on the natural, evolved properties of organisms, and that moral standing is dependent on attaining personhood at birth—a critical stage in gaining the status of a human moral patient. Human moral patients must be respected by moral agents at birth. The same is true to a lesser degree for all moral patients of any species. It was proposed in chapter 3 that rights are best left at the legal level because it is difficult to ground them adequately at either the natural or moral level. There can be no rights without duties and powers, and no duties and powers without laws.

The notions of animal welfare and cognition of both Regan and Singer are reasonable; they tend to give maximum allowable cognitive credit to animals. One should come down on the side of an animal if one has questions regarding its welfare or cognitive or linguistic abilities whenever these abilities are to play a critical role in moral decisions.

Equal Inherent Value   A critical assumption of Regan's rights stand is that any moral patient with *some* inherent value must be conceded to have an equal inherent value with moral agents, and this entitles the patient to equal protection from harm. This is because an individual should not be considered to be a receptacle of different amounts of inherent value, and one's inherent value is an absolute characteristic that either exists or does not. These assertions are questionable, and if so lead to the utilitarianism Regan considers to be "unsavory." Summer (1988) examined Regan's rights framework and found it not entirely insensitive to global cost-benefit considerations. Regan avoids such considerations only by stipulation, and violates rights whenever the aggregate costs become too great. Stipulated special considerations are used whenever it is difficult to support an abolitionist position regarding the use of animals in research. Sumner (1988, p. 170) argued, "Once a rights theory allows that the right not to be harmed can be overridden by a sufficiently favorable balance of benefits over harms . . . , then it cannot avoid making interspecific comparisons of harms and benefits." He suggested utilitarianism is being used to make decisions, despite the fact Regan prefers to consider groups of humans and animals to have the same basic rights and the same moral standing.

The concept of all-or-none inherent value is based on a two-value Aristotelian logic that does not admit shades of gray, and biological and psychological realities seldom if ever operate according to that logic. A useful analogy is provided by a commonly discussed all-or-none phenomenon in biology: The electrical transmission of a nerve impulse across a synapse (the functional junction between two nerve cells). The electrical firing of one cell by another appears as an all-or-none step function: It fires or it does not. However, the underlying reality is more subtle, because chemical events take place in a graded fashion, even though the cell does not discharge. Each subthreshold stimulus can raise the resting potential of a cell until what would have been but one more stimulus of insufficient strength will be sufficient to exceed the firing threshold of the receptor cell, and the all-or-none electrical effect is seen. Thus, the electrical phenomenon appears as an all-or-none response, but the underlying biochemical reality is graded.

Another example is pregnancy. One can assert a woman is either pregnant or she is not, and that there is no such thing as being a little bit pregnant. There are different degrees of pregnancy, however. It is a necessary condition for a sperm to fertilize an egg for pregnancy to begin. That occurrence signifies only a little bit of pregnancy because, as discussed in chapter 6 of *Human evolution, reproduction, and morality*, only a small percentage of fertilized ova survive the voyage to be implanted in the uterine wall. A large proportion of those implanted are spontaneously aborted very quickly. Throughout the course of pregnancy occasional spontaneous abortions occur. In one sense, then, a woman could be considered to be more and more pregnant as time progresses toward the time of birth. The occurrence of fertilization is a necessary normal condition for birth to occur, but not a sufficient condition, and the "value" of the pregnancy increases as time goes by.

Almost all biological and psychological abilities and achievements that have been described or measured vary both within and between species. If value is to be grounded on some physiological, behavioral, or psychological conditions (as Regan must do), it is reasonable to assume the inherent value of all individual organisms is not the same. It is more reasonable to ascribe levels of inherent value, certainly within a species. The evolutionary view is that more inherent value should be assigned to a young, reproductively able person than to a postreproductive elderly person, other things being equal.

Values (and rights, if that language is used) are relative; an individual possesses value when it satisfies relevant criteria, and when it no longer satisfies these criteria it no longer possesses that value. Summer (1981) gave an example of a faulty "natural kinds" argument: If one wants a juicy fruit it is not sensible to choose all mature peaches over mature pears. This is a bad decision even though peaches are juicer than pears. It is necessary to consider the characteristics of this particular peach and that particular pear; unluckily for us, this peach might be rock-hard and juiceless. It is necessary to consider individuals within the context of circumstances at any given time.

Regan's reading of the history of moral philosophy led him to conclude that utilitarianism dies hard. He wrote (1980, p. 95), "Just when one thinks it has been forced off the stage for good, one finds it loitering in the wings, awaiting yet another curtain call." As I noted, when he discussed the lifeboat dilemma he assigned a lower inherent value to a dog than to a person, and by doing so he sneaked in a loitering differential inherent value. I agree with him that utilitarianism dies hard, and suggest the reason might be that it is a sensible way to view morality, and that people routinely rely on utilitarian value when making ethical decisions. It is difficult for him to hold out coherently for equal inherent value in the utilitarian lifeboat that characterizes the world in which humans and nonhumans coexist.

Sorabji (1993) criticized Regan's violations of the principle of inherent value in terms similar to those developed here. He observed that special considerations always come into play and most of the time override the basic principle of inherent value. The way Regan employs them to override equal inherent value ". . . opens the floodgates to medical experimentation on animals, if it is necessary for saving the lives of humans, for whom death is a greater loss" (p. 213).

Evolutionary theory is the most powerful and universal synthetic theory regarding organic life, and it can be applied to understand phenomena ranging from geology, to plants, to earthworms, to human social systems. One of the basic assumptions of evolutionary biology is that utilitarian costs and benefits must be examined, and their balance (calculated in terms of ultimate reproductive success) must be determined to understand biological change. It would be surprising if the developed moral systems of humans did not embody rules that have been found essential to understand proximate evolutionary mechanisms. Many moral philosophers and social scientists (as well as evolutionists) adopted utilitarianism to understand a wide range of behaviors, and I suggest this occurs for the sound reason that reality works in a utilitarian manner.

I find no compelling statements leading me to agree with Regan's assertion that all animals have an equal inherent value merely because they all have some. It can be agreed all animals have some inherent value and that this value entitles them to respect, but it also can be said that this inherent value differs in kind and amount as a function of circumstances—indeed, what Regan calls special considerations.

The task is to determine the relative values appropriate to enter into utilitarian calculations rather than deny the existence of those values. It can be understood why Regan is hesitant to open this can of worms (given his aversion to letting utilitarianism have another curtain call), but it might be profitable for quantitative experts in the social sciences to attempt to estimate such values rather than to remain at the level of speculative philosophical argumentation, a proposition discussed in chapter 3.

When criticizing Singer's utilitarianism, Regan (1980) commented that Singer must prove that different treatment of animals brings about a positive balance of good over evil. To decide whether people should stop eating animals it would be necessary to examine such things as the effects on the economy in terms of costs, levels of productivity, maintenance and growth of existing resource-producing entities, and influences on people's lives. Regan believes it must be shown that better consequences "would" result, or at least be "very probable," if animals were used as food. He expresses disappointment that we have nothing approaching this kind of required empiricism because the necessary calculations are missing. He despairs in the face of the complexities involved in scaling values, and puzzles over whether one should take interests of a given race or sex into account at all, or should one take them into account but weight them equally or differently with those of a favored group. Or should one take all interests into account equally, but adopt laws and policies that give greater opportunities to members of favored (or disadvantaged) groups?

Regan correctly assumes it is necessary to scale values, and I would be the last to deny that a careful quantification of relative values should be undertaken in such situations. In chapters 5, 8, and 10 of *Living and dying well* I discussed problems encountered when developing quantitative scales to establish the relative value of various medical treatments.

Priority lists for health care have been established, and recipients who might receive organs for transplants have been ranked, tasks that have been accomplished adequately in several instances. Regan (1980, p. 90) remarks that if empirical data were available, they might show that ". . . the present speciesist way of treating animals might actually be justified, given [Singer's] version of utilitarianism." This is a serious challenge, and I believe scaling such values is a feasible undertaking.

Regan (1980) consistently asserts that rights of the individual trump those of collective interests. Although this is a cornerstone of his position, it remains little more than a stipulation of the "truth." In support, he cites a statement by Ronald Dworkin that rights of the individual trump goals of the group. After having stated this basic premise Regan presents an example that violates it. He asks us to suppose an individual has inadvertently swallowed a microfilm code that must be obtained to prevent a massive nuclear explosion in New Zealand. The individual sits safely in Arizona and refuses to consent to undergo an operation to retrieve the code and prevent the explosion. Regan finds it "not implausible" that the individual's right must give way to the collective interests of others. This might not be implausible to him, but others have objected to decisions of this kind on the grounds that they violate the essential principle that guarantees respect for an individual's freedom from harm; clearly it violates Regan's statement that individual rights trump collective interests. I wonder what his decision would be if the individual was to be killed to avoid a milder blinding of the New Zealanders rather than their death? According to his principles, the greater harm to the single individual would preclude killing the individual to save the eyesight of thousands.

Thomson (1990) discussed a dilemma she called transplant. In the basic version a transplant surgeon has five patients who will die if they do not receive organs; it is certain that the operation will be successful. One young man in excellent health and of the right blood type can be cut up to supply the part each patient needs. Thomson considers it impermissible to cut up the young man to save the five. To her, any moral theory that would permit the sacrifice of the young man is a disaster in dire need of revision. Yet, Regan maintains that the individual's right should give way to collective interests of others in the nuclear dilemma, presumably because the harm to the one is less than that to the many who might presumably die.

An even more benign version of transplant is closer to Regan's nuclear dilemma. A young man is peacefully reading a newspaper while seated on a park bench. It is known that, by cutting off his foot, a transplant surgeon can obtain enough tissue to save five dying people, and this can be done "painlessly" by anesthetizing him and removing the foot, and when he awakes he will have no pain—but also no foot. Once again, it seems intuitively impermissible to take the foot of the one innocent person without his consent, even though the harm to him is slight when balanced against the benefits to many. The freedom from harm principle has a powerful appeal, and it should be included as a basic element in any moral system. Most agree that, in an instance such as transplant, an animal could be sacrificed to save a human, and I propose in chapter 8 that such speciesist tendencies are strong, universal, and reasonable.

Thomson noted that most people would find it permissible to kick an innocent person in the shin to save the lives of five others. She justified this action by introducing what she called a trade-off: It is permissible to infringe a claim against harm if and only if infringing it would be sufficiently better for those who would benefit compared with the harm done to claim holders. The critical problem is to determine the relative sufficiency of each good, and once again, the scaling of sufficiency is at the heart of the matter. Thomson suggested that, in qualitative terms, the size of the required increment of goods varies with the stringency of a claim: The more stringent a claim, the greater the required increment of good. Rather than thinking in terms of one value having an absolute trump over others, the matter should be viewed in terms of some values being higher cards than others, and I believe this is a serious alternative to consider.

Once again it seems that Regan must invoke special considerations whenever a basic principle leads to an intuitively unacceptable conclusion, which I interpret to mean that the basic principles are not sufficient. He insists that the proper test should be between individual organisms rather than a consideration of aggregate values of all involved, but it seems easy to discard that propriety too often. I fear Regan occasionally becomes what Macklin (1988) called a closet utilitarian.

Dilemmas

Regan used the lifeboat dilemma to develop and illustrate his views, and his work strongly influenced the course of our empirical research (Petrinovich, O'Neill, & Jorgensen, 1993; Petrinovich & O'Neill, 1996; O'Neill & Petrinovich, in press) discussed in chapter 7 of *Human evolution, reproduction, and morality.* The lifeboat dilemma proposes that a number of individuals are in a lifeboat, but the capacity of the boat is exceeded, making it necessary to throw one individual overboard. The case Regan proposes involves four normal adult humans and a dog, with room for only four individuals. He concluded (p. 324): ". . . no reasonable person would deny that the death of any of the four humans would be a greater prima facie loss, and thus a greater prima facie harm, than would be true in the case of the dog."

This was based on the worse-off principle, which holds that less harm is done to the dog because it has fewer opportunities for satisfaction than any of the humans. Even if there were a million dogs they all should be thrown over to save humans because aggregate value is not morally relevant. Regan (p. 325) writes: "To decide matters against the one or the million dogs is not speciesist. The decision to sacrifice the one or the million is not based on species membership. It is based on assessing the losses *each individual* faces *and* assessing these losses *equitably,* an approach that is at once consistent with and required by the recognition of the equal inherent value and the equal prima facie right not to be harmed possessed by all those involved."

I find this solution intuitively difficult, and believe it involves backdoor speciesism. An animal will always lose in a confrontation with a human because almost inevitably it will have fewer opportunities for satisfaction. Using the worse-off principle in this manner justifies the outcome, and it always results in a normal human surviving and a normal animal perishing, other things being equal. This outcome may be satisfactory as long as application of the principle yields consistent results (given special considerations), but I think the position is based on a weak philosophical base and casts further doubt on the usefulness of the equal inherent value conception.

Humans engage in moral reflections, are morally autonomous, are members of moral communities, and recognize just claims against their own interest (Cohen, 1986). This state of affairs is totally different from that for animals of any other species. Animals engage in communal behaviors, but these behaviors do not have the characteristics of human communities. Midgley (1983) added that an essential element of social contracts involves reciprocity; fully responsible rational agents might at times accept duties solely to promote their mutual advantage.

Regan opposes using aggregate value theory to establish the impermissibility of animal farming and research in animals no matter how many people might benefit. Neither of these endeavors is permissible given the costs in terms of suffering and death of animals, and such suffering and death respect neither an animal's rights nor its equal inherent value.

I believe Regan's decisions generally are based on a covert assumption that a human has a greater inherent value than a dog, no matter how the justifications for the decisions are glossed, and to sanction killing the dog (or dogs) in the lifeboat dilemma introduces that utilitarian calculation with a human trump (or high card). If comparable human interests are involved they will always override those of an animal. It would be more satisfactory to face the implications of utilitarian aspects of the decision, rather than using them in this way and denying the fact.

We have no clear guidelines to decide when equal inherent value prevails and when a special consideration should be invoked. Some form of explicit utilitarianism might be preferable because it provides a more rational, consistent, and precise set of policies—all virtues that Regan espouses in discussing his rules. A utilitarianism with trumps is smuggled into the argument as Regan uses it to resolve dilemmas. It is bothersome that the fundamental rights principle can be overridden so easily, and I am concerned about who decides and in what instances it is permissible to override, as well as the bases on which these decisions are to be justified. The problem of equality arises any time the worse-off principle is activated because some calculation of comparability is involved to establish the relative magnitudes of harm based on potential attainments and satisfactions.

I will belabor this issue a bit more. Regan (p. 351) returns to the lifeboat and extends it to a case with four humans and a dog in which one of them is to be eaten for survival's sake. He proposes that the dog should be eaten. Later (p. 385) he says that if the boat contains one healthy dog and the humans all have a degenerative brain disease, it is not permissible to make the dog sick to test a compound that may possibly cure the disease. Yet, it is permissible to eat the dog in the interest of human survival. Presumably, he objects to making the dog sick because it is not certain the compound will cure the disease, even though the harm to the dog and to each of the humans is comparable. It is not certain, either, that feeding the dog to the humans will ensure their survival. It enhances the probability, but still they might not be rescued, and one might allow that conditional status to give the humans prece- dence. If the humans continue to face starvation it would not be permis- sible to kill one of them and feed him to the others; in fact such an act would be (and has been) grounds for prosecution for murder (Simpson, 1984). Once again, I sense an underlying speciesism: Humans are differ- ent from non-humans in a morally significant way.

I wonder if Regan would consider it permissible to cut up the dog and feed it to the humans if it was certain that doing so would cure the disease, given that it is permissible to cut up the dog to keep the humans from starving. I fail to see the difference between drowning the dog, eating it, using it to test a drug, or using it when it will cure a disease. These decisions seem arbitrary and inconsistent. The dog's rights do not depend on considerations regarding the animal itself, but appear and disappear as the special considerations change. He changes the basis on which the decision is made from example to example to avoid being trapped into approving animal research to benefit humans, an outcome that could be permissible if the concept of greater life satisfaction is allowed.

Consider another dilemma discussed by Regan (p. 387): This lifeboat contains four preeminent scientists on the verge of making discoveries that portend enormous health benefits for humanity; the fifth person delivers Twinkies to retail stores in Brooklyn. The four scientists have a degenerative brain disease and the Twinkie salesman does not. Regan would not use the salesman as the research guinea pig to evaluate a cure for the disease. Would it be permissible to invoke some special considera- tions to make it permissible to throw the salesman overboard, because he does not have the opportunities for satisfaction the scientists have? Or is there some kind of minimal threshold because the Twinkie salesman is human and that protects him from a calculation of this kind? Regan does not think it appropriate to sacrifice the salesman, nor did the participants in our research study who resolved similar dilemmas.

I fail to see why it is not possible to consider the level of relative satisfactions in this case, as Regan did when the dog was thrown over to drown. It could be argued that the Twinkie salesman will fail when he is compared against each scientist, on the same grounds as did the dog: Each of the scientists could be presumed to have a potential for greater satisfaction. To rescue the situation it is necessary to introduce another special condition; satisfaction and potential must be overridden to respect any individual's freedom from harm and freedom for respect. These concepts of freedoms ensure that the basic fundamentals of existence are honored. I fail to find any consistency in his arguments, and my intuitions are confused by the pattern of his decisions—he does not appear to have a consistent set of formal principles.

His resolution of another classic dilemma is also confusing: Fifty miners are trapped and will die, but they can be saved by blowing open a shaft that contains one trapped miner, who will be killed by the explosion. Regan (p. 302) invoked the miniride principle—it is permissible to override the right of the one in preference to overriding the rights of the many, given comparable harms. Here the decision is not based on aggregated harm, but on the fact that each of the fifty separate individuals has a right equal to the right of the one, and the rights of the fifty should not be overridden in the interest of the equal right of the one. He asserted that this principle does not involve aggregated value, but again, I fail to understand how it is more than a tortured conclusion to avoid the appearance of aggregation to support a solution acceptable to his intuitions, and to avoid any taint of utilitarianism.

For Jamieson (1990), Regan's handling of the miner's dilemma reveals a serious contradiction between the miniride and worse-off principles. He concluded that an appeal to consequences provides a more coherent solution; in fact, this dilemma really has three options: Kill one; kill fifty; or do nothing and let all fifty-one die. He asserted that Regan does not indicate how the principle applied in this instance. How should respect for the equality of the individuals lead us to kill one so that fifty may live? "Why shouldn't this respect lead us to kill none, rather than one or 50?" (p. 352).

Jamieson analyzed the worse-off and miniride principles by considering a couple of hypothetical examples in which their application leads to counter-intuitive results. John is crippled and Mary is not, and we must either cripple Mary or cause John to have a slight headache. If we apply the worse-off principle we should cripple Mary, since a crippled John with a headache would be worse off than either John or Mary would be if both were merely crippled. Assume a million people who are not crippled and one who is, and we must either give the crippled person a headache or cripple the million. The worse-off principle tells us to cripple the million—again, a counter-intuitive result.

He illustrated the basic conflict between the worse-off (which is framed in terms of comparative positions) and miniride (framed in terms of comparative harm) principles in the following way. Assume we must blind either six people or one. Because the harms are comparable, numbers count, and the miniride principle tells us to blind the one. He goes on to suppose the one is also deaf. If the worse-off principle is used we would be led to the intuitively unsatisfactory recommendation that the six should be blinded, because the deaf person, if blinded, would be worse-off than any of the six. It is not possible to make the two principles consistent by recasting them, and Jamieson concluded it would be more satisfactory to move in the direction of consequentialist theory.

Regan minimizes the importance of hypothetical life-and-death dilemmas because they involve bizarre circumstances. He maintains that outcomes of such exceptional cases as those involved in the lifeboat dilemmas should not be used to conclude much regarding ethical principles. Resolution of fantasy dilemmas, he says, cannot be fairly generalized to apply to unexceptional cases, because what may be done in such isolated, exceptional circumstances does not commit us to a similar view of real practices or institutions. I fail to understand why the solution of dilemmas can never be equated to solutions of daily problems in morality, as long as the formal substantive and logical principles are the same.

Much philosophical argumentation uses fantasy dilemmas and thought experiments involving hypothetical situations; the precise intent is to remove the ordinary constraints of everyday life to explore the implications of formal principles in depth, and to establish the precision of decision-making processes. As discussed in chapter 7 of *Human evolu-*

tion, reproduction, and morality, many problems that political policy makers have faced embodied characteristics of the unpalatable alternatives posed in fantasy dilemmas. For example, when the British government had to decide during World War II whether to use deception to divert German bombs from highly populated London to less populated areas, they decided it was morally impermissible to sacrifice a smaller number of innocent people to save an even greater number. Here is a clear instance of resolving a real dilemma where the numbers of individuals did not prevail and the miniride principle was violated.

Another instance was the British government's decision to engage in terror bombing of nonstrategic cities such as Dresden, rather than continue strategic bombing of military targets. The decision invoked the doctrine of double effect: The death of civilians in Dresden was foreseen, but not the primarily intended, effect of air raids that were considered permissible, because the end was to win a just war. When resolutions of fantasy dilemmas lead to intuitively or formally unacceptable outcomes, this might be due to weakness in underlying moral principles and the logic used to arrive at the decisions, rather than to artificiality of the method.

I defended the value of considering fantasy dilemmas in chapter 7 of *Human evolution, reproduction, and morality,* because they have the advantage of freeing individuals from realistic constraints that push respondents toward social conformity. In many episodes in history policy makers have had to resolve life-and-death dilemmas of the kinds involved in the hypothetical ones discussed. Examination of the resolution of these dilemmas—usually decisions made during wartime or after natural disasters—is instructive because it demonstrates that the kinds of issues embedded in hypothetical dilemmas are the same as those that have occurred in the past and undoubtedly will occur again.

A number of studies were conducted using fantasy dilemmas in the United States, China, and Taiwan (Wang & Johnston, 1995: Wang, 1966a, 1966b; Petrinovich et al., 1993; Petrinovich & O'Neill, 1996; O'Neill & Petrinovich, in press). The patterns of results consistently supported expectations based on evolutionary theory and behavioral ecology models (discussed in chapters 2 and 3). It is arguable that human behavioral decisions of the types projected in the dilemmas are strongly influenced by biological and ecological factors, and involve biological universals that are influenced by ecological conditions that face the members of different cultures.

Regan believes that decisions made to resolve fantasy dilemmas cannot be used to justify eating animals or raise them as food in factory farms, because the available alternatives make it unlikely any humans will starve if they forego eating animals. He (1975) suggests three general conditions that must prevail if one is to approve of any practice causing an animal nontrivial pain: (1) The practice prevents, reduces, or eliminates a much greater amount of evil; (2) there is no other way to bring about these consequences; and (3) there is good reason to believe these consequences will occur. It is permissible to eat meat if circumstances are such that required nutrients cannot be obtained from other sources (as he points out correctly, this is not the case for much of Western society), again invoking the worse-off principle. Meat eating could be permissible if ". . . the deterioration of our health would deprive us of a greater variety and number of satisfactions than those within the range of farm animals" (p. 337). When humans such as Eskimos live in a subsistence economy, Regan considers it morally permissible for them to kill and eat animals to avoid starvation, and keep themselves clothed and housed.

I will not discuss Regan's position further at this time. In the next chapter more implications and problems with the rights view are considered after Peter Singer's utilitarian-based animal liberation theories are presented. I do this because utilitarianism is an obvious alternative to the rights view, Singer clearly articulated this position, and Regan and Singer aired their differences in print.

Legal Status of Animals

To gain a comprehensive view, the legal status of animals should be considered. This was clearly summarized by the animal activist and legal scholar, Gary Francione (1995, p. 4): "As far as the law is concerned, an animal is the personal property, or *chattel*, of the animal's owner and cannot possess rights." The fundamental premise of property law is that animals, as property, cannot have rights that stand against human owners, and legal regulations regarding animals facilitate the most efficient exploitation by the owner—meaning any animal interest can be overridden if the consequences are sufficiently beneficial to humans. Francione deplored this state of affairs, and contended that to override Regan's belief that there is a duty not to harm individual organisms, laws must be based on moral issues beyond an appeal to consequences.

Laws regulating the use of animals do not apply to rats, mice, or birds, those used in industry, or to horses or farm animals used in agriculture, even for agricultural research. Rollin (1992) imagined an example of twin male lambs, one of which goes to an NIH-funded biomedical research project, and the second to an agricultural research project. If they both are to be castrated, under current law the NIH lamb will receive anesthesia and postsurgical analgesia, and the operation will be done under aseptic conditions. The agricultural lamb could have its testicles removed under primitive field conditions with a knife, and without anesthesia, analgesics, or asepsis. He considers this unacceptable, and there certainly is no consistent legal protection of animal welfare.

Even ships, municipalities, and corporations have more legal rights than animals (Rollin, 1992). Legally, human interests always come before those of animals, and the extensive catalogue of prohibitions against mistreating animals does not take cognizance of behavioral or psychological cruelty. All legislation is aimed to protect human interests and property, to prevent human brutalization of animals, and to protect animals against dramatic atrocities.

The law requires animal property not be wasted by killing or causing suffering when legitimate economic purpose exists (Francione, 1995). To this extent, animals must be treated "humanely," which comes down to ensuring they are used efficiently. Courts do not address the interests of animals as a factor in litigation. The legal test for cruelty to animals is not based on the actions perpetrated, but on whether they result in some human benefit and use commonly accepted methods. He discussed a case involving severe neglect of horses. The owners claimed the horses were intended to be sold and slaughtered for dog food, thereby exempting them from anticruelty laws based on agricultural use. The owners were convicted, the court deciding that they had not proved that severe maltreatment involved methods common to the industry. If they had met that test, the convictions would likely have been overturned.

The doctrine of legal standing is an important factor that can exclude animals from legal rights. Children, the elderly, and mentally incompetents do have legal rights and legal standing, and their interests can be articulated by court-appointed guardians (Francione, 1995). Although these individuals may be unable to use the courts without assistance, a guardian can protect their legal interests. Animals, however, are considered property and thereby have no rights to protect, and humans cannot have significant legal interests in animals owned by others.

Francione overstates the claim that children have legal rights. As Forer (1991) noted, the term "child" loosely refers to every person from birth to the age of eighteen years, although courts engage in considerable evasion that leads on the one hand to denying children of legal rights, and on the other to treating them as adults. An example is a California case where a juvenile referee decided that a six-year-old boy who was accused of smashing a baby's skull during a burglary was not competent to stand trial for assault. This decision was rendered on the grounds that the boy was not capable of meaningfully assisting his attorney, having an attention span of three to four minutes at most, and had trouble distinguishing between fact and fantasy. The deputy district attorney promised to monitor the boy and press for a trial if and when the court finds him competent and able to assist in his defense. In numerous cases children under the age of eighteen have been tried as adults, and requests by prosecuting attorneys to do this are increasingly frequent.

The legal standing of research animals has been considered by the courts. The Animal Welfare Act (AWA) was examined by a federal court and it was concluded that Congress did not intend the goal of humane treatment of research animals to come at the expense of progress in medical research (Francione, 1995). The court held that the Secretary of Agriculture was required to establish standards regarding the humane handling, care, treatment, and transport of animals, but was explicitly prohibited from regulating the design and performance of research in any way; those decisions were considered to be within the province of the research facility. Francione considers it a proper role of animal advocacy groups to interfere both in the relationship of animals as property and a research institution as owners, ensure that owners use animal resources efficiently. The legal challenge, as he poses it, is that animals are not being used efficiently and therefore are being wasted as a resource. If this view is accepted, a research project with any flaws in design or conduct, that is ill-conceived, or is likely to result in no significant advances should be prohibited because animals are being wasted. A question arises regarding the ability of jurors to make determinations in such cases in anything approaching an informed manner.

Throughout history laws have permitted animals to be prosecuted and executed for various crimes, such as mangling a child or being possessed by the devil. These prosecutions often seemed to be in the interest of a simple principle of retaliation, and sometimes to reverse some bad turn of fortune for members of the human community. Animals have been spared execution, however, if the owner's property interest can be shown to be compelling. Francione (1995, p. 108) summarized the legal status of animals as follows: "There can be no doubt that our legal treatment of animals is goal-based on at least two levels. Legal welfarism states that the overall goal governing animal use is to provide maximum benefits to people from animal exploitation. The goal of obtaining benefits from animal use is supposedly tempered by a second goal seeking the 'humane' treatment of animals, and their protection from 'unnecessary' suffering." The problem remains to reach agreement regarding the meaning and limits of the terms "humane" and "unnecessary."

Some of Francione's views do not agree with those of Tannenbaum (1995), who considers the basic American law dealing with animals to be sensible and serviceable, rather than manipulative and heartless. He holds that animals are not just one kind of personal property, as Francione stated, but are what he called a seminal kind of personal property, in the sense that they represent the first items of personal property common people possessed. Most items of property belonged to the Church or the king and were kept safely away from disputes over possession. People could possess cattle, a category that included oxen, cows, sheep, goats, donkeys, mules, horses, and chickens, which were important to promote survival and constituted wealth. Establishment of the Anglo-American law of personal property began with litigation over the right of possession of such cattle, in the broad sense as described, with the first chattels being these animals. Thus animals were not just one kind of personal property, they were among the earliest objects included as personal property, and hence, were the subject of litigation.

Cattle came to be used as money, and if one was deprived of cattle as property, or if its value was destroyed, the owner was entitled not to the original property or one of the same kind, but to its monetary value. This led to a distinction between real property—an object that could be replaced in kind—and personal property—something that cannot be replaced in kind, but can be measured in terms of monetary value.

The point of this distinction is that owning a piece of property does not give one "sole and despotic dominion" over it; it only means one is ordinarily more entitled to possess or use it than anyone else is and if the property is taken or devalued it must be replaced in kind or monetary compensation provided for its value. This viewed property not as a thing, but as a set of legal relations that govern the use of things by persons.

Tannenbaum reported that under the Anglo law that became part of United States common law, animals were classified into two categories, wild and domestic. Everything not classified as domestic was considered wild, and domestic animals were those that had been tamed, bred, and used for farming, food, and draught. They were "useful" in terms of economics and benefits—those same animals to whom the earlier term "cattle" was applied. All wild animals were considered to be the property of the king under the terms of the Magna Carta, and anyone wanting to possess or use them could be given permission or license by the king to do so. In American law, wildlife is owned by state and federal governments in lands they hold in trust for the people. Household pets, such as dogs and cats, are classified by law as domestic animals because they are tamed and kept for pleasure, curiosity, or entertainment, even though they are not used as either produce or producers.

The early legal status of animals was as property without interests; it was not a crime to cause considerable suffering to one's own animals, but prosecution could be brought for injuring or harming those belonging to someone else. Under the law that injury was considered to be done to the owner rather than the animal: A cruelty statute was enacted to punish individuals if, with malicious intent they beat or tortured any domestic animal. It was amended to include all animals, and to allow for prosecution on grounds of negligent cruelty. The statute explicitly exempted properly conducted scientific experiments and investigations performed under the authority of a medical college or university.

This concept of cruelty is a matter of statutory rather than common law, which gives state legislatures virtually unbridled discretion to define cruelty, to decide which animals are covered by cruelty law, and to determine who may be prosecuted for cruelty (Tannenbaum, 1995). Because states can prosecute the owner of an animal, the legal status of animals as property does not permit an owner despotic dominion over this property.

Cruelty has been defined as the infliction of unnecessary or unjustifiable pain, distress, or discomfort upon an animal, for example, by failing to provide one's dog or cat with sufficient food or water, or leaving it outside in the cold or in a hot automobile on a summer day. One cannot be prosecuted for failing to play with a pet or not making it happy, however. This interpretation protects animals and creates legal duties regarding them. In Tannenbaum's view it affords legal rights for animals and protects interests.

Tannenbaum is emphatic, however, that the possession of legal rights does not confer legal standing. This is important, because activists want animals to have legal standing so that they can sue owners, veterinarians, and scientists. This goes beyond current law and represents an extension of the legal rights animals now have.

Francione's view is that cruelty laws are archaic because they are intended not to protect animals but to foster better behavior by people toward people. To Tannenbaum, this view is incorrect, and laws protect animals because animals themselves are considered worthy of protection. Laws do require a balancing of human and animal interests, but give weight to animal interests. However, animals will probably never be viewed by most people as the moral equals of humans. Cruelty laws have been applied to prohibit activities such as dog and cock fighting, which some people still want to conduct. Tannenbaum agrees that Francione is correct when he claims cruelty laws are not always sufficiently respectful of animal interests, and some activities, especially those involved in meat production, scientific procedures, and entertainment (e.g., rodeos and horse racing), should be subjected to careful ethical analysis. I propose in later chapters that such an ethical analysis has happened and still is happening.

Tannenbaum recommended that cruelty laws be amended so that, rather than prosecution as misdemeanors, the most serious kinds of animal abuse and neglect would be felony convictions, and judges should be sensitized to the importance of imposing meaningful punishment in these cases. In addition, the public, especially children, should be educated about the evils of animal cruelty. Animals would still be property, but they should be treated fairly. Consideration of the legal status of animals strengthens my belief that the notion of rights should remain at the legal level, and that it is adequate to protect the interests of animals.

8

Animal Liberation and Speciesism

One of the most articulate and prominent advocates for the animal liberation movement is Australian philosopher Peter Singer. His book *Animal liberation* (1975) is an important and widely cited treatment of the issues involved in the ethical use of animals by humans. It really is two books in one cover (as is the 1990 revision). A large part of it is a political tract urging political and civic action, encouraging people to become vegetarians, listing animal liberation organizations, and (in the 1975 edition) providing meatless recipes to assist those who want to become vegetarians or vegans, those who eat no animal flesh and no eggs, milk, or foods made from milk: Interspersed throughout the political and activist arguments is a utilitarian philosophy. Singer published another book, *Practical ethics* (1979), that presents the philosophical treatise in a more systematic, organized manner, without the polemic tone of *Animal liberation*. In the revision of *Animal liberation* (1990a) he responded to criticisms of the 1975 edition, discussed the idea of speciesism further, and celebrated the success of the animal liberation movement. All pages cited refer to the 1975 edition unless otherwise noted. I chose this edition because it is the one that has had the maximum impact; changes between the 1975 and 1990 editions are noted, and new material in the latter is cited whenever appropriate.

I discuss the philosophical ideas on which Singer's books are based, especially his preference utilitarianism. Special attention is given to the idea of speciesism, a central idea to many of the ideas of both Singer and Regan. Because the theories in the two editions of *Animal liberation* have both philosophical and practical aspects, I discuss the practical issues in later chapters when I examine specific issues regarding animal research, alternatives to animal research, vegetarianism, animals as pets, the role of zoos, and matters of public policy related to these issues.

Animal Liberation

Animal liberation, subtitled *A new ethics for the treatment of animals*, has become the authorized manual for the animal liberation movement. The paperback copy of the 1975 edition I have was distributed by People for the Ethical Treatment of Animals (PETA), one of the most active and vocal of these organizations.

Singer (1979) views classic utilitarianism as a universal position regarding ethics that emphasizes a self-interested decision-making process seeking to maximize pleasure over pain. He prefers a form of utilitarianism that respects the preferences of any being affected by an action or its consequences. This principle should consider ". . . a person's interests to be what, on balance and after reflection on all the relevant facts, a person prefers" (p. 80).

It is important to regard concerns such as having hopes, plans, and future goals when considering the value of a life (Singer, 1990a). Depriving an organism of fulfillment of any of these aspects of life might produce a greater loss to individuals that possess them than to ones that do not. These preferences must receive consideration without concern for an organism's species membership, which could lead to the conclusion that it is permissible to choose in favor of a normal human being over an intellectually disabled one. By this rule, in some circumstances animals with demonstrable preferences to fulfill their life's goals would prevail over members of the human species who cannot have such preferences. He summarized his position as follows (1990a, p. 21): "Normally this will mean that if we have to choose between the life of a human being and the life of another animal we should choose to save the life of the human, but there may be specific cases in which the reverse holds true, because the human being in question does not have the capacities of a normal human."

His preference utilitarianism means that ". . . an action contrary to the preference of any being is, unless this preference is outweighed by contrary preferences, wrong. . . . The wrong is done when the preference is thwarted" (1993, p. 94). Taking the life of a person will normally be worse than taking the life of some other being, because persons are highly future oriented in their preferences. When considering a fish struggling to get free of a barbed hook in its mouth, the struggle indicates no more than a preference for cessation of a painful state of affairs. This does not suggest that fish are capable of preferring their own future existence to nonexistence, only that a preference utilitarian would prefer a method to kill the fish instantly without first causing pain or death by using a hook and line.

Sentient beings have an interest to experience as much pleasure and as little pain as possible: "Sentience suffices to place a being within the sphere of equal consideration of interests; but it does not mean that the being has a personal interest in continuing to live" (p. 131).

Equality is accepted as a basic ethical principle on which all universal ethical judgments must be grounded, and it is to be based on an individual's interests. A central thesis is that equality must be extended to animals other than humans; the first chapter of *Animal liberation* is entitled "All Animals Are Equal . . . ". He appeals to the same premise that Regan accepts: All animals can feel pain, and this awareness provides them with the same interest (for Regan, "right") to be free of any pain we would ascribe to humans.

Capacities to feel pain and to suffer are shared by human and nonhuman animals, and this shared capacity is of central importance to Singer. He, as does Regan, believes that all animals have an equal capacity to suffer, and accepts this fact as adequate to establish equivalent moral standing. It should not be assumed that animal suffering is less important to them than human suffering is to us. "But pain is pain, and the importance of preventing unnecessary pain and suffering does not diminish because the being that suffers is not a member of our species" (p. 232). However, in another context (1981, p. 120) expansion of the moral circle ". . . does not mean that a human being and a mouse must always be treated equally, or that their lives are of equal value. Humans have interests . . . that mice are not capable of having. It is only when we are comparing similar interests—of which the interest in avoiding pain is the most important example—that the principle of equal consideration of interests demands that we give equal weight to the interests of the human and the mouse." This statement creates more problems than it resolves, because it is necessary to weigh similar interests that humans and other animals have (e.g., pain avoidance) against those peculiarly human interests (e.g., enjoying a long and vigorous life, providing goods, enriching the human condition, and all the goodies that characterize a rich autobiographical life), and he never clearly specifies when one interest should override another to develop a consistent scheme of relative value.

Singer's consequentialism (1990b, p. 49) is expressed when he considers one can ". . . hold that an act is right if and only if its consequences are better or at least as good as the consequences of an alternative act open to that agent." "As long as we remember that we should give the same respect to the lives of animals as we give to the lives of those humans at a similar mental level, we shall not go far wrong" (1990a, p. 21).

I find his discussion of the relative interests of humans and animals equivocal: At times interests are equal, but at others humans have greater interests. This is not a minor consideration. If the former is acceptable, then animals always must receive equal treatment to that received by humans; if the latter is accepted, normal human interests would always prevail, or it would at least be necessary to specify a hierarchy of interests.

Singer popularized the concept of speciesism, a term coined by Ryder in 1970 and maintained that it is present whenever interests of one's own species are allowed to override greater interests of members of other species. He allowed for the possibility that it could be appropriate to place interests of some individuals ahead of those of others, although all interests should be given equal consideration. Assignment of relative interest should not be based on species membership alone, however. If that is the sole criterion for preference, evaluation of an organism's status is based inextricably on speciesism, which is impermissible. The critical point is not that equal treatment should be guaranteed, but that each organism should be given its due consideration.

To justify any weighting of the value of one organism compared with another, it is necessary to specify qualities that justify a differential moral evaluation, and such evaluations must be applied universally. Singer highlighted this point to emphasize the importance of avoiding any taint of speciesism. He stated (1975, p. 9) that speciesism is "identical in pattern" to the evils inherent in racism and sexism: "The racist violates the principles of equality by giving greater weight to the interests of members of his own race. . . ", and "The sexist violates the principle of equality by favoring the interests of his own sex. Similarly the speciesist allows the interest of his own species to override the greater interests of members of other species." And later (1979, p. 76): "To give preference to the life of a being simply because it is a member of our species would put us in the same position as racists who give preference to those who are members of their race."

The test of individual moral standing, he insisted, must not be made by merely listing qualities that typify humans (e. g., language ability and superior mental capacities) and assigning all other species a lesser moral value using this definitional gambit. When discussing Regan's views in chapter 7, I suggested difficulties are encountered whenever attempts are made to assign different quantitative strengths or make qualitative judgments to determine relative value. Problems arise whenever it is necessary to consider marginal human cases compared with normal individuals of other species. I devote the next section to speciesism, because Singer is correct that resolving this issue is of central importance both to his views and to those of anyone who disagrees with them. He believes the case in favor of speciesism has been asserted rather than argued convincingly, and because of this, they should be rejected. The issue to be joined is whether Singer's case is made convincingly, or whether it is vulnerable to rejection on the same grounds he uses to reject the views of his opponents. Finally, the charge of speciesism is not akin to sexism and racism, and attempts to prove otherwise are neither compelling nor convincing.

Speciesism

Singer (1990b) agrees with Regan that certain characteristics allow some animals to live fuller lives than those without those characteristics, and that the characteristics should carry strong moral weight. The pressing issue is to identify such characteristics and determine how they can be applied universally to all nonhuman animals, to human embryos and fetuses, as well as to intellectually defective and disabled humans. Singer

(p. 10) wrote: "Because there is an overlap between the capacities of human and non-human animals, there is no way of drawing a line that will leave *all* human beings above the line and *all* nonhumans below it." He concluded that rationality is not always the essential feature of humanity that provides a sufficient basis to distinguish between beings such as dogs and profoundly retarded human beings. Yet, we tend to extend both respect and moral consideration to the retarded human that we deny to the most intelligent dog. I agree with this observation, and believe it represents a gray area that should be explored; this is where the test of individual characteristics becomes important to avoid speciesism as Singer defines it.

Equality of All Animals

The case for equality of suffering and pain by animals of all kinds, as well as the importance of realizing life's potential is stated by Singer over and again in *Animal liberation*, and he writes with a degree of satisfaction (p. 256): "So, throughout this book I have relied on rational argument. Unless you can refute the central argument of this book, you must now recognize that speciesism is wrong, and this means that, if you take morality seriously, you must try to eliminate speciesist practices from your own life, and oppose them elsewhere. Otherwise no basis remains from which you can, without hypocrisy, criticize racism or sexism." This is a severe indictment of any who would disagree with him, making it important to provide an adequate counter-argument. It is necessary to examine his central thesis in detail to decide whether it has been developed sufficiently to support such a strong conclusion. I say it has not been, and that we are left only with emotional assertions and appeals to sentiment that do not meet the test of adequate rational debate. I also contend that there are reasons to consider species identity as one of the most important defining biological characteristics that determine moral standing, which should be included whenever the relative value of different individuals is considered. Although I believe the charge of speciesism is not sustained, I do not believe it is necessary for Singer to stand or fall for that reason. His preference utilitarianism is sufficient to sustain a great deal of the philosophical position he wants to establish.

Animal Suffering

Most agree that animals of many species have cognitive abilities that could indicate awareness and consciousness (see Hauser, 1996). Most contemporary experts who have examined the issues also agree that nonhuman animals are able to experience fear and panic, and that they have at least first-order intentions (Hauser, 1996). The point at issue is whether humans and nonhumans differ in the degree and kinds of suffering and awareness of which they are capable, and if so, if these differences have moral significance.

Singer begins *Animal liberation* with the statement that all animals are equal, reiterating his position several times throughout the book. However, he also compromises his position throughout. For example, he agrees (p. 75) it could be justifiable to perform an experiment on retarded humans, "If it really were possible to save many lives by an experiment that would take just one life, and there were *no other way* those lives could be saved. . . ." This opens the door to claims of degrees of inequality, in this case between retarded and normal humans, that could well be extended to animals of other species. Imagine that several cognitive tests have been made to estimate the intellectual and emotional levels of a mentally retarded human and a chimpanzee, and for every test the chimpanzee outperforms the human. Would he consider it permissible to experiment on the retarded human or to sacrifice that human for parts or medicinals to save our closest phylogenetic neighbor? I doubt that he would, and I am sure such action would violate many people's moral intuitions. I suggest the species barrier is an almost insurmountable (and reasonable) one in the moral domain.

Later (p. 232) he writes that anyone who has not made a thorough study of animal pain cannot possibly know that suffering is less serious in animals than in humans. Inability to prove the negative is a weak basis on which to conclude that the suffering experienced by different individuals differs (or does not), and lack of evidence seems to demand more research with both humans and nonhumans to decide the issue. In any event, the position cannot force agreement that there are no differences in suffering, especially because large individual differences in degree of experienced pain are found between different animals of the same species, including humans. Large differences also exist among different animal species in almost every aspect of sensory, emotional, and cognitive behavior that has been studied, and they are related to anatomical and physiological differences. It is impossible ever to know the precise quality of experience as it exists in the mind of an animal of another species, just as it is impossible ever to know the quality of experience as it exists in the mind of another human.

". . . When capacities for suffering are greater, we need to have greater concern for the beings with the greater capacities for suffering" (Singer, 1990b, p. 46). Once again, this opens the way to suggest that all animals are not equal. A case in point is his statement that animals with a hope for a fulfilled future would suffer more through deprivation of that hope than would those not having the ability to foresee a future. Singer is careful to point out he has never claimed there are no significant differences between normal adult humans and other animals.

He maintains it is preferable to eat plants because they do not experience pain (they do respond to tissue insult with defensive and avoidant behaviors, although he doesn't want to acknowledge it). Because plants do not have a central nervous system he finds it difficult to imagine why they should feel pain, and decided such a belief is unjustified. He goes on, though, to say that if plants do experience pain, and if we must inflict pain or starve (p. 249), "Presumably it would still be true that plants suffer less than animals, and therefore it would still be better to eat plants than to eat animals." His initial strong position is weakened progressively, and it can be held that all animals are not equal, and it is even possible that plants have a (lesser) degree of moral value because they can respond aversively to stimulation.

As mentioned, Singer (1990b) agreed that beings able to live fuller lives might deserve a higher degree of consideration (p. 45): ". . . there is nothing speciesist about believing that mammals require greater moral concern than a number of other species . . . because they have a greater capacity for suffering." He continues (p. 46). ". . . when capacities for suffering are greater, we need to have greater general concern for the beings with the greater capacity for suffering," and ". . . we are justified in using animals for human goals, because as a consequentialist I must also hold that in the appropriate circumstances we are justified in using humans to achieve human goals (or the goal of assisting animals)."

I do not believe he successfully defends the premise that all animals are equal in their capacity for suffering or pain, and thus he concedes they are not equal in terms of interests. Thus, an assumption of equal inherent value does not provide sufficient grounding for philosophical principles regarding the ethical treatment of animals, and if it cannot support those ethical principles, Singer's position is weaker than he cares to admit. He does agree that different organisms possess different capacities for suffering as well as a different scope of interests, and that a greater capacity and scope signals a greater moral value, which means all animals are not equal.

Concept of a Biological Species

The concept of speciesism as Singer uses it is bothersome from a biological perspective. Although it is complicated, the species unit is basic to understanding evolutionary change, as discussed in chapter 1. Species come and go, they breed with other members of their species; they breed only rarely with members of other species, and if they do, viable and fecund hybrid offspring are seldom produced. The species concept is basic to biology because it focuses on actions of interbreeding individuals sharing characteristics that permit them to adapt to the demands of their environment. These demands permit the development of characteristics that can be quite different from those possessed by members of other species. Those other species often developed from a different phyletic lineage and have different physical, physiological, and behavioral characteristics. Behavioral tendencies evolved that enhance the likelihood offspring will survive and themselves be able to reproduce, thereby continuing the parents' lineage. The biologically crucial unit of the reproducing species line embodies qualities that have moral relevance as well, such as the tendency to favor family members, kin, neighbors, community members, and members of one's own species.

Humans, as well as all other social animals, are speciesists (Nicoll & Russell, 1991). Animals of all species show a clear preference for their own kind: They associate and mate with their own species; they fight alongside their own kind against members of a foreign species to secure resources; and they defend the young of their own species. Any species that did not show preference for its own kind would become extinct.

Rachels (1990) discussed Robert Nozick's view that a member of any species may legitimately give members of its own species more weight than it gives to members of other species. Nozick commented that lions, if they were moral agents, could not be criticized for putting other lions first. In fact, we do not condemn animals (which are moral patients) for killing animals of other species, ascribing this to their animal nature. We accept infanticide in other species, realizing that evolved biological tendencies contribute to the ultimate reproductive success of parents. However, when an animal kills a human, it is sometimes considered justifiable to kill the animal, presumably to deter its killing more humans, but probably in retribution as well.

Another difference is that, whereas there is always a hierarchical difference between humans and nonhumans, two or more animal species sometimes form mutually beneficial associations, and these mixed-species flocks cooperate while foraging or defending against predators. The human species is the least speciesist of all because it seems to be the only one that displays a moral concern for the welfare of other species. The species concept is of paramount importance within the biological universe.

Language and Species

Although most animals (certainly mammals and birds, and some would include certain insects) engage in communicative acts that extend beyond simple reflex responses, the types of signals differ greatly, and the syntax of the communication systems of most animal species is, at best, incredibly simple compared with human syntax. It is these syntactic abilities that make it possible for human moral agents to understand what is entailed in concepts of right and wrong. I find it morally uninteresting that a chimpanzee can be taught a communication system that has some of the characteristics of human language. Any known primate language system is, as Narveson (1987, p. 32) phrased it, ". . . pretty thin stuff compared to that of normal humans." This observation is true even after animals have been given years of training, and becomes especially important when it is realized that no training is necessary for a budding human to acquire a language system; it develops spontaneously, requiring only exposure to a language community at the proper developmental time.

The human language system is capable of mediating the concepts on which the ability to phrase and understand principles of morality depend; chimpanzees spontaneously develop a language system, but it does not permit the phrasing and understanding of moral principles.

As linguist Derek Bickerton (1990) pointed out, we have no evidence language developed gradually, in the sense of a natural linguistic mode intermediate between primitive communication systems (what he calls protolanguage) and true language. The movement from protolanguage to true language took place rapidly in evolutionary time, seemingly without intervening stages. In at least two instances the development of true language has been observed directly: That of human children, and the change in a single generation from a primitive pidgin language system, which lacks syntactical structure, to a Creole language with the same structural characteristics as any other natural human language. Bickerton uses these two cases to show that language is a direct expression of a species-specific biological characteristic developed in relatively recent time, evolutionarily speaking. He maintains that, in human syntax, the structure of communication is mapped onto phrase structure according to a hierarchy of thematic roles that is universal in all known human languages.

Animals of many species (vertebrate and invertebrate) have abilities that indicate "intelligence" in the sense that they are able to form associations between stimuli and responses, and stimuli and other stimuli. Only humans develop a language system adequate to consider points regarding such things as moral philosophy. As noted in chapter 6, only humans seem to have the second-order intentionality adequate to support the concepts of morality, and it is language that makes possible a great deal of the acquisition and transmission of moral systems.

The Emotional Contract

Although language is necessary for humans to claim their rights (and I have stated often that rights should be a legal concept only), I do not accept the premise that it determines a person's moral value. I proposed in chapters 3 and 6 that language supports cognitive structures that grant the status of being a moral agent with duties and responsibilities. I also said that the essential requirement to be a human moral patient depends on emotional bonding between persons, not on language. In chapter 9 of *Human evolution, reproduction, and morality* I addressed the centrality of the status of personhood at length, and suggested that personhood is a condition that can and usually does exist for members of every species within their own species.

A meaningful biological basis for speciesism can be posited and it does not extend across species boundaries. It is the special relationships among members of a given species, such as within kinship lines and community circles, that form and regulate what I refer to as the biologically supported social contract that grounds morality. The process of emotional bonding between the neonate and members of the basic reproductive unit provides what Singer (1987) demands in terms of minimal characteristics to justify favoritism for members of one's own species. If my viewpoint is accepted, speciesism becomes a basic aspect of biological reality on which the human social condition is founded.

Some aspects of the evolutionary ethics position espoused here were accepted by Singer (1981), who agreed that the core of ethics has a biological basis that is common to humans everywhere. This core is "inherited" from our prehuman ancestors, a point compatible with the notion that emotional bonding between a neonate and members of the social community is an adaptive characteristic. Singer also agreed that, whereas particulars of ethical codes among different cultures are diverse, common elements underly the diversity, among them kin selection and reciprocal altruism. He wrote, "The proposal that we might risk lessening the happiness or prospects of our own children, to however slight a degree, in order to save strangers from starvation strikes many people as not merely idealistic but positively wrong" (p. 32). He believed this preference can be understood in terms of human evolutionary history.

Elsewhere he stated that kinship obligations are strong because they are part of evolved human nature, and to violate those obligations seems unnatural (1979). I believe it is just as understandable for us to favor the interests of our species over the welfare of animals of other species for the same reasons we favor our own kin and members of our community. He also concluded that a norm of reciprocity is universal and reasonable, especially among humans who can reason and communicate so efficiently: "A rational ethical code must also make use of existing tendencies in human nature" (1981, p. 155). I heartily endorse that conclusion.

Feminist Arguments

Midgley (1983) proposed that a necessary part of human social nature is emotional rather than rational, a position stressed by several feminists who have discussed the human moral condition (e.g., Gilligan, 1982; Collard, 1989; Donovan, 1993; Gruen, 1993; Slicer, 1991). When preference for one's own children and kin is viewed in terms of emotional bonding, no further justification is required. It is a deeply embedded part of evolved human social nature. As Midgley noted, this preference promotes special considerations people have for those of their own species, and it is found in all human cultures and is not a product of culture, as is the case with race prejudice. A tendency toward speciesism begins as an essential aspect of biological kinship, and the emotions involved in the bonds are subsequently elaborated by the abstract, rational structures humans build.

Feminists object to the rational nature of theories that philosophers such as Regan and Singer offer in defense of animals on the grounds that they devalue, suppress, or deny emotions. Some hold that moral choices should be based on a need to recognize and affirm the significance of moral feelings, and it is important to rely on direct sensory stimuli—seeing, smelling, and hearing the results of moral decisions—rather than on rational thinking (Kheel, 1996). Donovan (1993) does not like the utilitarian quantification ("mathematization") of suffering because she believes it is used to make it legitimate to sacrifice animals.

The alternative rational processes is to emphasize caring for another, especially a child who requires preservation and time for growth. This injunction to care includes eliminating needless suffering wherever possible, especially suffering by those who are conceptually (and, I would stress, biologically) connected to one's own (Curtin, 1996). Although Curtin is a "contextual moral vegetarian," he would kill an animal to provide food for his son if the son was starving, and would prefer the death of a bear to the death of a loved one. One need not treat all interests equally or pretend that one has no relationship to any of the parties involved.

Adams (1996) condemned the primary texts of Regan and Singer because they overvalue rationality and disavow a legitimate role for emotions in theory making, and one does not have to eliminate emotional content from legitimate moral philosophy. My position is in essential agreement. One should consider the most salient point in human moral standing to occur at birth, and recognize the proximate emotional mechanisms that bond the neonate and caregivers to one another. These feminist ideas regarding mechanisms critical to the definition of moral standing, that define being a person in the human moral community, are compatible with my ideas regarding personhood. I discussed in detail in chapters 5 and 6 that proximate mechanisms evolved to ensure that a neonate will be accepted and responded to positively by caregivers. I also pointed out how, from an evolutionary standpoint, these proximate mechanisms would increase the likelihood a neonate will survive, be nurtured, and become a reproducing member of the human community.

I part company with Adams when she draws a sharp and absolute distinction between reason and emotion, between man and woman, white and "colored," mind and body. She believes these dichotomies represent the power of an ecofeminist analysis of racist, paternalistic dualism, but I believe such dualisms do violence to the texture of reality. We do not live in a polarized nature—each of these dimensions may exist, but they represent continua, and not two-value events. Morality has evolved emotional components, but they become overlaid by strong and important rational ones. It is never a case of emotional versus rational, just as it is never a matter of nature versus nurture. Both components always influence the moral community, and both have an independent input to the moral system—but that input is never in isolation—with one distinct from the other.

I believe that emotional mechanisms producing bonding provide the biological bases for sociality and are the basis on which to distinguish between human and animal moral patients. This base concerns the identity of the neonate as a member of our biological species, and this membership places it in a special category entitling it to treatment as a member of the social community. Beyond this level there should be a rational test for moral agency, a category that probably is exclusively inhabited by humans, and the criteria to be met involve the ability to understand rules, duties, obligations, and causality, and to have a ToM.

Empirical Study of Speciesism

The importance of speciesism as an element in human moral intuitions was attested to in our research program (e.g., Petrinovich, et al., 1993; Petrinovich & O'Neill, 1996) that was discussed in chapter 7 of *Human evolution, reproduction, and morality*. Respondents in our studies did not use the worse-off principle whenever dilemmas involved saving the life of a human in preference to another animal. A human was always favored, even if the choice was between saving the last five remaining members of an endangered highland gorilla species or a young adult human. Another dilemma involved a choice between a young boy who had but one year to live and a young gorilla. Yet another involved a seventy five-year-old human man and a nonendangered adult gorilla. In all instances, the human was favored.

I presume Regan could insist that the five endangered gorillas should be saved rather than the human by employing the worse-off principle. Or would he invoke special considerations regarding the concerns of family and friends of the human, each of whom might suffer more than any of the gorillas given greater levels of satisfaction and a deeper sense of social loss that human relatives can experience? Or would a special consideration be introduced so that the remaining period of life for humans, even the seventy five-year-old man and a youth with one year to live, would provide more satisfaction because of the ability of humans to do such things as savor poetry, philosophy, and music (perhaps even produce them), to contemplate the universe, to interact with and instruct offspring who will perpetuate the family lineage, and in general enjoy the richer satisfactions of life that are available to a human? What if the remaining life of the seventy five-year-old man was only one year, one month, one week, or one day—would the time remaining make a difference? If the old man is someone who can contribute substantially to the health and welfare of the planet and its inhabitants, would this lead to a special consideration that is sufficient to override the worse-off principle? For the youth with one year to live, would the pleasure his relatives would experience due to his presence during that year call for a special consideration? It is not clear which of these alternatives might influence Regan's decision, and he has suggested all of them as special considerations in various contexts. The basic principle of equal inherent value is incapable of bearing definitive moral weight, and subsidiary special considerations seem to be doing all the work. The overwhelming decisions made by respondents in our research on moral intuitions favored a human in all of the above examples. The pattern of choice does not reflect any concept resembling the equal inherent value of all beings as developed by both Regan and Singer.

The examples to this point involve the all-or-none harm of death, and it is instructive to consider ones in which where death is not involved. What would be the proper thing to do if the lifeboat could accommodate four humans and a dog, providing the legs of one of the humans were amputated below the knees, with the person surviving? My intuition is that it would not be permissible to amputate the legs of an unwilling human to spare the life of a dog, and results I reported with O'Neill (1996) support this intuition. However, the worse-off principle would permit the amputation because the human is harmed less than the dog, given that the dog would be killed and the human only suffers. A straightforward argument against speciesism is not as strong as it appears at first glance. People favor members of the human species under a wide variety of special circumstances, and this factor, as propounded by Singer, is readily (and often) overridden when resolving fantasy dilemmas, and in historical instances where survivors had to choose whom to eat. Neither equal inherent value nor speciesism appears strong enough to qualify as fundamental moral principles.

Differences Among Speciesism, Sexism, and Racism

A point made by both Singer and Regan is that the proper test to ground values or rights should be based on characteristics of individual organisms. Some say that chimps should be accorded full moral standing because it is possible they possess enough cognitive characteristics to meet the test of reason. This is convincing to some, at least as it provides a reasonable presumption that chimps might have enough reason to acquire a moral standing equal to certain classes of human moral patients. But, as discussed in chapter 7, this presumption is not based on a compelling body of evidence.

Midgley (1983) addressed speciesism and racism in an enlightened and constructive manner. She considered Singer's equation to be too loosely construed, noting that race in humans is not a significant grouping at all. It is never true that one must know a person's race to know how one should arrange conditions to accommodate that person (only in matters related to cultural traditions that might differentially affect members of different human societies of whatever race). It is essential to know the species of an animal to know how to treat it. She phrased it as follows, "A zoo-keeper who is told to expect an animal, and get a place ready for it, cannot even begin to do this without far more detailed information. It might be a hyaena, or a hippopotamus, a shark, an eagle, an armadillo, a python, or a queen bee" (p. 98). Such things as species, age, sex, and cultural traditions are more important characteristics that determine how one should treat a being than is race, and this is true for animals of any species, including humans.

Devine (1978) expressed a similar view, that racial (and sexual) categories are not biologically real in what he called a profound sense. The physical differences in appearance are real, and are exploited by racist and sexist societies to support a certain social ordering. However, neither the differences between races not those between the sexes represent such profound differences as species membership.

In the interests of justice it is necessary to treat people with respect for their individual qualities and needs, and race is not one of those characteristics that meaningfully dictates basic needs or determines quality of treatment. Species membership, on the other hand, is highly significant, and simply because it indicates meaningful differences, recognition of such differences does not have a prejudicial basis (Midgley, 1983). In addition, neither the special interests parents feel for their children nor our tendency to rescue those closest to us sooner than we would strangers is an indication of prejudice. The basic evolutionary importance of human emotional bonds and ultimate importance of kinship has been stressed throughout discussions of the biologically significant emotional contract.

It is alleged by many in the animal welfare movement that speciesism is the same as racism, and slavery is used as a case in point. Racism is undesirable, and racist beliefs have been used to sustain the institution of slavery. Sperling (1988) cited humane societies that were established in both the United States and Britain in the nineteenth century after the abolition of slavery. She considered this temporal connection to be the result of reformers applying methods developed by abolitionists to focus and mobilize public opinion against slavery. This timing provided a strong historical precedent to link reforms regarding human slaves and animals.

Although human slavery is considered impermissible by everyone except avowed racists and despots, the slavery of animals is considered permissible even by many in the animal welfare movement. Writers such as Singer and Regan seldom discuss the moral permissibility of having animals as pets or as companions. Singer (1993) approached the subject of pets after developing reasons to oppose the use of animals for food and in research, and suggested that other areas should be considered; however, he dismissed the subject (p. 68): "Since the philosophical questions raised . . . are not very different . . . , I shall leave it to the reader to apply the appropriate ethical principles" In the revised edition of *Animal liberation,* he mentions only in appendix 2 that it is possible to obtain vegetarian diets for dogs or cats, rather than feeding them foods that contain animal products. In the preface to the 1975 edition he admitted he was not interested in writing a book about pets because he was not inordinately fond of dogs, cats, or horses. He enunciated this position to establish that his beliefs were not driven by the emotions of an "animal lover," but were based on philosophical beliefs that led him to want animals to be treated as independent sentient beings, not as means to human ends. His positions on animal slavery are vague and equivocal.

Expressing opposition to people keeping pets would not be politically wise given that many supporters of the animal movement have pets. It would also be difficult politically to argue against such practices as using seeing-eye dogs to assist the blind, or introducing animals as companions for elderly or depressed people, even though these animals exist in a state of slavery in the strict sense of a being owned as property and subject to the will of another.

Although practical politics can be appreciated, philosophical implications should not be sidestepped in a cavalier fashion. If racism is impermissible, human slavery cannot be justified on the basis of the race of the slave (or any basis, for that matter). If speciesism is considered to be the same as racism, enslaving animals as pets, guides, or companions cannot be justified without invoking the fact that they are not of the human species—in short, speciesism. Something is amiss here—the permissibility of having and using animals in such benign ways has to become another special consideration, set afloat to rescue sinking philosophical arguments. I believe a more consistent philosophical position can be developed from a straightforward utilitarian stance. Singer's preference utilitarianism could be used to contend that pets prefer to be kept comfortably, and that guide dogs genuinely prefer to assist their owners, especially in view of alternatives available to them. Singer might find this difficult to support, especially because he does not accept the fact that animals in zoos and in certain kinds of research settings have a degree of comfort making it permissible to maintain them in these ways. The question is, can a utilitarian justification be permissible in the instance of pets, but not in conduct of animal research to benefit humans? The analogy between racism and speciesism is questionable, and discussions might proceed more sensibly if the tired charge of speciesism is dropped, with the central issue being how to assess the relative value of certain practices and outcomes.

Few would insist that the reason most players in the National Basketball Association are black is the result of racism favoring blacks, even though they are a minority of the United States population. This preponderance of black athletes exists, in large part, because of characteristics of anatomy (e.g., height and skeletal structure) that are more common in blacks whose ancestors originated in certain regions of Africa. These physical and physiological characteristics were adaptations to ecological demands. Their continuing presence enables these men to excel at basketball, providing a classic example of secondary adaptations that originated to serve functions other than the one they now favor. Blacks are premier basketball players because they were tested one-on-one and excelled in spite of the racism that exists in society. To avoid the charge of racism and sexism, each individual must enjoy the opportunity to compete, and this is not analogous to the situation regarding speciesism.

A clear instance of injustice is provided by examining the early days of professional baseball. Blacks were not allowed to compete with whites, even though it was clear to experts who watched the play of those in the segregated leagues that black players were at least as competent as whites.

Only recently have blacks been permitted to compete on an even footing in many sports, and they clearly meet those competitive tests exceedingly well. Speciesism is on a different level than racism and sexism, and the assertion they are all the same does not hold, but rests on emotional and self-serving appeals.

Differences between sexism and speciesism are also of interest. Whereas the distribution of physiological and mental characteristics for male and female humans, reveals a high degree of overlap (except for matters intimately related to reproduction), there are many differences between the sexes. Such differences, make it improbable that any woman will ever be a professional football player, for example. Features required to play American pro football (with kickers, punters, and coaches possible exceptions) can be met by only a small number of individuals at the very extreme of such characteristics as size, strength, speed, ability to stand pain, and speed of recovery from injury, a combination found only in men. Thus the fact there are no female professional football players is probably not due to sexism. This is not the case for golf and tennis pros, softball, volleyball, or basketball, or for police, firefighters, and combat soldiers, endeavors in which abilities of women at acceptable extremes surpass those of successful males.

The proper test is to allow all individuals an equal opportunity to compete, and it is likely that many females would be able to achieve at a higher level than most males in many endeavors they are not permitted to engage in, and that some would perform as well as many successful males. Not to be judged on ability is clearly an instance of sexism, but I do not think this is analogous to comparisons made across species. Each species has a special emotional attachment to those of its own kind, and no overlap in those critical aspects of emotional bonding establishes the personhood determining moral standing in the human community. In terms of language and cognitive abilities, no species overlaps any normal human distribution (with the possible exception of some of the great apes, especially chimps, although the case is not strong).

A high degree of overlap occurs between different groups of humans in just about any physical and behavioral characteristic. For this reason, it is essential that individuals not be stuck into arbitrary categories on the basis of surface features (such as skin color or sex) without giving them an opportunity to compete on an equal footing. Inevitable inequality in abilities among individual humans should be recognized. The importance of equality of opportunity also must be recognized—and must be guaranteed in a just society. The natural lottery deals a different hand to every individual, but the social lottery should be conducted with complete regard for equal opportunity.

Humans and animals have little overlap, especially in cognitive abilities relevant to moral agency (most especially in language and in meeting the tests for ToM; see chapter 6). I suggest the cognitive differences between most humans and chimps are as great as those between women and professional football players in "football stuff." The important question is to meet the challenges that both Regan and Singer made; it is necessary to consider individual cases where overlap exists between humans and nonhumans. At the high end of the animal distribution we should encounter few problems. It should be possible to agree on appropriate behavioral tests as indicators of whatever characteristics are considered to signal full moral standing. These tests would include such things as self-consciousness, comprehension of rules and causation, a sense of individual continuity over time (which is an indicator of a biographical life, discussed in chapter 4 of *Living and dying well*, Petrinovich, 1996), and ability to understand the minds of other individuals, which is an indicator of a full sense of intentionality. If agreement cannot be reached at the basic level of characteristics of moral agency, there is little hope that satisfactory agreement will be reached regarding full morality.

As suggested earlier, it is possible that great apes, especially chimpanzees, might meet some of the criteria that signal possession of a high capacity to reason. The reasonableness of assuming cognitive continuity is suggested because of behavioral, physiological, and evolutionary similarities among animals of different species. Animals of species other than humans should be considered in terms of the same criteria that establish moral agency for humans, and it is necessary to consider individual animals, rather than to stereotype all members of a given species. The reason for such a procedure is to determine whether *any* overlap can be found between humans and other animals in characteristics accepted to justify full moral standing. In short, it is necessary to agree on criteria, to agree on methods of evaluation and classification, and to make the observations.

Marginal Cases

One problem is to decide how the lower end of the human distribution should be dealt with when overlap is present between individual humans and animals. These marginal cases constitute a gray area that tests the adequacy of basic moral principles. For example, Regan (1975) rejected the notion that humans have the natural right to be spared underserved pain because all, and only, humans reason, make free choices, and have a concept of their identity. Some humans, such as infants, the severely mentally deficient, and the senile, cannot meet these conditions any more than animals can. He wrote (p. 13), "What one would want here are detailed analyses of these operative concepts together with rationally compelling empirical data and other arguments that support the view that all non-human animals are deficient in these respects." He proposed the existence of some morally relevant feature of being human that is possessed by all human beings and only by human beings. I contend that human neonates possess such morally relevant species-specific features, and they are the emotionally based social contracts between species members.

To Singer (1990a), human fetuses, infants, and brain-damaged individuals possess no morally relevant characteristics to a higher degree than adult nonhuman animals. If humans have special relations with such marginal beings, they must be justified on other than an affectionate regard; morality should not be tied too closely to our affections (Singer, 1979). On the contrary, these affections represent an evolved tendency toward emotional bonding in the service of differential reproductive success; they are an essential part of the biological predispositions that promote a cohesive community, and this affectionate basis is highly relevant to morality, conferring the status of a human moral patient on neonates as well as on the cognitively disabled. When matters are cast in terms of evolutionary biology we can meet the test that those humans influenced by our actions have a moral claim not grounded on sentimentality, but on respect for the basic aspects of the human social contract.

Careful consideration is necessary to decide what characteristics confer moral agency on an organism. I suggested in chapter 6 of *Human evolution, reproduction, and morality* that these characteristics should include at least four aspects: The existence of memory, the ability to categorize, the ability to make causal analyses, and the ability to solve the kinds of problems involved in evaluating costs and benefits of plans. In chapter 6 of the present book I added the possession of a complete ToM. To move to a stage where policy issues can be discussed meaningfully, prior discussions should address the adequacy of these characteristics to confer agency. If no agreement is reached at this level, the consistent views of those who support different positions should be understood in order to recognize the nature of, and reasons for, the dissenting views. A separate attempt should be made to establish observable indicators for each characteristic agreed to be relevant, and this information should be integrated. When these tasks are completed, the agreed-upon relevant characteristics for moral agency will at least be understood, behavioral indicators for each identified, basic agreements and disagreements understood and reasonably debated, and relevant observations and tests done.

In the same way, the characteristics and manifestations that confer the status of moral patient on a human organism should be agreed upon. The intermediate stage of personhood determines that status, and I developed and defended the importance of that stage in chapter 9 of *Human evolution, reproduction, and morality*, and discussed it in chapter 3 of the present book. It might well be that certain human organisms, such as anencephalics, lack the requisite characteristics to be considered human persons; if so their status may not place them on equal moral footing with animals. Consensus regarding the desirability of adding this stage of personhood might enable people to arrive at more satisfactory agreements (and honest decisions to disagree) than now exist.

Attacks on Psychological Research

Almost all contemporary physiologists, animal behaviorists, and psychologists accept the fact that animals are sentient (in the sense of being aware of experience), can feel pain, and can suffer. A common ploy used by those who oppose psychological experimentation in animals is to attack the position of the classic Behaviorists, a school of psychology that dominated experimental psychology for much of the first half of the twentieth century. Rollin's (1992) arguments provide an example of how such attacks on the Behaviorist straw man are conducted to insist that contemporary behavioral psychology is a case of bad science. He accused the fields of experimental, behavioral, comparative, and "sometimes" physiological pscyhology of being guilty of mindless activity that causes great suffering. He wrote that behavioral psychology was an intellectual sham that impedes understanding of the behavior of dogs, cats, rats, and mice. His extreme disapproval of these fields led him to write (p. 176): "Nowhere are researchers further removed from theory, nowhere are researchers less engaged in trying to develop a picture of some aspect of the world, nowhere are researchers less concerned with the morality of what they do." He said that no theory connects rats and humans (could I suggest the theory of evolution?). He doubted whether psychology has any theory at all, and B. F. Skinner was an exemplar of the state of psychological theory.

The problem is that the field of psychology historically has suffered an embarrassment of theory that too often is not supported by an adequate data base, and some of the reactions of Behaviorists were in the spirit of opposing such free-wheeling concepts. I am referring to some of the early personality and social psychology theories, in which the ratio of data to theory was much too low. The hypothetico-deductive theories of learning (e.g., Hull, 1943) were careful attempts to develop a formal model that could be directly tied to operationally defined constructs. Formal learning theories of this type did not succeed, mainly because the theoretical edifice was too general, the assumptions providing universal laws that were to apply to all animals in all situation were incorrect, and the data base was too narrow to support such grandiose models.

Although theories such as Hull's suffered from what Rollin (1989) referred to as acquiescence to positivism's demand that only observables be permitted in science notable exceptions to hidebound positivism appeared in the form of Tolman's (1932) purposive behaviorism and Hebb's (1949) neuropsychological theory. Attempts to ground personality theory using the formal learning principles of the Hullian type (e.g., Miller & Dollard, 1941; Mowrer, 1960) did not succeed because they were based on both personality and learning theories that were flawed fundamentally, not because they involved observables.

It is hardly apt to suggest Skinner's operant conditioning program as an exemplar of American psychological theory. He held an explicit antitheoretical view, maintaining that theory was not necessary to the progress of behavioral science, expressing the beliefs that the science of psychology should be based only on empirical regularities (see Skinner, 1950).

All of these scientific approaches to understand the rich interplay of factors regulating complex behavior surely were more than mindless activity that led to dead ends. Failures of some of them produced the realization that certain avenues of inquiry indeed were not productive, but at the same time the way was opened for a more satisfactory wave of theory building. I am reminded of the oft-quoted statement by Darwin (1871, p. 909): "False facts are highly injurious to the progress of science, for they often endure long; but false views, if supported by some evidence, do little harm, for every one takes a salutary pleasure in proving their falseness: and when this is done one path towards error is closed and the road to truth is often at the same time opened." Because psychological theories were not correct and led to dead ends does not mean the attempts are worthy of contempt. Hull's theory was a bold attempt to apply to psychology the formal methods of hypothetico-deductive theory that had proved so successful in the science of physics. Because its reductionism failed is no reason the attempt should be scorned.

Most contemporary theories in experimental psychology, such as those discussed in chapter 6, emphasize cognitive factors. They reject the extreme positivism of classic Behaviorism and respect the richness of behavioral processes. They allow for multiple, probabilistic, and vicarious strands of causation, and examine behavior in terms of vicarious functional achievements, rather than of molecular responses. This view was supported most cogently by Brunswik (1952), and I developed them further in the interest of incorporating a more evolutionary and ethological perspective (Petrinovich, 1973, 1979).

The theory of evolution provides tools that will enable psychologists to develop adequate theories of behavioral function in terms of adjustments that must be made to adapt organisms to the demands of ecology. Incorporating evolutionary mechanisms into the explanatory scheme led psychologists to devote attention not only to the proximate processes that cause behavior, but also to ultimate factors at the level of differential reproductive success (see Daly & Wilson, 1988; Barkow, Cosmides, &

Tooby, 1992; Hauser, 1996). It is time for philosophers to stop beating the dead horse of classic Behaviorism and address the structure of contemporary theories that attempt to deal with the complexities of behavior. I will return to the issue of the permissibility of psychological research in animals at greater length in chapter 11.

Philosophical Comment Regarding Singer's Arguments

Singer's philosophical arguments, as well as his political and ethical stands, are acclaimed by most animal welfare advocates. His positions on the evils of speciesism and equality are used to justify the political agenda of the activist faction. For example, Francione (1995, p. 97) referred to the "sophisticated and persuasive arguments" of Singer and Regan, both of whom, in his opinion, demonstrated that speciesism is no more logically or morally defensible than any other form of prejudice. More recently, however, Francione (1996) scorned the positions of Singer and Regan because they do not call for total abolition of all uses of animals by humans.

Feminist Josephine Donovan (1993) characterized Singer's *Animal liberation* as an ". . . admirable and courageous book . . . that largely galvanized the current animal rights movement" (p. 171). Orlans (1993) credited the recent rise of the animal rights movement to the 1975 edition of that book, stating that it changed the way many look at animals. DeGrazia (1996) considered the book, more than any other work, to have brought questions about the moral status of animals into intellectual respectability. Ryder (1989) credited Singer with providing the animal protection movement with its new intellectual leadership through his cool and unemotional contribution, and concluded that the American conscience regarding animals might have "continued to slumber" without publication of the book. Undoubtedly, Singer provided the philosophical leadership that fueled the animal liberation movement.

Philosophers treated Singer's ideas with respect, although some disagreed with the implications of his preference utilitarianism. Rachels (1990) contributed a thoughtful discussion of his ideas and considered the concept of speciesism at length. He suggested two versions of this concept. The first he called *radical speciesism*, which holds that even relatively trivial interests of humans should take priority over the vital interest of nonhumans. He believes this is the version of speciesism Singer describes and opposes:

Rachels suggested a more plausible version that he called *mild speciesism:* When the choice is between a relatively trivial human interest (such as experiencing a transitory thrill) and a more substantial interest of a nonhuman, we should choose in favor of the nonhuman. He added that if interests are comparable, preference should be given to the welfare of the human—or in baseball parlance, the tie goes to the runner (human).

Rachels also suggested a *qualified speciesism:* Species membership should be considered to be correlated with other differences that are morally significant. The interests of humans could be more important, not simply because they are human interests, but because humans have morally relevant characteristics other animals lack. He rejected this view, worrying that the same arguments could be used to defend racism. To be sure, the arguments are difficult: Xenophobia has led to incredibly inhumane treatment of humans by other humans, and can be considered an undesirable side effect of the evolutionary bias most social animals have to favor kin over others. Humans in particular have a bias to favor members of their own social group who might have kinship ties, and who might be able to reciprocate when helped. In this light, xenophobia would be an undesirable outcome of tendencies to express love and engage in care of one's own in the EEA.

Whereas these tendencies could have undesirable consequences in terms of producing human inequality, it is possible to establish social conventions and legal barriers to counter inequalities created between individuals who have comparable characteristics. Rachels suggested that if a person is capable of acting to consider another person's interests and refuses to do so, we are released from similar obligations to that person; accepting such a state of affairs might be a first step toward understanding and remedying existing social inequalities.

Rachels held that humans can have greater moral weight if they possess some essential quality, but not merely because they are human. In 1993 he stated that it does not follow that all animals must be treated as equal to humans, for differences between humans and some animals may justify a difference in moral status. I agree, although disagree about what those differences are and where the line should be drawn, and suggest the one essential quality conferring status as a human moral patient is being a person in the human social community.

Animals of other species clearly have welfare interests that should be respected. Mild speciesism can be defended on utilitarian grounds, with deaths of animals justifiable whenever they are necessary to save humans. Our data regarding moral intuitions indicate that most people accord a priority to humans, and as I have noted several times, both Regan and Singer resort to mild speciesism when discussing moral dilemmas requiring a choice between sacrificing an animal or a human. Problems arise and must be faced regarding where a line should be drawn between permissible and impermissible choices, and I consider such problems when discussing specific issues regarding the use of animals by humans in later chapters.

Rachels (1990) contended that cruelty to animals is wrong, but he did not imply that it is never justified to inflict pain on an animal if a *good* (his emphasis) reason is found to cause suffering. He adopted the type of cost-benefit analysis that characterizes most evolutionary processes. He noted: "While Singer was a reformer, Regan was an abolitionist" (p. 218), and he tended to side more closely with Singer. To Rachels (p. 222), species membership itself should be a relatively unimportant primary quality, and he favored moral individualism according to which individual characteristics of organisms are of greater importance than the classes to which they are assigned. The heart of his position resides in an insistence on equal concern for the welfare of all beings, with distinctions made only when relevant differences justify differences in treatment. This position he asserted, is in the spirit of Darwinism. I agree, but add a caveat that the concept of species membership also qualifies as an entity to enter into the balance sheet.

Rodd (1990) expressed a view similar to what I suggested when she observed that claims for nonhuman animals to have rights have become firmly associated with absolute opposition to all use of animals in biomedical research. Animals ought not be harmed merely to provide things humans find pleasant, but she found it difficult to insist that animals have an absolute right not to be harmed to the extent that humans should forego preservation of themselves and the lives of other humans to prevent such harm.

According to Regan (1983), Singer's preference utilitarianism frames the wrongness of killing animals in terms of their preferences (desires) to go on living rather than dying. Singer regards self-conscious beings as individuals leading lives of their own, and not merely as receptacles that contain quantities of happiness. The status of being self-conscious is important because conscious beings (they do not necessarily have to be self-conscious) are replaceable receptacles of value. Regan objects to this view because it allows an optimal aggregated balance of satisfaction of preferences. He believes (pp. 214–215) that Singer has allowed all the undesirable aspects of aggregate utility to become basic to his theory, and this violates the essential notion of equality.

The crux of the differences in the philosophical principles of Regan and Singer is that Singer considers it basic that an animal's interests ought to have equal consideration with like interests of humans. Regan considers moral rights to rest on the concept of the inherent value of all beings and that inherent value is equal for all. Although the principles are different, they both arrive at a common goal—that animals are to be accorded equality of treatment.

Sorabji (1993) objected to the one-dimensionality of the philosophies, both Regan's idea of inherent value and Singer's preference utilitarianism. Instead, more concern should be given to the particular situation and characteristics of the individuals in those situations, such as close family ties, friendships, and vitality. In short, he suggested it is not possible to reduce all considerations to one set of basic principles, that a moral pluralism is preferable and is necessary to include all the various cases one must consider when making moral decisions. The view I propose is in the spirit of Sorabji's suggestions.

When decisions must be made that involve only humans, the principles of kinship and community prevail, and in most circumstances should help promote a just and moral society. However, as the philosopher James Fetzer (1996) reminded, humans who respond on the basis of kin selection and reciprocal altruism are not invariably ethical. Social cooperation and preference for those similar to us have, throughout human history, led to monstrous policies that harmed many who were regarded as outsiders. As Fetzer succinctly stated, cooperation is not morality. He emphasized the often neglected point that the traits produced by evolution of characteristics through natural selection are not moral behaviors, but a capacity for moral behavior. Evolved traits lead to commitment to respect the intrinsic value of enhancing reproductive success of individuals who are members of the species, but some tendencies, such as favoring kin and neighbors, can promote xenophobia with its distrust of and harm to strangers.

Rodd (1990) concurred with these general views, noting that strong moral intuitions exist for good reasons; in evolutionary terms they might have been developed for reasons that are no longer applicable: "If we have a powerful feeling that certain kinds of action are wrong, then the idea that this feeling is likely to exist because it has been important during evolution gives some support to the validity of the intuition . . . the theory claims that we have ethics instead of instincts because we need to think rationally about our actions," (p. 239). This statement embodies the essence of many of the arguments regarding moral intuitions and their relevance for ethics that I have presented throughout this book.

Fetzer (1996) considered compatibility with the laws of biology to count as a necessary condition for morality, but not as a sufficient condition. He concluded that the usual evolutionary view of morality is incomplete, and I agree. Because of the incomplete nature of a purely evolutionary ethics it is necessary to add a principle emphasizing the necessity to respect the basic freedoms of human beings—what I called a rational liberalism in chapter 6 of *Human evolution, reproduction, and morality.*

To circumvent problems that could arise due to unbridled chauvinism it is necessary to ensure that all moral agents retain the freedom to make decisions, and that decisions regarding their welfare are the result of voluntary actions by competent and rational persons. This concept of voluntary decision making, coupled with freedom from harm and offense that is equally due all moral agents, should avoid much of the evil that could result if total reliance is placed on evolutionary currency alone.

9

Morality and Animal Research

An issue that has occasioned disputatious discussion, activism, and political jockeying is the permissibility of animal experimentation conducted in the interest of understanding and manipulating biological and psychological characteristics of various species. Animal rights activists have long targeted vivisectionists for scorn, and many books and conferences through the years expressed varying degrees of objection to basic research using animals. Equally strong defenses were made by prominent academic and commercial interests, which often stressed the importance of tradition and utility, as well as the search for knowledge, accompanied by emotional appeals regarding the value of biomedical research to alleviate human and animal suffering. Many defenders believe that interests of humans always trump those of the animals whose welfare is jeopardized by research.

Some opponents advocate absolute abolition of all research whenever it jeopardizes the interests and welfare of any sentient creature. Others object only to research that uses primates and some mainly decry research that involves the most common mammalian pets. For those taking either of the last two positions, these animals are not only sentient, but possess emotions and a level of consciousness entitling them to be considered morally comparable with humans.

Abolitionists are adamant that all animal research should be stopped, and they conduct active informational campaigns replete with statistics and vivid pictorial representations of horrible acts of violence against animals. Some encourage and engage in acts of civil disobedience, and condone violence against individuals and institutional facilities of which they disapprove. These campaigns are accompanied by active political lobbying at local, state, and national levels.

Many antiresearch proponents object to certain types of procedures and to investigations involving certain objectives they regard as trivial. Some animal advocates, believe that animal experimentation is never justified, but consider its immediate abolition to be an unrealistic goal, and acknowledge that responsible experimentation for medical purposes should be done as long as no alternatives are available and the knowledge sought is absolutely essential (see *The animal rights handbook*, 1990, for a brief expression of these views). Moderate reformers propose including animal welfare advocates as members of IACUCs and allowing them to evaluate procedures and observe their conduct (especially surgical procedures). It has been suggested that animal welfare representatives should be allowed to veto research proposals that use procedures they consider harmful to animals.

I discuss the claims of disputants who represent the poles of the issue, evaluate the facts as they are presented by the disputants, and in chapter 10, place the conflicting views in a perspective that considers principles of moral philosophy. I begin with a brief history of the antivivisection movement, including opinions of those who insist all animal research should be abolished. Then, views of those who take a more moderate rights position are discussed, followed by the even more moderate animal liberation position. A segment of the research community contends that it is justified to conduct any animal research that could potentially benefit humans.

I have chosen this format not only to highlight and evaluate the substantive arguments, but to clarify underlying philosophical, medical, and moral theses on which the positions are based. Throughout, I consider relevant facts, and address specific arguments in light of these facts. Moderate views have been proposed by those who find merit in some suggestions of all the disputants. These represent a philosophical and practical middle course, one that, unfortunately, is unlikely to find a cordial reception in either polar group. The situation often epitomizes Alexis de Tocqueville's observation that people often would rather believe a simple lie than a complex truth.

This chapter stresses the issues discussed in part I, which presented basic biological, evolutionary, and philosophical aspects of moral, scientific, medical, and economic issues. These issues are always involved, either implicitly or explicitly, when practical issues are raised related to the permissible use of animals as research subjects. Especially important are questions concerning the general nature of scientific research, what benefits might justify the costs of a research project, how to decide what the potential value of research might be before it has been conducted, and how to determine whether a study has led to advances in pure or applied science.

The Research Abolitionists

History of Legislative Actions

The permissibility of using animals for anatomical and physiological research has been discussed over the centuries (see Smith & Boyd, 1991). Physiological studies of sensory, motor, and autonomic activity of animals were reported as early as 500 B.C. and animals were used to test toxic substances as early as the second century B.C. By the nineteenth century, theological objections were raised to using dead human bodies for anatomical studies, and animals were used widely as an alternative for both anatomical and physiological investigations.

In Britain, attacks on the morality and value of animal experimentation began as early as the midnineteenth century. Opposition has never solely been concerned with animal welfare; as much unease has been expressed about possible positive and negative consequences of animal experimentation to influence human well-being (Elston, 1997). By 1850, experiments using living animals were an integral part of teaching and research activities in British medicine, and in 1876 scientific and medical associations were able to defeat a bill that proposed to govern this practice. The mild control measure that passed at that time remained in effect for the next 110 years.

The core of the Victorian antivivisection movement was composed largely of affluent upper- and middle-class women who believed that much of the declining morality of British society was due to demoralizing and brutalizing effects of exposure to experimental physiology. Women occupied important leadership positions in the Royal Society for the Prevention of Cruelty to Animals (RSPCA), which was not the case in traditional humane movements (Sperling, 1988). For many of these Victorians, the moral implications of developments in physiology and bacteriology were as disturbing as Darwin's theory of evolution had been (Elston, 1992). In short, science was threatening to usurp religion; specifically, faith in God's healing power was being undermined. The attention of these individuals tended to be directed toward practices of the working class that involved animals. These were the targets of both the American movement and its British antecedent, the earliest cases of arrests in the United States were of working-class individuals (Sperling, 1988).

The position of antivivisectionists was similar to that of present day left-wing opponents to research—that society is obsessed with health and tends to move too quickly in the direction of increasingly dangerous medical interventions, whereas attention should more properly be given to alternative methods of healing and to social factors that produce human disease. While the left wing demands more social engineering, the right wing places emphasis on individual responsibility for health practices.

In 1986, new legislation was enacted in the United Kingdom (UK) in the form of the Animals (Scientific Procedures) Act. This act controlled animal experimentation, and according to Elston, modern antivivisectionists began to couch their arguments in the secular language of science rather than in terms of religious imagery. They called for reorientation of research toward prevention, specifying either health education or social engineering rather than microbiology and toxicology. The National Anti-Vivisection Society insisted that "real science" should involve the study of human beings and their diseases, and that animal experiments tell us only about animals, not about people.

The strength of the animal welfare movement varies in different countries. MacKenzie (1992) reviewed legal regulations in several European nations, ranging from those in Switzerland, where strict animal welfare laws are enforced and there are national efforts to ban animal experiments entirely, to Spain, Greece, and eastern Europe, where animal welfare hardly is represented in the law. The European Commission tried to establish uniform rules regarding animal experimentation, proposing common standards for testing procedures, especially with regard to testing the safety of chemicals. The commission proposed to eliminate duplication in animal testing through abolition of different national licensing authorities, and elimination of the practice whenever alternatives become available. A directive was issued to protect animals used for these and other scientific purposes, calling for use of the smallest possible numbers of animals, and insisting that experiments should cause minimum pain and be carried out in species having "the lowest degree of Neurophysiological sensitivity" (whatever that might mean). Only Germany, Britain, and The Netherlands have enacted these provisions into national law. France and Italy have prepared the required legislation, but Spain, Portugal, and Greece are opposed. Countries in eastern Europe have few rules governing the care of experimental animals, with only Poland and Czechoslovakia having drafted their first laws to protect the animals. Although Hungary has no related laws, its scientific standards are considered comparable with those in the West. Some Western countries, as well as Japan, are commissioning animal tests to be done in Hungary in order to cut costs (MacKenzie, 1992).

Regulations in the United States are "remarkably weak" compared with to those in Britain (Gavaghan, 1992). Legislation in the United States specifically excludes research practices from regulatory control, and covers only warm-blooded animals; British law includes fish, amphibians, and reptiles. Regulations adopted everywhere apply only to animals used in experimentation, and not to agricultural animals.

Research regulations of the USDA require that, to accomplish scientific goals, laboratory procedures must cause a minimum discomfort, distress, and pain. The principal investigator must consider alternatives to procedures that cause more than momentary pain, and procedures must be performed using appropriate sedatives and anesthetics unless their omission can be justified for scientific reasons. All IACUCs must be established to review all federally funded research proposals, and USDA regulations require a minimum of three people on the committee, one of whom must be a veterinarian familiar with laboratory animals, and another someone from outside the institution. The NIH guidelines stipulate a minimum of five members on institutional review committees, one a veterinarian, one a nonscientist from within the institution, and one from outside it.

An extensive survey of legal requirements in several countries can be found in Smith and Boyd (1991), a book that is the report of a working party of the Institute of Medical Ethics in Britain. Examination of these requirements indicate a wide range of regulations, enforcement provisions ranging from strict enforcement to voluntary compliance, and considerable variation in species falling under the regulations. The working party concluded "Laboratory animal protection laws are all based on the premise that, in certain circumstances, it is morally acceptable to use animals in scientific procedures for the benefit of humans or other animals" (p. 275). The laws of most countries permit weighing costs and benefits to evaluate the merit of proposed research. Although United States law explicitly refrains from interfering with the design and conduct of research, various professional learned societies, as well as a number of scientific journals, adopted guidelines regarding experimental techniques and care procedures that can be considered ethical. The scientific establishment has begun to respond to demands of animal welfarists, and it is equally clear that most welfarists consider the responses inadequate for a number of reasons (explored in chapters 10 and 11).

Some who object to animal research insist on total abolition of any procedures that negatively affect the welfare of subject animals, both human and nonhuman. The position proposed by Regan (1983) supports abolition, whereas the stance adopted by Singer (1975) only tends in this direction. Francione (1996) suggested a strongly abolitionist position, the goal of which is to apply animal rights theory to eliminate the basic evil of considering animals as property. He rejects the positions of Regan and Singer on grounds that their methods of welfare reform assume and reinforce the property status of animals. He stated (p. 188) that animal advocacy groups are ". . . more like bourgeois charities than revolutionary organizations." In addition, those who work within the system for reform are misguided, and the only morally permissible actions are those that help abolish the institutionalized exploitation of animals.

Anti-Vivisectionists   Abolitionists will accept nothing less than the cessation of all research using animals. Some of their arguments are based on positions in moral philosophy, some on theological beliefs, and others appeal to emotional responses to animal suffering. The antivivisection movement in both Britain and the United States adopted extreme positions, and published provocative material aimed to evoke strong emotions through slogans, photographs of appealing pets, tragic laboratory settings, and animals that have undergone mutilation in experiments.

One such pamphlet bears the title, *Vivisection is scientific fraud* (Ruesch, 1979), which is part 7 of his book *Naked empress, or the great medical fraud.* The pamphlet starts with a banner headline on page 1 that reads, "A Government-sponsored School of Violence/ An endless Source of Profits and new Diseases/ THE MODERN BARBARITY palmed off as Science through the venality of the mass media and industry-beholden politicians." It ends with a statement that the United States is the world leader in vivisection, informing readers (p. 47): "If you don't like this kind of 'medical research', write to some of the people responsible for assigning those Federal grants for animal experiments." They provide addresses of the heads of two federal granting agencies, and of the chairmen of Senate and House appropriation committees. The pamphlet has twenty three pages of photographs of animals (mainly nonhuman primates, dogs, and cats) who have undergone experimental procedures, with an occasional scientist viewing an animal with an air of objectivity, satisfaction, or apparent amusement. These photos have captions such as, "These scared little primates are being turned into dope addicts. . . . ," "This screaming monkey . . . flees from the needle . . . to test a new 'miracle' drug [Methadone] on him. But in man the anti-dope becomes in turn a dope. . . . It's like calling in Satan to drive out the Devil," ". . . the overgrown child at the controls [the experimenter] watches in breathless fascination how he can cause the monkey to lift an arm by pushing a button," and ". . . this latest demonstration of vivisectionist sadism and idiocy."

The photos are followed by three pages of statements by physicians and physiologists selected from a collection of close to a thousand similar ones gathered by Ruesch. Typical comments are, "It has been demonstrated that results from animal experiments are in no way applicable to human beings," "No experimental worker can provide a single fact about human disease," "There really exists no logical basis for translating the results of animals to man," and "In the United States today the only cause of polio is the polio vaccine. . . ." These quotations are offered to support the claim that animal experimentation is not only useless, but is harmful for medicine. This series of statements is followed by another twenty two pages of photographs, including some of children deformed by thalido-mide. Some of these statements are discussed in chapter 10 when the value and contribution of experiments with animals to the progress of biological and medical science are considered.

The pamphlet is loaded with emotional appeals, graphic displays of dead and suffering animals, and overblown rhetoric. All in all it is a fine piece of propaganda aimed at enlisting political and financial support toward the goal of abolishing all animal research, and ultimately any use of animals by humans for food, services, or entertainment.

Javier Burgos founded a group called Students United Protesting Research on Sentient Subjects (SUPRESS) whose intention is to further the aims of Hans Ruesch. In a pamphlet issued in the Spring of 1991 (*supress*, 1991), the group announced that it is the "**New** Anti-vivisection Movement," and that it openly supports the aims of the Animal Liberation Front (ALF) by speaking on its behalf and endorsing its call to violent activism. In this pamphlet the group's views are presented along with appeals for financial support. The emphasis is on denouncing strongly those who endorse animal rights, and on encouraging readers to direct financial contributions to them rather than to groups that advocate measures they believe compromise the goal of complete abolition of animal research. Their criticisms of other groups are based on the position that the concept of rights is a moral one, whereas the antivivisection position should be based on scientific fact. They wrote (p. 16): "**Vivisection is a medical and scientific issue** and it must be tackled as such" (emphasis in the original). They asserted that the largest and wealthiest animal rights organizations insist on discussing morality, ethics, religion, and philosophy, while they should expose the scientific fraud that is part and parcel of all experimental research with life. Their scientific agenda is based on an insistence that animal research has had no beneficial effects for mankind (that it has been harmful); that interspecies similarities (p. 4) ". . . are spectacularly superficial"; that "Vivisection is, if anything, a pseudo-science"; that "One derives a broad, general body of knowledge not by enquiring broadly or generally, but by narrowing the field of enquiry while enquiring variously, then assimilating and correlating the results of those many enquiries [insistence on the use of induction rather than deduction]; that (p. 8) it is a ". . . totally fraudulent premise that one can understand human anatomy, physiology [or neurophysiology] by studying non-human animals. Any real scientist knows that non-human animals are not only different from man but also from each other, meaning that each species is a different entity and thus, information cannot be extrapolated from one to another"; and (p. 13) that ". . . animal experimentation and eating animals **are the two main causes of human suffering and death.**" In the material that follows I challenge assertions that appeals to philosophy are absurd and useless, disagree that interspecies differences make the results of any animal research not generalizable to humans, and suggest that deduction, rather than induction, is the better method for science to follow.

SUPRESS insists that all scientists who disagree with its position are motivated by greed because they benefit from, and depend on, billions of dollars from research foundations. It asserts that these vast sums allow scientists to control the media, which extol their virtues and herald their accomplishments, leading the general public to engage in hero worship. It is not possible to respond to such a broadside of allegations regarding the integrity, intentions, and gullibility of all who disagree with them. I agree that the argument should be joined at the level of medical and scientific issues, but recommend attention be devoted to some of the niceties of reasoned philosophical debate, and that positions be subjected to the scrutiny of factual evidence, logical consistency, and universal applicability.

The Arguments of Michael Fox   The vice president of the Humane Society of the United States, M. W. Fox (1990), published *Inhumane society*, which contains a more detailed version of many of the notions set forth by Ruesch and Burgos. Fox, too, considers most biomedical research to be useless, says that much animal research is unnecessary and irrelevant, and believes that corrective actions to prevent degenerative diseases should be primarily social and political.

He believes the reason results of animal experiments cannot be generalized is that the totality of body-mind-environment interconnectedness has been broken by conditions that exist in all laboratories, making their conclusions unscientific and counter to progress in medicine. "Although admittedly [vivisection] contributed to the advancement of medical knowledge, it now impedes further significant medical progress" (p. 96). Fox dismissed animal tests of toxicity, considering them ". . . to amount to little more than a public relations campaign to dispel public concern and, at best, give a false sense of security" (p. 61).

One of his basic premises is (p. 64) that ". . . if the pain and suffering to the animal would be greater than the amount of pain and suffering that a human might feel under the same experimental conditions, then the experiment should not be permitted." Because we cannot ascertain how much an animal is in pain and how great its suffering (nor can we for different humans, incidentally), we should not perform experiments on animals. With this neat assertion the game can be declared over, even though the conclusion does not qualify as an argument. In fact, if knowing the exact level of pain is the criterion to determine the permissibility of animal research, more research should be done to determine the quality and severity of pain in response to various treatments in both human and nonhuman animals.

Fox, as do many other antiresearch activists, invokes evolutionary theory to support a continuity to mental experience, which means that research on beings with such similar qualities is impermissible. In other instances, the existence of evolutionary *discontinuity* is used to hold that differences between humans and other animals are so great that no generalizations can be made across species, and research on animals is impermissible because the inability to generalize renders it useless. The tactic seems to be to pick whichever alternative suits the claim being made at the moment. I consider the concern regarding similarities and differences several times in the material that follows.

One difficult notion expressed by Fox as well as by numerous other writers is that peer review of research proposals, which is done in almost all cases in which public funds are involved, is inadequate because it does not represent prevailing societal values. Rollin (1989) stated that because most biomedical research is funded by public money, the scientific community cannot remain aloof from public concerns, and the moral assumptions of the community should shape the form of science.

I suggest that outcomes of peer review might accurately represent societal values, especially when questions involve the development and application of medical diagnostic procedures and treatment methods.

Members of the general public have as strong an interest in adequate health care as does the scientific community. Several polls over a number of years indicate the general public predominantly supports animal research to study health problems (Orlaus, 1993). In 1985, 81% agreed animals should be used for studies of cancer, heart disease, and diabetes, with only 12% disagreeing; 61% agreed animals should be used to study allergies. In 1989, 77% agreed that the use of animals in biomedical research is necessary for progress in medicine, with only 17% disagreeing. It appears the general public is not as opposed to these practices as abolitionists would have it.

More important issues regarding whether scientific research should be governed by society's values or by its quality as judged by scientists, bear on the merit of theoretical questions, the adequacy of procedures used to address them, and possible practical consequences that might result. If these are the important issues, a rigorous peer-review system would always be an essential and irreplaceable part of the scientific process. Careful and strict review by scientists is a better way to evaluate the merits of research than relying on votes by members of society at large or following poll results that reflect its values. Society has input at the level of the political forums that set public policy and funding, and that seems to be the proper level.

Fox found it difficult to justify research expenditures to study the heritability, diagnosis, and treatment of genetic diseases, especially using inbred animals, noting that people are not inbred. Langley (1989) considered it immediately obvious that using inbred, genetically similar animals is unlikely to improve the relevance of tests to outbred, genetically dissimilar humans. Fox suggested efforts would be better spent to seek ways to prevent suffering by cleaning up the environment. I suspect, however, given that millions of people are sick at present, the morality of not developing treatments for existing maladies in order to concentrate all effort toward preventing further disease in future generations can be questioned. Those who suffer might want their morbidity to be ameliorated and the quality of their existence enhanced. Benson (1978) remarked that it might not be morally permissible to prescribe that others must sacrifice their life or health in the interest of sparing animals. He likened this to saying to individuals who owed their eyesight to a treatment whose development involved the sacrifice of animals that they should have chosen to be blind.

Diseases and disorders might be prevented more easily if their causes and symptom patterns were understood and used to guide efforts at environmental interventions. It is not a case of either-or: Most reputable biomedical experts would not disagree with either the medical or environmental approach to public health problems, and many would prefer that each be applied in conjunction with the other. Although either-or arguments are popular, this is not a zero-sum game in which any resources taken from one activity will be devoted to the other. There are many competing priorities, and it is just as likely that funds siphoned from medical research would be directed toward defense or highway funding rather than automatically spent on environmental approaches to public health.

Fox (p. 98) endorsed the basic position outlined by Regan that all life has equal inherent value: "Thus the life of the ant and the life of my child should be accorded equal respect." He adopted this view on the premise of a basic sanctity of life, and explicitly rejected utilitarian principles. Later, however, he amended his stance, acknowledging that animals do not have equal rights because their needs, wants, and interests are different from ours, a qualification that is similar to that made by Singer, as discussed in chapter 8. He held that giving the rights of all animals equal consideration does not necessarily imply they should be given equal treatment. I find his ideas too dense to provide much of a handle on the problem of determining morality in any given situation. To me this all smacks of Regan's special considerations being brought in whenever needed to rescue basic principles from leading to unthinkable conclusions.

Sanctity of life is central to Fox's ideas. He wrote (pp. 227–228), "Denial of our duties toward all creation culminates in dominion over God, and the values and rationalizations that lead to this pyramid of power with humanity at the top is the biological fascism of the anti-Christ." He concluded (p. 243): "So I close this book in a declaration of war against the anti-Christ; against the powers of human evil evident in our corrupt and selfish proclivity to abuse the powers over life we have achieved."

In 1986 he stated (p. 170): ". . . since science does not deal with ethical issues and is purportedly an objective and amoral discipline, we must, it would seem, turn to religion and moral philosophy for some direction and answers." Devotional inspiration will lead one to recognize the sacredness of the world, and morality of compassion gives equal and fair consideration to all of creation (1990). Although these sentiments may be admirable, they do not provide an adequate grounding for the morality that should regulate secular society, nor do they offer an acceptable basis for those with a different theological position or who reject all theologies.

Although explicitly rejecting utilitarianism, he suggested that certain human needs and interests could be satisfied at the expense of animals' rights and interests, and that a balance should be established that is neither exclusively human centered nor animal centered; both should be given equal and fair consideration. This statement admits utilitarianism because it leaves room for balancing needs and interests of some against those of others. Fox rejected utilitarian justifications because they are not objective, always being biased by subjective self-interest. If it is accepted that members of our own species have developed an emotional bond with their infants, this would provide the necessary objective grounding for the moral justification Fox seems to desire. Although he heaps condemnation on both the biomedical establishment and agribusiness for using animals to attain the goals of science and realize economic profit, he treads lightly on philosophers who maintain informed utilitarian positions, specifically exempting Peter Singer's preference utilitarianism from criticism.

Although Fox said that the life of an ant and the life of his child should be accorded equal respect, two paragraphs later he allows that one may love an animal, but love one's own child differently, ". . . because we are naturally more connected and emotionally involved with our closest relations who need us more than rats and other creatures normally do." If we have a responsibility to support those beings who need us most, Fox's view could lead one to insist that the welfare of my child could be neglected as long as that child is above the minimal threshold for a satisfactory life, and that I should use my resources to assist other creatures, such as rats, providing they need me more in terms of their survival and welfare. This view most would find indefensible. I doubt Fox would demand that I not use a product obtained from a rat's organs if it would treat, and perhaps cure, my own child's serious illness, even if the procedures caused the rat's death.

Fox (1990, p. 224) insisted that illegal acts to liberate animals are ethically justified, and legal grounds should support such actions, just as they do justifiable homicide in self-defense. A similar argument is made by members of antiabortion groups to the effect that violence against, and even killing of, abortionists is justified to "stop the murder of unborn children." It is not possible to maintain a reasonable and just society if it is permissible for people to take the law into their own hands, or make an idiosyncratic interpretation of the meaning of the law whenever they want to justify any well-intended interventions they believe are required by some higher authority.

Animal Rights

The SUPRESS group rejects rights statements because they deflect discussion from their main goal—to demonstrate the fraud of scientific research using animals. They prefer to base their position on a utilitarian cost-benefit analysis of the research enterprise.

Philosophical aspects of the animal rights movement were discussed in chapter 7, when the theories of Tom Regan were examined. Here I concentrate on some of Regan's specific comments. He noted quite correctly that in many cases of scientific research the interests of animals were not counted at all, or were counted less than the comparable interests of human beings (1980). This fact provided him reason to think that animals are being treated immorally, that such treatment must be stopped, and "grotesque 'scientific research'" should not be allowed.

With regard to toxicity testing of drugs, he suggested it might be preferable to allow human moral agents to take new drugs, provided they voluntarily chose to do so, rather than violate the rights of animals (1983). Human volunteers could choose to run risks, but animals (and all moral patients) lack the capacity to make such choices. If animals have inherent value, new drugs should not be tested on them in respect of this inherent value. If human volunteers who give informed consent are to be subjects for toxicity testing, he worried that this informed consent may not be truly free. Thus using volunteers should not be encouraged, because it could lead to deceptive or coercive means to obtain consent; in addition, the poor and uneducated might volunteer, especially if remuneration was involved, thereby exploiting the least powerful members of society.

Rollin (1992) also entertained the idea of replacing animals as research subjects by human volunteers. He thought it more defensible morally to test a drug that could possibly check a raging epidemic on child murderers awaiting execution, because their right to life has already been preempted by society; prisoners who wish to serve as volunteers in experiments in a desire to atone should be allowed to do so.

The British working party (Smith & Boyd, 1991) noted increasing numbers of epidemiological studies in biomedicine that proceed after obtaining informed consent of volunteers. Healthy human volunteers are also allowed to take part in testing pharmaceuticals, diagnostic procedures, and cosmetics, and in certain physiological studies without prior animal tests. Human participation is increasing, even though the UK has no special legislation regulating human subjects in research. It seems apparent that replacing animal research by human volunteers is possible, but that, too, raises serious moral problems.

Regan contended that alternative methods be developed to test toxicity, methods that do not harm moral agents or patients. Not many scientists would disagree regarding the desirability of alternative testing procedures, and several that have been developed and replaced heretofore standard procedures are discussed in chapter 10. However, given the fact that effects of compounds often are different in the test tube (in vitro) than in living organisms (in vivo), it probably will be necessary to continue testing with living organisms before new agents can be considered safe or effective as medical treatment. Questions have been raised regarding the permissibility of doing in vivo tests in animals after a compound has been found to be safe and efficacious by in vitro tests before prescribing it for humans. We can accept Regan's notions regarding the undesirability of permitting tests to establish whether cosmetic products are toxic, especially if those products duplicate existing ones, but reservations remain regarding the extension of his views if an agent is urgently needed to treat human sickness. Here, our old friend cost-benefit analysis of relative value resurfaces.

The rights view leads to insistence that the move be from the in vitro procedure directly to humans who suffer from whatever malady the treatment is intended to ameliorate. Regan considered animals as sub-jects-of-a-life and not reducible to their utility for human interests, even important ones. Because animals are unable to make choices, human agents should not make choices for them, which led him to conclude that animal testing is never permissible.

Regan acknowledged that one might accept views against toxicity tests using animals, but drew a line when it came to basic scientific research: It is not permissible to harm a single rat, even though the aggregated human benefits would be great. He based this position on the rights argument that the rat should not be considered to have value as a receptacle; doing so accepts the impermissible utilitarianism. He (1983, p. 384) also spoke of ". . . the by-now well-established difficulty of extrapolating results from animal tests to the species *Homo sapiens*." He maintains that much research is known to be a waste of time before it is undertaken, and wanted to sidestep the process of challenging specific ways animals are used in research to directly challenge the general prac-tice. He made this challenge referring to the principle of equal inherent worth, considering it impermissible for scientists first to look conscien-tiously for nonanimal research alternatives, and resort to the use of animals if no alternatives are found. His position is based on the belief that such an approach does not go far enough: Animals should never be used.

Regan upheld his case by describing a lifeboat dilemma in which the boat contained four normal adults and a dog. The contradictions in-volved in his resolution of such dilemmas were discussed in chapter 7, and that discussion should be consulted for details. He considers permis-sible to throw the dog over or eat it in order to save the four humans; permissible to drown the dog or cut it up and eat it in order to save humans; but not to use the dog to test a drug or cure a disease. I find an arbitrary inconsistency in his decisions regarding a number of the dilem-mas he described, and no consistent adherence to a set of formal princi-ples. Regan engaged in elaborate maneuvers to avoid any type of consequentialist reasoning, and these maneuvers did not take him suc-cessfully through the utilitarian minefield.

He believed that using the many benefits that flow from medical science is not wrong, provided the knowledge was obtained through treating a sick animal (or human) to improve the treatment of other animals (or humans). This position is not coherent: Earlier he stated that difficulties in extrapolating results from animal tests to humans are insurmountable, whereas now it seems possible to make such extrapolations if the data were obtained without intentionally harming laboratory animals. The strength of his case depends on the intentionality involved; how the means were gained, without considering benefits, or even the procedures.

Regan (p. 387) wanted to deflect "the tired charge of being anti scientific" by stating that the rights view is not against research if it does not harm animals, or put them at risk of any harm that would diminish their welfare opportunities. He expressed doubt that a benign use of animals in research is possible, or if possible, whether scientists could be persuaded to perform such procedures, concluding that research should not make use of any moral agent or patient. I believe scientists would prefer alternatives to whole animals whenever possible and still answer vital research questions. Stephens (1989, p. 164) quoted a National Academy of Sciences (NAS) report that supported alternatives using invertebrates, lower vertebrates, microorganisms, cell and tissue culture systems, and mathematical approaches. The NAS is a highly respected body, its members are elected, and it has been considered a think tank of the United States government. The report expressed concern that alternative methods were not being funded at an adequate level, while traditional mammalian animal models were over funded. This hardly reflects an intransigent defense of the status quo, at least by this most respected group of scientists.

Regan (p. 358) regarded those who believe it is unlikely that alternatives will be found to in vivo research to be ". . . unscientific at the deepest level," concluding that scientists should redirect "the traditional practices of their several disciplines away from reliance on 'animal models' toward the development and use of nonanimal alternatives." Although it is logically possible that in vitro alternatives to many in vivo procedures can be developed, few exist at present, and it would be necessary to forego progress in biomedical understanding and treatment for a number of years while alternatives are sought.

It would be especially difficult to progress if, as Regan suggests, no experimental research is done using either human or nonhuman animals.

I consider his rights view to be inconsistent to the point of incoherence, that some of his statements regarding factual matters are not correct, and that acceptance of his views would bring the progress of biomedical science to a screeching halt (suggestions I flesh out in chapter 10). It is fair to conclude that Regan's views would lead to the abolition of all animal research, and that such abolition is his goal. I believe the charge made against him by SUPRESS and Francione are not fair. His goals are similar to theirs, but his rhetoric employed reason rather than emotional appeal, and he attempted to develop a consistent philosophical grounding rather than inflame passions. Rollin (1992, p. 12) expressed it well: "In a democracy, . . . incremental change should surely proceed by rational dialogue and consensus, not through hysteria, bullying, and crisis management."

Animal Liberation

Singer's position is not strictly abolitionist because his utilitarianism permits cost-benefit analyses. When benefits are great enough, he considers it permissible to conduct research on animals, and even on retarded humans. Part of what makes it wrong to kill normal human beings is interference with a life plan, and we should question the practice of making nonhuman animals lead miserable lives so they can be eaten at less cost than if allowed to live relatively happy lives (1987). The problem remains to determine how a rational calculus of moral value can be established that will apply to humans and nonhumans, be they plant or animal. Once such a system is determined, how can one apply it universally? I contend that an ethics based on evolutionary principles might provide an adequate beginning to support such a calculus.

Singer (1975, p. 78) believes it would be permissible to conduct research, "If it really were possible to save many lives by an experiment that would take just one life, and there were *no other way* those lives could be saved." In the revised edition of *Practical ethics* (1993, p. 67), he approves such research ". . . if one, or even a dozen animals, had to suffer experiments in order to save thousands." In the revised edition of *Animal liberation* he concludes there can be no absolute answer to the question of whether an experiment is justified. Instead, utilitarian calculation of costs and benefits should be done (1990). Singer believes an animal experiment should not be done unless it would be justifiable to use a brain-damaged human for that experiment. In *Practical ethics* (1993), he asks whether it would be permissible to perform experiments on orphaned humans (orphans, to avoid important complications of the feelings of human parents whose wishes must be respected) who had severe and irreversible brain damage. Such humans would be less intelligent, less aware of what is happening to them, and perhaps less sensitive to pain than normal animals of many other species. To avoid speciesism, he holds that researchers should prefer to experiment on these humans. I do not disagree with his analysis, suggesting it would be permissible, and perhaps preferable, to perform crucial experiments using those humans in the interest of enhancing generalizability of results, because they would be made from human to human.

He believes that torturing a human being is almost always wrong, but not absolutely: If torture was the only way to discover the location of a nuclear bomb that would destroy New York City, it would be justifiable; if a single experiment would cure a disease such as leukemia, that experiment would be justifiable. He doubts such benefits would be possible in actual life, and questions how we should decide when an experiment is justifiable. I believe he should also consider who the "we" are that should be empowered to make these decisions.

"Among the tens of millions of experiments performed, only a few can possibly be regarded as contributing to important medical research" (Singer, 1990a, p. 40). One can only wonder how he obtained such an astronomical figure of the number of experiments—perhaps the same source Francione (1996, pp. 7–8) used to estimate that "Hundreds of millions of animals are used in experiments in which they are burned, scalded, blinded, and otherwise mutilated." Singer follows his statement with a discussion of a series of animal experiments he considers to have been useless, most of them behavioral research. He asserts that experiments serving no direct and urgent purpose should stop immediately, and those that are allowed to continue should, whenever possible, seek to replace animal experiments with alternative procedures. Once again, the question of who is to judge that an experiment does or does not serve an important interest remains, and an even more critical question is whether there is any place for experimentation intended to provide a more complete understanding of organic functions—be they physiological or behavioral—that are of interest because their only aim is to advance basic theory.

Some of his specific objections are relatively trivial ones regarding terminology, such as the word "extinction." He finds the word objectionable because it enables the indoctrination of the "normal, non-sadistic young psychology student" (presumably by sadistic professors) to proceed without anxiety being aroused (1990a, p. 51). Such terms are often used because they are a shorthand that supports scientific communication, provided they are defined by operations producing the presumed states; they are useful because they allow us to avoid the surplus meaning of common language usage. He finds the term "avoidance" to be acceptable because it is an observable activity, yet in other contexts he freely uses words to denote unobservables such as desire, preference, and fear when he wants to uphold his case.

He cites a number of examples to support the conclusion (1990a, p. 51): ". . . the logical consequences of this view of 'scientific method' is that experiments on animals cannot teach us anything about human beings." He correctly insists on caution when making generalizations based on results obtained with a sample to characterize the nature of a general population. Generalizations must be drawn with great care and subjected to independent cross-validation. The claim that animals can teach us nothing about human beings is clearly false if the basic evolutionary principle regarding the continuity of species is accepted. A couple of pages after the preceding statement, he notes that either an animal is not like us, in which case there is no reason to perform an experiment, or else it is like us, in which case we ought not to perform any experiment that would be "outrageous" if performed on one of us. This statement, similar to that made by Fox, embodies the excluded middle—you are either like us or not—that beggars the reality of the complexities of both evolutionary continuities and discontinuities that characterize all physiological and behavioral processes. Some mechanisms and processes have been conserved throughout the course of animal phylogeny, and others represent true phyletic discontinuities.

According to Martin Daly (personal communication, 1997), it must be morally impermissible to use squid giant axons to study neural mechanisms because they contain the same type of sodium pumps as humans have; and it is useless to experiment with devices such as crash-test dummies because they are too dissimilar to humans to tell us any-thing—or are they too similar, in which case it would be immoral to use them.

Singer presents a bleak view of the moral character, honesty, sincerity, and intentions of members of the scientific community. In addition to indoctrinating nonsadistic students, he finds them guilty of indoctrinating students gradually, beginning with the dissection of frogs in school biol-ogy courses (1990a, p. 70). Many proponents of animal liberation char-acterized the training of students to become biological or psychological researchers to be a process of dehumanization, whereby their initial humane and kindly characteristics are systematically overcome and re-placed by the view that animals are preparations to be applied to further research endeavors.

An often-quoted "experience of an American psychology graduate student conducting experiments on rats" was recounted by Rollin in the 1981 edition of *Animal rights and human morality* (he did not include it in the 1989 revision). The anecdote runs that an instructor dispatched a rat by dashing its head on the side of the workbench, breaking its neck. When the student expressed horror, the professor "fixed him in a cold gaze" and said, "What's the matter Smith, are you soft? Maybe you're not cut out to be a psychologist!" (included in Langley, 1989, p. 198; Rowan, 1984, p. 95; Luke, 1996). Langley commented that this anecdote is an illustration of how "Natural sensitivity and respect for other animals in young biologists are all too often scorned and caricatured as squeam-ishness by senior researchers" (p.198). Luke quoted it (p. 98) to show that men who would be scientists must establish hard callousness, and women who would be scientists must be like men. Such a catchy anecdote drives home the point, but it hardly qualifies as an argument unless a serious defense can be made that it happened at all, and that it is typical of psychologists, or it was just an action by a deranged individual who happened to be a psychologist.

Ryder (1989, p. 254) likened the training of students to ordeals that primitive tribesmen undergo at puberty to emerge as "men": ". . . the student scientist conquers his or her initial revulsion at seeing animals cold-bloodedly taken apart and graduates as part of an 'elite' . . . in as much as science competes with religion as a source of power and meaning, its qualified exponents take on, whether they like it or not (and many like it) some of the social connotations previously reserved for the priesthood."

Sperling (1988) commented that videotapes have been circulated by animal activists to illustrate the horrors of research, and they often picture researchers as callous abusers making fun of injured animal subjects. She suggested that such jokes and callousness at times might not reflect unfeeling cruelty, but a way to deal with the anxiety aroused by severe procedures. As she noted, this kind of black humor is familiar to anyone who has worked in medical settings that involve the manipulation of the human body, or as I experienced in medical school anatomy classes when human cadavers were dissected for the first time. There is no evidence that animal researchers keep pets less often than others in their community, or that they are cruel to those they have. There is no evidence that those who engage in biomedical or psychological research with animals are doomed to slide down the slippery slope to sadism, child abuse, and genocide any more than those in the nonresearch community. One irony in this tack often taken by animal liberationists was mentioned by Rowan (1984); the leaders of Nazi Germany came very close to banning all animal research, and before the war animal welfare groups lauded these. It is just as (un)reasonable to reverse the game by claiming it is inevitable that banning animal research will lead us to slide down the slope to fascism and genocide.

In his zeal, Singer makes strange value judgments throughout the chapter entitled "Tools for Research" (1990a): "The philosophers and historians who publish to improve their career prospects do little harm beyond wasting paper and boring their colleagues" (p. 74). I would ask what of the influence some philosophers had on excuses dictatorial totalitarians trotted out to justify their horrendous actions? The pen is as influential as the scalpel. In another place (p. 41) Singer observes that the situation in the United States is much worse than it appears, because it has been estimated that in Britain only about one-fourth of experiments find their way into print; thus probably an even lower proportion are printed in the United States, given the higher proportion of minor colleges with researchers of lesser talents in the United States than in Britain. This kind of statement was deplored by Russell and Nicoll (1996) who accused Singer of demonizing American scientists.

Singer accused scientists of conducting trivial, obvious, or meaningless experiments that offer no prospect of yielding vital new knowledge (1990a p. 50); of doing mindless animal testing (p. 57); of rejecting new methods not making use of animals in order to obtain publications, promotions, awards, and grants through the use of accepted modes of research (p. 72); of being bogged down in petty and insignificant details because the big questions have been studied already and solved, or have proved too difficult (p. 73) (shades of Ecclesiastes—there is nothing new under the sun); and of being philosophical ignoramuses (p. 76), who can do exactly as they please in their research (p. 76), who do not attempt to assess the necessity to justify inflicting pain (p. 76), who inflict pain for trivial purposes (p. 77), and who do animal studies that often hinder the advance of understanding of diseases in humans and their cure (p. 89); and that knowledge gained from animal experimentation has made at best a very small contribution to our increased lifespan (p. 91). Altogether, enough of an indictment that, if sustained would justify incarceration or deportation of the entire bunch of immoral folks—or at least a public flogging.

Certainly we have much to be concerned about regarding standards that often prevailed in the care of laboratory animals, and Singer deserves credit for having brought these matters to the fore. Considerable attention has been paid by those in the scientific community to issues concerning the welfare of laboratory animals, and considerable discussion and research have been published regarding how to determine the physical and psychological well-being of laboratory and zoo animals (see Dawkins, 1990).

Singer's estimates concerning the value of animal research are unduly negative and pessimistic, and not altogether fair. Given the large number of published studies on research in animals it is a simple matter to search that literature and pick examples of what seem to be useless, inadequate, and questionable studies that caused animal suffering. Much of this picking and choosing is focused on procedures, whereas emphasis should be on the quality of theoretical questions and the adequacy of procedures to address those questions. One can just as easily comb through the literature and select ground-breaking research programs that alleviated suffering of humans and animals, benefited most people living today, and produced a better quality of life for all on the planet, yet all of which involved various degrees of animal suffering. This list could then be presented as justification to allow scientists to do whatever they wish, given their immense contributions. Box scores do little to shed light on either the underlying moral issues or the good and bad practices of animal research.

The practice by both pro- and antiresearch groups to scan the literature to find papers that can be held up as good or bad exemplars is unfortunate, because the intent—and the outcome—of these exercises usually is to confront rather than lead to productive debate (Morton, 1989). One could just as well comb the philosophical literature and find that dictators and demagogues used these writing to justify their despotic practices, and on that basis, propose that all philosophy be banned.

Research with animals (and humans, for that matter) is sometimes done badly (how many mistakes are permissible before we condemn the entire scientific enterprise?) or seems not to have any direct application. These facts, however, do not provide sufficient reason to stop all research, or to characterize those performing biological and psychological research as having inadequate moral and scientific standards and values. The scientific community tended to be aloof and arrogant for much too long, but it instituted sweeping changes by establishing animal care standards (under considerable political pressure) and created mechanisms to provide adequate institutional oversight. Funding agencies and journal editors instruct peer reviewers to ensure, as far as possible, that animals are treated according to established standards. A number of scientists have undertaken the difficult task of trying to understand the motivation and fitness of animals, and to characterize those things essential to the welfare of animals both in natural and confined circumstances (e.g., Dawkins, 1990). The issues are complex, and it is as difficult to define and understand well-being in animals as it is to understand the quality of their consciousness. I agree with Frey (1990, p. 22): "To tell scientific and medical researchers that animal suffering is ethically significant and that it must be taken into accout is, I think, preaching to the converted." Even though one will always find a few bad apples in the scientific barrel, as Singer (1990a) agreed, Frey's statement is reasonable.

Singer was able to list only a few of the tens of thousands of experiments performed annually in the field of psychology (and where did that figure come from? The land of hyperbole, I would guess). He believes these experiments have ". . . no prospect of yielding really momentous or vital new knowledge" (1975, p. 44), and that much research labeled "medical research" is motivated by a "general goalless curiosity" that turns out to have been "quite pointless" (see pp. 51–52). He went so far as to write (p. 81): "Those who are genuinely concerned about improving health and have medical qualifications would probably make a more effective contribution to human health if they left the laboratories and saw to it that our existing stock of medical knowledge reaches those who need it most." I believe the progress realized to apply the findings of genetics and new discoveries regarding basic cell function, with the goal being to understand and treat such things as cancer and AIDS, casts doubt on the wisdom of his suggestion

Singer moves back and forth between developing serious philosophical arguments to being an effective propagandist. The factual bases underlying many of his claims are weak and his arguments overdrawn. Many have not examined Singer's reasoning regarding speciesism and equality of animals, and rely on his assertions to deny the value of all animal research.

Regan (1983, p. 393) concluded: ". . . the harm done to animals in pursuit of scientific purposes is wrong," and the radical political wing extends the polemic to state that "vivisection" (which includes all research with animals) is scientific fraud: "Vivisectioners claim that they can learn about human diseases by experimenting on four-legged animals, and yet diseases kill more people every year . . . Help us kill vivisection before it kills you" (report on a Television commercial in the *LA Times*, 5/24/90). And there is always the lunatic fringe: "As I sit with my beautiful cat looking at me with trusting eyes, I recall revulsion at the unspeakable photo of the tortured cat. . . . I'd like to meet one of the individuals who inflicts such pain and stick electrodes in *his* skull" (letter to the *LA Times*, 5/27/90).

These statements suggest that the debate regarding the value and worth of animal research moves quickly from notions regarding proper moral values into the arena of propaganda and political action that borders on hysteria and terrorism. We should focus on Singer's (1975, p. 255) appeal to reason rather than respond to emotional calls to mount the barricades. He believes he has argued the case against speciesism and not merely asserted it, and that his rational views should prevail over those of his opponents. In chapter 8 I contested the claim that speciesism is based on blind prejudice, and concluded his theory does not have the intended force.

Beyond philosophy, many of the polemics reviewed above are to promote a political agenda. One has to hopscotch through *Animal liberation* to separate serious philosophical propositions from political nostrums, and often it is necessary to examine Singer's other writings to understand their philosophical bases. If he is unable to sustain the charge that speciesism is philosophically incorrect and impermissible, his ideas lack force, and the central question concerns the relative values that should be used to make cost-benefit analyses.

The Research Community

From the Bunker
Early interactions between animal researchers and animal activists were documented by Dewsbury (1990). Physiologists and psychologists have been under attack by antivivisectionists since the Victorian era. The London Society for the Prevention of Cruelty to Animals was founded in 1824, and at Queen Victoria's command became the RSPCA in 1840. The first significant act to provide protection for all vertebrate animals was the Cruelty to Animals Act of 1876, which required licensing experimenters, provided for inspection of research facilities, and limited the use of animals in teaching. Because it did not abolish all vivisection, the antis were not satisfied. The British scientific community began to admit that a new law was needed to replace the 1876 act only when it became obvious in the 1970s that lobbying by animal welfare advocates made it likely that new legislation was bound to be drafted, whether scientists liked it or not (Langley, 1989).

Charges have gone back and forth between researchers, who claim that animal research is justified because of its importance to secure medical advances, and to accumulate new knowledge, and antivivisectionists, who challenge all vivisection for any purpose and insist on its abolition (Dewsbury, 1990). In the United States several states passed laws in the first half of the nineteenth century forbidding cruelty to animals. The American Society for the Prevention of Cruelty to Animals (ASPCA) was founded in 1867. Finally, the medical community took the threat to research seriously, and the American Medical Association (AMA) formed the Council on the Defense of Medical Research in 1908. Criticisms by antivivisectionists led the American Psychological Association (APA) to form a committee on animal experimentation in 1925, which has become the present Committee on Animal Research and Ethics.

Charles Darwin, with his usual scientific insight, did not defend animal research on the basis of its immediate applicability, but held that experiments must be done even if no immediate good can be predicted (Dewsbury, 1990). He justified this view by appealing to the history of science to support the belief that physiology cannot possibly progress except through experiments on living animals. He appealed to the importance of building a strong basic understanding of the organismic world, as such enhanced understanding will support future applications—a defense of the power of deductive methods in science.

Eminent Harvard psychologist and philosopher William James maintained that it was more important to pursue basic science than to attempt to produce immediate benefits to human health. Dewey went even further, proposing that scientists are under definite obligation to experiment on animals to save human life and to increase human vigor and efficiency, and that such research is preferable to subjecting humans to possible harmful experimentation (Dewsbury, 1990). Pavlov, whose research is still criticized by antivivisectionists, justified his classical conditioning research by arguing there is no other way to become acquainted with laws of the organismic world except by experiments and observations on living animals.

Rowan (1984) concluded that biomedical researchers do not help their cause by arrogantly insisting on their right to study whatever they wish in whatever manner they deem appropriate. He characterized this insistence as a plea for academic license, not academic freedom. Researchers tended to ignore, as much as possible complaints regarding practices that use animals, and urged that standards of animal care be left to individual discretion, until they were forced to take a responsible position by the public, politicians, and institutional administrators.

The initial tendency of the scientific community was to defend established positions and fight against any concessions (Orlans, 1993). Scientists provided encouragement for further pressures that would lead to further retreats, rather than seriously and objectively examining the issues to arrive at reasonable accommodations. The first line of defense against any suggested reforms was to obscure the issues and to portray reforms as an attack on biomedical research, if not on science in general.

Many animal advocates complained that research animals should not be obtained from pounds. With the rapid growth in funds for biomedical research in the 1950s and 1960s, the demand for research animals increased. Scientists focused on the euthanasia of millions of unwanted dogs and cats in the nation's pounds and shelters each year. They made no real attempt to negotiate with the humane movement (Rowan & Rollin, 1983). Instead, they imposed their will through political actions, which led to increased hostility, conflict, and mobilization of an effective political counter-offensive.

When the clash of examples cited by the two sides became intense, scientists could no longer succeed through appeals to their unquestionable judgment and superior wisdom. They finally organized to exert political pressure to influence public opinion in favor of research. Much of this political posturing was characterized by Orlans as stonewalling, automatically denying all charges, insisting everything is perfect, and attempting to block all access to information until compelled to produce it.

An even more subtle strategy was used to avoid painful discussions of animal ethics. Arluke (1992) described his experience when invited to speak at a conference of animal researchers. He called the talk, "The Experimenter's Guilt," but was told that was too controversial and "Stress Among Researchers" would be more palatable. A popular journal invited him to publish the talk, but insisted that the term "stress" was too extreme and inaccurate, preferring "uneasiness," which he used. When asked to speak on this subject at a research center of a major pharmaceutical company he was told he could not use "uneasiness" in the title because it would inflame research directors. They suggested "How Researchers Deal with Their Feelings." His cynical conclusion was that he has decided simply to call future talks "Untitled."

The battles have continued for decades, but have intensified in recent years, perhaps because both sides learned to use the media with greater effectiveness. The antivivisection movement presents vivid portrayals of animal abuse, raises huge sums of money, and is able to distribute materials rapidly to influence opinion. The research establishment, which depends heavily on public funding to support its studies, has begun to respond in kind with its own media blitz featuring such things as pictures of children in leg braces who were crippled by polio, and AIDS victims pleading for increased research support to find a way to save their lives. Universities and medical schools, at which much of the research is done, are subjected to public and political pressures that influence all of their funding, and their response often is intended to minimize controversy rather than to develop any consistent moral position.

The animal liberation movement has gained momentum in recent years. The leading animal liberation group, PETA, grew from 18 members in 1981 to over 250,000 in 1990, claiming a membership of 350,000 in 1991, with assets approaching $10 million (Baldwin, 1993). In that same period the Humane Society of the United States (HSUS) increased its membership ten-fold to about one million (Orlans, 1993). The combined membership in 1982 of three of the large national groups with animal rights platforms, Friends of Animals, the HSUS, and the Fund for Animals, was 446,000 (Sperling, 1988). The annual operating budget of the major animal welfare groups was estimated to be about $50 million, and they are staffed by hundreds of zealous personnel assisted by large numbers of volunteers (Nicoll & Russell, 1990).

The attitude of many scientists was characterized as a siege mentality, leading them to behave in ways that can be characterized using the metaphors of barricades, behind which they retreat to the security of their labs, and parapets, above which they do not want to expose their heads for fear of reprisals (Birke & Michael, 1992). Some of these fears are quite real, given the threats, destruction, and injuries that the ALF has promised, and delivered in many instances. The ALF took responsibility for breaking into a USDA-licensed California facility that supplies laboratory rodents. Their press release demanded life and liberty for all species, and they promised to continue the struggle for a compassionate and nonviolent society until the last laboratory is razed. They justified this contradiction on the grounds that they consider the laws protecting the right to torture, maim, burn, and electrocute animals should be overridden to adhere to laws of morality and nature.

Actions of the ALF have been very costly to the research enterprise (Orlans, 1993). The Association of American Medical Colleges estimated the costs to have been $3.5 million and 15,000 staff hours between 1985 and 1990, and that the installation and maintenance of security systems to protect research facilities cost another $5.5 million over that period. Tactics of destruction, intimidation, and violence undermined the early effectiveness the raids had in winning public sympathy for the animal rights crusade, and Orlans expressed the hope that raids have run their course, having served the purpose of generating publicity.

Research Animals

Numbers, Species, and Purpose

In many discussions, the numbers and kinds of animals as well as the intended purpose of studies often are cited. However, the discussions sometimes are not comprehensible, because the tendency is to conflate studies used to screen drugs and cosmetics or to investigate toxic effects of new compounds with those that serve basic and applied biomedical and scientific purposes. The number of animals used in basic biomedical research is quite small relative to those used for pharmaceutical and cosmetic research and testing. Rollin (1992) suggested that six distinct activities should be distinguished, and that (p. 137) "It is thus quite important to be clear about which activities one is referring to when discussing 'research on animals' since arguments relevant to one area will clearly not fit one or more of the others." The six activities he listed were basic biological research, applied basic biomedical research, development of drugs, therapeutic chemicals, and biologicals; testing of various consumer goods for safety, toxicity, irritation, and degree of toxicity; use in educational institutions; and use of animals for the extraction of products.

Orlans (1993) presented official data for The Netherlands in 1987. This report indicated that 42% of all experiments qualified as fundamental research, 47% was for vaccine or drug production and testing, 6% for toxicity testing, 4% for education and training, and 1% for other purposes. She examined the best estimates regarding laboratory animals in the United States and reported that 40% were used for biomedical research, 26% for drug testing, 20% for product safety testing, 7% for teaching, and 7% for other purposes.

Various estimates were provided by those with different agendas, but few seem reasonable. The UK working party (Smith & Boyd, 1991) cited Home Office statistics regarding the number of scientific procedures carried out, not the number of animals used. This statistic leads to overestimation of numbers because several procedures are sometimes performed in one animal, especially in toxicity testing. In 1989 the Home Office recorded 3,315,125 procedures carried out under the authority of 3,276 project licenses, with 70% of the licenses at universities and polytechnics, 13% at research institutes, and 12% at commercial organizations. When percentages of procedures are examined, the picture is quite different: 61% were at commercial organizations, 23% at universities, and 10% at research institutes. Eighty-four percent of animals used were rodents—53% mice and 27% rats. Birds accounted for 8%, reptiles and amphibians for 0.3%, and mammals other than rodents for 5%. This last category consisted of rabbits 65% of the time, with sheep, dogs, pigs, cattle, nonhuman primates, cats, ferrets, horses, donkeys, and mules being used less than 2% of the time. Seventy-nine percent of all procedures had an applied purpose, mainly to develop and test medicines and veterinary products.

According to the working party, in Britain the number of animals used decreased from about 5.5 million in 1976 to about 3.3 million in 1989. They speculated that the decrease was due to the greater prominence of microbiology in biomedical research and the general use of in vitro systems, particularly, the pharmaceutical industry's increased reliance on in vitro procedures and computer models. The increased costs of buying and maintaining animals also was a factor, as were increased sensitivity and caution on the part of researchers faced by attacks of antivivisection groups.

Rollin (1992) estimated that 200 to 225 million animals were used for research annually throughout the world, although Ryder (1989) presented

lower worldwide estimates of between 50 and 150 million. Rollin estimated the United States accounted for about 100 million of these: 50
million mice, 20 million rats, and 30 million others, which included
200,000 cats and 450,000 dogs. The USDA reported that, in 1994, only
32,610 cats and 101,090 dogs were used in research. Orlans (1993) cited
estimates that 25 to 30 million vertebrate animals are used each year in the
United States, and official sources place that figure at around 25 to 30
million, more than 80% of which are rats, mice, and birds (Hampson,
1989). Nicoll and Russell (1990) presented figures regarding the number
of animals consumed in the United States in 1988: 96.5% of animals were
eaten for food (only birds and mammals, not including many millions of
fish), 2.6% by hunting, 0.4% killed in pounds, 0.3% for research and
teaching, and 0.2% for fur garments.

Figures for Britain indicate a decline in the number of procedures that
involve pain from 5.2 million in 1978 to 3.2 million in 1990 (Orlans,
1993). Control of animal pain during experimentation significantly increased during that period. A report by the Tufts University Center for
Animals and Public Policy estimated the number of animals used in
research in the United States had declined more than 50% since 1968
(Hilts, 1994). About 50 million or more animals were used each year
before 1970, and only 20 million in 1992. The same drastic drop was
reported by countries in Europe that keep accurate figures. The United
States Department of Defense reported that their animal use (which
included rats and mice) dropped from 412,000 in 1983 to 267,000 in
1991. Through the 1980's, animal use at the pharmaceutical company
Hoffman-LaRoche Inc. dropped from 1 million a year to 300,000. The
National Cancer Institute reduced its annual use of animals by 95%,
from 6 million to 30,000, through extensive development of in vitro
screening procedures (Orlans, 1993).

Hodos (1983) surveyed the types of animals used in neuroscience
research by tabulating species used in 1971 and 1981. He published his
findings in the journal *Brain Research*, which publishes a broad spectrum
of neurophysiological research and can be considered a good indicator of
trends in the field. In 1971 cats were ranked no. 1 (42% of articles), no.
2 was rodents (22%), and no. 3, monkeys (10%), with tissue cultures
(0%) ranked 11. In 1981, rodents were no. 1 (59%), tissue cultures no. 2

(9.3%), invertebrates no. 3 (7.3%), with cats having dropped to a three-way tie for no. 5 (5.6%) with monkeys and rabbits. Although these estimates vary considerably, they all support the conclusion that relatively few animals are used for basic research, and most of them are rats and mice. The numbers used in all research procedures has been steadily declining in recent years due to increased performance of in vitro methods and tighter controls at national and institutional levels.

The number of animals used in research is small compared with those involved in agriculture. Singer (1990a) estimated that over 100 million cows, pigs, and sheep and 5 billion poultry are raised and slaughtered each year in the United States. In Britain, estimates are that 1 billion animals, excluding poultry, are slaughtered each year for their meat: about 100,000 per day (Ryder, 1989). Ryder's personal estimate was that, in 1986, 400 million chickens were reared in Britain, 480 million in France, 170 million in Germany, 280 million in Italy, 230 million in The Netherlands, and about 2 billion in the United States. In addition, over 12 million pigs were slaughtered annually in Britain.

Regardless of the differences in these estimates, they point to the fact that immense numbers of animals are involved, and the numbers support the idea that the greatest harm to animals occurs in agriculture, an area that has very few regulations of the kinds that exist for research laboratories. These figures make it difficult to accept the claim made by Rollin (1992) that the greatest potential for the diminution of animal suffering can be found in the realm of animal experimentation. I suspect his interest is to press the case against animal experimentation to make it more dramatic, reflecting his belief that we are not likely to stop using animals for food.

The battle lines were described, the positions of the disputants illustrated, and some of the claims by both sides discussed. I also presented data regarding the number and species of animals used to gain an understanding of the magnitude of the problem regarding animals in research. In the next chapter specific claims made by the disputants are examined in the light of evidence that can be brought to bear. In chapter 11 I discuss the use of animals in basic research, especially psychological research, and consider issues regarding the use of animals in education. I suggest what I consider the most acceptable philosophical position and examine it in the light of the issues.

10

Research Is . . .

In this chapter I examine arguments made against animal research: claims that animal research does more harm to humans than it does good, that alternatives to animal research are available and should be used, and that safeguards to protect animal welfare are not adequate to the task. Different categories of animal research are discussed and regulations to provide oversight of animal research described. In the next chapter attention is directed to issues of scientific philosophy as they affect the choice of research methods. These issues are relevant when considering denunciations of animal research that have no immediate applied aim. Questions regarding the permissibility, uses, and abuses of psychological research with animals has received especially harsh condemnation, and they are examined.

The purpose of such discussions should be to recommend policies regarding the permissible use of animals, and to improve the lot of animals without impeding scientific progress. Strong positions are taken regarding some issues to stimulate constructive open debate, but not in the spirit that they define the only appropriate moral view.

Value of Research

Opinions regarding the value of science range from the belief that science is the only way to achieve true knowledge, to arguments that science is a dehumanizing trivialization of the human condition. Most of us land somewhere between those poles, believing that science moves steadily toward an increasingly accurate picture of an underlying reality, while appreciating the strong residue of conjecture in all scientific endeavor.

This middle position is based on the importance of recognizing the contexts of discovery and of justification discussed in chapter 4.

When people debate the permissibility of conducting research with animals, they often apply three general types of criticisms. One is the ad hominem argument (personal attacks on an opponent to support the conclusion he or she is wrong) in which the character, honesty, and intentions of scientists who participate in such research is impugned. This strategy has been applied by philosophers such as Regan, Singer, and Rollin, and is widely adopted by animal welfare activists such as Fox. On the other side many in the scientific community characterize animal liberationists as radical discontents, sentimental animal lovers, and anti-intellectuals who are cruel in their willingness to deny the benefits of medical discoveries to suffering people. Several ad hominem statements were identified and discussed in preceding chapters, and as with many like them, they are raised less to contribute to a debate than to pursue a quarrel.

Walton (1992) examined the nature of several kinds of emotional arguments and concluded that they should be admissible in critical discussions because they can have a positive influence by opening new and valuable approaches that permit critical questioning; in this way they can steer discussions in a constructive direction. They often have the negative effect, however, of leading too quickly to conclusions that favor particular biases. He distinguished between a quarrel and a debate: A quarrel he characterized as a personal exchange between two sides, whereas a debate is an exchange between two sides with the goal being to win over or persuade a third party. The ad hominem approach makes it too easy for both sides to settle into defensive positions for the purpose of quarreling, without openness to the possibility that the point of view of the other side may be reasonable. Instead, the motivation of those on the other side is challenged, and that only incites more intemperate quarreling.

Walton believes ad hominem arguments can be useful when directed to influence a third-party audience to defeat arguments of opponents. The intent is to demonstrate that participants on the other side have bad characters, are dishonest, or are unreliable, all of which legitimately would disqualify them as credible participants in collaborative dialogue.

This approach can shift the weight of evidence toward one's own side, and lead to reasonable questions that must be answered by opponents, provided the questions are relevant to the proceedings. However, this tactic is fallacious when the intent is to close down the sequence of legitimate dialogue that was to have occurred. Ad hominem allegations should be examined carefully to decide whether or not they have a germ of truth, and if so to establish the impact and extent of their truth. Without compelling evidence that they are correct and do have a bearing on the disputed points, they should be recognized to rest at the level of quarrel, rather than contributing to debate. At that level they can inflame people to mount the barricades and overthrow evil opposition, but they can be dangerous impediments to reasoned debate.

A second type of criticism by opponents of research concerns the nature of science. It is often effective because the general public and policy makers have inadequate knowledge regarding problems in evaluating scientific progress, and are oblivious to the essential nature of scientific method. Some maintain that, because of an element of subjectivity in science with regard to what is chosen for study, how it is studied, and in what settings it is studied, science is no more objective than any other speculative human pursuit. Langley (1989) challenged the view that basic research is value free, dealing only in truths and hard facts; he preferred to emphasize the subjective matters and ethical choices involved in the pursuit of science. He cited, with approval, a statement made in 1978 by the president of the Royal Society, Lord Todd: ". . . there are questions which should not be asked and research which should not be undertaken" (p. 206). The danger is that it is always a serious concern as to who is to make decisions to prohibit certain lines of inquiry, who establishes what should be asked, and on what basis such decisions should be allowed.

The views of Feyerabend, a self-styled epistemological anarchist, were discussed in chapter 4, and they frequently are cited by those who characterize science as a political enterprise rather than as a source of objective knowledge. A strong subjective influence is present in all science, but the particular strength of science is provided by the development of public procedural steps to test the justifiability of alternative statements regarding reality. After assertions regarding such reality have been made, objective scientific methods can be brought to bear. Scientific method requires that all steps of logic involved are public and explicit, procedures used to make observations are specified and justified, results are presented and analyzed in an objective manner, and conclusions based on these steps are logical, clear, and (one hopes) compelling. The strength of this procedural style is that subjective choices are made clear to all, and the adequacy of the objective procedures can be evaluated by any qualified observer. The problem is that most objections to science are based on a (willful?) misunderstanding of scientific method, accompanied by failure to appreciate the complexities involved in establishing and evaluating scientific theories

The third type of criticism does not challenge the general credibility of scientists or of scientific method, but charges that certain lines of inquiry and experimentation are instances of bad science. In chapter 9 numerous statements were cited to the effect that animal research has contributed nothing to the progress of medical science, that it has impeded progress, and that it is bad science. Even a cursory examination of the facts give the lie to those assertions. I will not review the primary literature to discuss the progress of medical science, but rest content describing a few achievements that have been denied by opponents of animal research.

Categories of Research

When the subject of research is broached confusion often surrounds what is being discussed. It was noted in chapter 10 that Rollin (1992) suggested six activities that should be kept in mind. Among them were basic biology, applied basic biomedical research, and the development of drugs and extraction of products from animals. These three aspects are discussed now; toxicity testing is considered later.

Basic Biological and Biomedical Research

At the most fundamental level are research advances identifying the characteristics and locus of receptor sites for drugs. This knowledge made it possible to identify sites in the cell where certain classes of drugs produce their effects. An instance in which such knowledge has led to important advances is the study of conditions under which, and how, a number of neurotransmitters are released from nerve endings to permit transmission of nerve impulses to receptors on other cells. This understanding was produced using both animal tissue and intact preparations, and resulted in the development of drug therapies for disorders such as peptic ulcers, and neurological and mental diseases such as depression and schizophrenia. With detailed knowledge of the physiology of renal function and of water and electrolyte balance, the artificial kidney was developed, which would not have been possible without such basic knowledge. Kidney dialysis is necessary to keep patients alive who could benefit from transplantation of a new kidney, and it was estimated that about 30,000 people are currently in this category (Petrinovich, 1996).

Surgical techniques to implant organs successfully depend on advances in understanding immunology to cope with rejection of the transplanted organ by the patient's immune system. It is estimated that 35,000 people in the United States are on the national waiting list for organ transplants, and that as many as 32,000 to 73,000 per year are not even placed on the waiting list for hearts. An estimated 150,000 patients are receiving Medicare benefits for kidney transplantation. The overall one-year success rate in the United States is about 85% for kidney, heart, liver, and lung transplantation, and the five-year success rate is about 50%, figures that are comparable with those for other surgical and medical treatments (see Petrinovich, 1996, for a review of those statistics).

Organ transplantations have saved and enhanced the lives of large numbers of people for considerable periods of time. Most of the procedures were developed by applying methods discovered in laboratories where animals, especially mice and rats, were used extensively. The benefits to thousands of people are large; the costs in terms of the lives of thousands of animals also are large. It is at this point that a utilitarian cost-benefit analysis is appropriate. I believe the general public is willing to support such research and consider the cost in animal lives to be acceptable. I am sure the medical research and treatment communities contend that the benefits are worth the costs, and that antivivisectionists and many, if not most, animal liberationists disagree. In fact, Fox (1990, p. 78) claimed that, ". . . if the environment and our food, air, and water were cleaned up, along with our dietary habits, food-processing procedures, and agricultural practices, there would be little need for dramatic organ transplants or life-saving open heart operations." I am sure most people would consider it reasonable to sacrifice thousands of animals in the interest of saving the lives of their own children or immediate kin. Often what starts as a discussion of absolutes moves into a gray area, and absolute principles regarding permissible costs are overridden by concerns involving the welfare of the human community.

Cancer Research Other advances in basic biological science that have astounding implications involve increased understanding of processes of cellular proliferation and identification of genetic mechanisms regulating those processes. Much basic genetic research was done in fruit flies, mice, and rats, and the results (even with flies) were generalized to understand mechanisms involved in the development of human cancers. Human fetal tissue could be used to great advantage to develop therapeutic measures, because a human host readily accepts this tissue, but existing laws make it difficult, if not impossible, to perform these procedures.

One exciting finding is the identification of a gene, BRCA1, that could account for one-half of cases of familial breast cancer, which are about 10% of total cancer cases (see Petrinovich, 1996). This large complicated gene has been studied extensively, and drugs were developed that successfully treat cancer in rodents. Just eighteen months after the isolation of the gene, it was suggested it could be at fault in 90% of all breast cancers and also involved in ovarian cancer. Studies of the gene's function in mice demonstrated that it inhibits tumor development by slowing or stopping growth of tumor cells in vivo (Holt et al., 1996).

Because inhibition is specific to tumorous tissues it might be possible to develop a "magic bullet" that affects only cancerous cells, leaving healthy noncancerous ones unaffected. Tumorous mice injected with functioning copies of the gene survived, whereas those injected with mutant copies all died of huge malignancies. The mechanism by which BRCA1 functions is being investigated further (Jensen et al., 1996) with the hope of producing chemical agents that, administered orally or intravenously, could inhibit growth of breast cancers. This discovery represents a significant medical advance, because breast cancer is the most common form of cancer in women, affecting 182,000 women and 1,000 men in the United States each year, and killing about 46,000 women and

300 men each year (Maugh, 1995). It is estimated that one woman in nine will develop cancer sometime in her life, so it is possible that these developments can prevent suffering of a substantial number of humans.

Another gene, BRCA2, inhibits breast cancers in both women and men, as well as prostate and laryngeal cancer (Wooster et al., 1995). Its identification should allow more comprehensive evaluation of families at high risk of developing breast cancer, and make it easier to study the roles of environmental and lifestyle factors that modify risks in gene carriers.

The gene believed to cause the most common form of human cancer, basal cell carcinoma, as well as a rare inherited disorder that can result in multiple cancers, was found after years of basic research on fruit fly genetics (Johnson et al., 1996). An estimated 750,000 cases of basal cell carcinoma occur in the United States each year, and it is especially common on sun-exposed skin of middle-aged or older people of northern European ancestry. The gene was first isolated in fruit flies, later in mice, and then in humans. It is a tumor suppresser that is mutated by the sun, or transmitted in damaged form in the case of the rare inherited type.

All of these studies testify to the power of basic research that capitalizes on known genetic similarities in gene functioning in species ranging from fruit flies, to mice, rhesus monkeys, and humans. Because of these similarities, suggestive findings obtained with the rapidly reproducing fruit flies can be examined in mice, and those that seem promising in that rapidly reproducing mammalian species can be further pursued using nonhuman and human primates. This strategy is economical in terms of time and money, both to produce greater understanding of basic mechanisms and to develop biomedical applications of this understanding. Cross-species strategies permit detection of evolved mechanisms that are conserved across species, and make it possible to understand critical differences among species.

Consideration of such research studies indicates that basic biomedical research has been highly successful in advancing understanding and could lead to development of treatments to remedy physiological deficits. Understanding advances in basic science might be more productive than engaging in the ritual half-full, half-empty arguments regarding similarities and differences among animals of different species. Findings such as those discussed support informed positions regarding the relative costs to research animals and benefits to human cancer sufferers. I find the balance to be overwhelmingly in favor of the large number of humans, and suspect the general public, which provides the research funds, would as well. Animal welfare advocates should stop quarreling about animal models and concentrate their energies to demand improvements in animal care, development of alternative procedures where those are possible, and better training of research personnel in biotechnology and bioethics.

Applied Biomedical Research

Francione (1995, p. 171) expressed doubt regarding the value of animal research, suggesting that, because so many unsolved medical mysteries remain relative to the number of medical successes, ". . . there is strong evidence that animal experimentation has retarded medical progress, not facilitated it." Fox (1990) believed reduction in sickness and death from major infectious diseases was not accomplished through animal research, although he offered nothing beyond this assertion. One attitude characteristic of the antivivisectionists is that new technologies involved in modern medicine are antithetical to nature, with disease considered to be the result of dis-harmony with nature. Only by restoring the homeostatic balance with nature can health be achieved, and this is preferred to medical intervention of any kind.

The UK working party report (Smith & Boyd, 1991, p. 27) listed an extensive number of medical advances realized through animal research that would have been unlikely without using animals. These advances included research on aging (including Alzheimer's disease), AIDS, anesthesia, autoimmune diseases, basic genetics, neurosurgical procedures to treat behavior disorders, diseases and defects of the cardiovascular system, childhood diseases, cholera, convulsive disorders, diabetes, gastrointestinal tract surgery, hearing, hemophilia, hepatitis, infectious malaria, muscular dystrophy, nutrition, ophthalmology, organ transplantation, Parkinson's disease, treatment of pulmonary disease and injury, prevention of rabies, radiobiology, reproductive biology, surgery of the skeletal system, treatment of spinal cord injuries, toxoplasmosis, trauma and shock, yellow fever, and virology. Research in all these areas contributed to the alleviation of suffering and basically depended on animals.

Sulfa drugs were discovered by testing mice that had been inoculated with pathogenic bacteria, a research program that led the way, a few years later, to the development of penicillin. The diphtheria antitoxin was one of the first major therapeutic advances that owed its development largely to animal research, and it was produced and standardized using animals (Rowan, 1984). With this antitoxin the prospect of dying after contracting diphtheria was cut from 40% to 10%. Antiseptic surgical techniques were improved through animal research, and Rowan noted that without them, elective surgery would still be the exception rather than the rule, because mortality rates would so high they would make surgery a life-threatening rather than life-saving choice. Animal experimentation also played a critical role in the discovery and production of antibiotics.

As did the UK working party, Rowan cautioned that research projects should be reviewed carefully to evaluate the quality of procedures and likely benefits in terms of relieving suffering, and that those benefits should be balanced against costs in terms of animal suffering. Although such a balancing is possible, it is unlikely that pro- and antiresearch advocates will agree. However, disagreements could be based on an evaluation of research evidence, rather than wild charge and counter-charge.

The working party concluded that it is doubtful even the most radical champions of animal welfare would abandon all that has been learned from animal research when it is weighed against the amount of suffering that would result for human beings and other animals if such knowledge did not exist. They did not argue that current benefits provide a moral justification for a continued unquestioning use of animals in biomedical research. Realized benefits are great enough to justify costs, but attempts still should be made to minimize costs to research subjects.

Development of Drugs and Extraction of Products

Animals are often used to extract products for biomedical research and therapy (Rowan, 1984). Many hormones, such as insulin, are extracted from dead animals in the slaughterhouse, and many other types of cells are grown in blood serum obtained from slaughtered animals. Many antivivisectionists claimed that insulin therapy is not successful because people still die of diabetes, and the frequency of the disease has increased during the twentieth century. Rowan rejected this claim, noting that in 1974 it was estimated that 130 million diabetics had their lives prolonged by insulin. In addition, extension of normal life span through conquest of infectious diseases and increases in the standard of living both resulted in a higher frequency of maturity-onset diabetes.

Animals are used to produce a wide range of antisera, vaccines, and antibodies that are essential in research, diagnosis, and therapy. For example, smallpox vaccine is produced on the skin of calves or sheep, and diphtheria antitoxin is produced in animals. Rabbits are widely used as antibody factories to produce antibody sera, although this technique is now being replaced by cell cultures. Rowan estimated that between 1% and 5% of all laboratory animals are used each year to diagnose diseases such as tuberculosis, dipththeria, brucellosis, and anthrax, and to determine pregnancy, although alternative in vitro methods are being developed for most of these purposes.

The World Health Organization estimated that vaccination against six common diseases prevents the deaths of 3.2 million children worldwide each year (Russell & Nicoll, 1996). A number of statements made by animal liberation advocates regarding the negligible value of research represent inability to understand biomedical science, deliberate distortion of findings, or blatant misstatements regarding data. These tactics are unfortunate because they tend to harden lines of dispute, fuel suspicions both of researchers and their opposition, and lead to political power moves that progress on the weight of might makes right.

Fox (1990, p. 88) stated that chemotherapies, antibiotics, and other drugs and vaccines developed from animal research, ". . . really had no significant impact and were put into use when infectious diseases were already disappearing from the population, thanks to advances in public health and preventive medicine instigated by humanitarians and social reformers of the nineteenth century." Sharpe (1989, p. 110) also attributed increases in life expectancy to improvements in public health, ". . . with medical measures playing only a relatively small part." Most would agree that improved public health measures, enhanced sanitation, and preventive medicine should be encouraged as much as possible. It is difficult, however, to accept the contention that "at most" animal experiments had only a marginal effect on reducing death rates. Fox blithely went on to announce that communicable diseases are now something of the past, and that the "new set of diseases" (cancer, stroke, obesity, heart, disease, bronchitis, emphysema, alcoholism and drug addiction, diabetes, high blood pressure, sterility, birth defects, and genetic disorders) are difficult to cure and are all largely preventable.

One of the more fantastic statements was made by Finsen (1988, p. 210) to the effect that, "Given the proper education of the public, anyone can voluntarily avoid contracting AIDS. Those who voluntarily expose themselves to risk have no grounds to demand that others who have not done so (namely, experimental animals) should run serious risks in order to either produce vaccines or cures for them." She suggested human volunteers should be infected with AIDS and attempts made to see if a vaccine might save them. Her comments have a moralistic tone I find obnoxious, and they are similar to those I heard from people early in the AIDS crisis, when many believed that only homosexuals contracted the disease through "sinful" sex. These attitudes rapidly changed when it was understood that heterosexual transmission not only was possible, but was becoming one of the common avenues of transmission. With the realization that heterosexual members of their own families could be affected, many in the moralistic heterosexual community insisted that more public funding be devoted to AIDS research.

Polio Vaccine   An instance of distortions of biomedical research is provided by Collard's (1989, p. 69) construal of the history of the polio vaccine. She wrote that monkeys were used to grow polio vaccine "in their nervous system" in initial stages of the research program, a ". . . practice that was abandoned for lack of results in 1949, when Enders found the alternative that worked better." First of all, a minor matter, the virus is grown in a monkey kidney cell culture, and monkey kidney cell cultures are still used for this. One alternative is to produce the vaccine on human cell cultures, but the virus yield is too low to make it a viable alternative. Several other alternatives have been explored, but either have not been economically feasible or have too many safety problems (van Wezel, 1981).

Rowan (1984) presented a detailed review of the history of the polio vaccine. It supports the notion that the intense interest of the biomedical establishment in eliminating polio led companies to engage in and to tolerate cruel animal abuses. The ban India placed on the export of primates in 1944 was lifted because the animals were needed to produce and test polio vaccines. It is estimated that, between 1953 and 1960 well over a million monkeys died, many of them during transport from the field to laboratories—the race was to be the first to develop an effective vaccine. The incredible waste was overlooked at the time and excused by the sense of public urgency, although polio was never a major killer.

As noted, the virus to produce the vaccines is grown in monkey kidney cell cultures. Without going into detail, a cell tissue culture alternative has been available for many years to test the safety of the Salk vaccine, but the cautious attitude of vaccine producers (resulting from the 1955 Cutter disaster in which 60 of 120,000 children and 89 members of their families contracted polio after receiving the vaccine) delayed the use of this alternative procedure. This disaster was the result of a flaw in the manu-facturing process that was easily solved by an improved filtering method. At present the incidence of polio due to the vaccine is only 1 in 1 million doses (Hilleman, 1995). Rowan commented that it has been difficult to adopt alternative methods to produce and screen polio vaccine because of a fear of consequences of change, bureaucratic inertia, and economic considerations, all of which contributed to a failure to exploit available alternatives.

Although some antivivisectionists still claim that the only cause of polio is the oral polio vaccine, and that the best way to catch polio in the United States is to be near a child who recently had taken the Sabin vaccine, the relationship between the decline of polio in the United States and the introduction of vaccines indicates otherwise. Before the introduc-tion of the vaccines (1950–1954) the average incidence of reported polio was 24.8 per 100,000 population; after the introduction of the vaccines (1964) it was 0.1 per 100,000 (Koch & Koch, 1985).

It would be better to consider facts in such episodes as those typified by polio vaccine research, and to pursue actions that might lead to adoption of reasonable alternatives instead of relying on distortions of the biomedical facts. The biomedical establishment engaged in highly questionable practices in the initial search for an effective vaccine. The scientific race (with its immense economic implications) drove these practices, and most experts agree that such unethical practices should not be permitted and that safeguards should be instituted to prevent their recurrence. It is better to examine the record to exploit the lessons provided by that record if the aim is to benefit animals, rather than engage in distortions for ideological purposes. Discussion should revolve around questions of how to minimize costs to animals, and whether even those minimal costs justify benefits to humans and other animals. In the instance of polio, it could be held that the benefits did not occur for enough people to justify the cost in terms of monkey lives, even assuming that preventable initial abuses in transport had not existed. On the other hand, the public and politicians responded with strong emotional reactions to pictures of children struggling to survive in an iron lung, and media hype and high-pressure fund raising were based on insistence that no child should so suffer.

Some, however, probably would not be moved by such appeals. For example, Fox (1992) questioned the use of animals to develop chemotherapy on the grounds that it only averts a few thousand of the 400,000 deaths from cancer that occur each year in the United States. The actual case may be somewhat different. Russell and Nicoll (1996) reported figures provided by the American Cancer Society that 90% of people diagnosed with cancer in 1913 died; in 1960 the figure was 70%; in 1970, 60%, and in 1990 only 50%. These figures suggest that basic cancer research has had a high pay-off in terms of survival rates and probably decreased human suffering. For many, that level of human benefit would justify considerable animal costs. It is possible that questions regarding costs and benefits can be debated reasonably if the available information is accepted and implications are considered in light of that information.

Thalidomide Most are aware of the tragic fetal malformations produced when thalidomide, a drug prescribed widely in Europe in the 1960s as a sedative and hypnotic, was taken by pregnant women and resulted in severe malformations in their infants. This case has been attacked frequently as failure of the animal drug-testing program (e.g., Singer, 1990a). Singer presumed that the drug had been extensively tested on pregnant dogs, cats, rats, monkeys, hamsters, and chickens, with no deformities resulting (although deformities did occur in rabbits).

Therefore, he concluded that extrapolation from one species to another is a highly risky venture, and cited ". . . decades of mindless animal testing" (p. 57). The general issue regarding extrapolation of results obtained on one species to others has been alluded to several times, and is discussed below.

Sharpe (1989) characterized animal experimentation as failed technology, citing the thalidomide disaster as an instance in which animal testing probably delayed warnings of the damaging effects of the drug on the fetus. The record, however, indicates that thalidomide had not been tested for birth defects, only for effects on female reproduction. Sharpe based his claim on the fact that an obstetrician "strongly suspected" the agent caused unusual malformations—a rather weak evidential claim.

Animal welfarists regularly maintain that thalidomide was thoroughly tested on pregnant animals, but such was not the case (Rowan, 1984). Testing was not required at the time the drug was introduced, and the European manufacturer did not perform premarket tests in pregnant animals. When defects in human infants began to be reported, animal testing was started, and regulations were established to require more thorough animal tests whenever fetal development might be affected.

The scientific community has realized for many years that animal tests, especially for fetal malformations, are not reliable predictors of human risk. Factors such as subtle differences in maternal, placental, and fetal metabolism can produce profound differences in the response of developing tissues and organs at different times during gestation. Monkeys are more sensitive to teratogenic effects of thalidomide than most other animals, and humans are more sensitive than any other animal.

The thalidomide episode led Millstone (1989) to conclude that, although one should be wary of placing too much reliance on them, animal studies should be improved rather than dismissed. One improvement would be to do the testing more carefully, in a wider range of species to detect possible harmful effects of new chemical substance. If harmful effects are found, the substance should not prescribed to treat humans or other animals until reasons for the effects are understood and the generality of effects across species has been established. It can be contended that substances should be used routinely by humans only after preliminary screening with animals fails to produce harmful effects. After screening procedures that fail to find any adverse effects with other species, tests should be done in monkeys, followed by limited testing in humans. Even though such a system of guidelines could be instituted, questions remain regarding costs to individuals who are tested relative to benefits to those who require treatment. I note once again that resolution of such questions might proceed more satisfactorily if facts could be established.

Toxicology

Animals are used most extensively to test the toxicity of such things as cosmetics, toiletries, drugs, and pesticides, with most tests done by the pharmaceutical industry. This has raised serious questions. According to MacKenzie (1992), in 1990, 3.2 million animals were used to test pharmaceuticals in the European community. Only 276,674 were used to test products other than pharmaceuticals, and only 4,365 to test cosmetic ingredients. Opponents of animal research often cite excesses in toxicological testing to indict the entire research community. In fact, some of the most emotional appeals are directed against testing toxicity of cosmetics, although the number of tests done is small and they are being eliminated. Toxicological testing usually belongs in a separate category from biomedical research, with an overlap when new drugs produced as a result of basic research are ready for premarket testing to establish their safety.

A general problem arises when animals of certain species are selected for toxicological studies (Sharpe, 1989). Usually the selection is done on the practical bases of cost, breeding rate, litter size, ease of handling, resistance to infection, and continuing tradition. Sharpe suggested that phylogenetic relationship would be a more proper basis for selection, but I believe that similarities of physiological systems would be even better. The UK working party (Smith & Boyd, 1991) insisted that toxicologists understand the physiology of any species of animal used in testing to justify extrapolation from that species to others. This means that the physiology of all species used in a testing program must be understood.

Performing toxicological tests to determine the safety of new products developed through biomedical research is a relatively noncontroversial issue. If development of the polio vaccine can be justified morally, then testing the safety of the product should be as well. General issues, however, regarding the kinds of tests and the possibility that alternatives can be developed still must be resolved.

Toxicity Test Procedures Rowan (1984) estimated it costs about $1 million for a comprehensive battery of toxicological tests to assess human risk, although he suggested that a suitable battery of screening tests could be developed costing no more than $50,000 to $100,000 if more care were taken to select procedures. Scientists are reluctant to change the procedures, preferring to continue what has been done traditionally, and fearing that omission of some test might result in liability claims should adverse reactions be found that the omitted one might have detected.

Of the general procedures used, the median lethal dose LD_{50} the dose that kills 50% of the animals is one of the most questionable. There is nothing magical either physiologically or statistically about the choice of one-half, it seems to have just grown up as a standard end point—and death is an easily recognized end point. It was estimated that at least sixty to eighty animals must be used per test to obtain a reliable estimate of the location and standard deviation of the LD_{50}. Another point, the approximate lethal dose (ALD), would be sufficient to establish a reasonable point of toxicity and to identify the effects of sublethal dosages. The ALD is determined by administering graduated dosages to single animals, each dose increasing by about 50%. If doses are sufficiently close together, and a suitable starting dosage is chosen, only six to ten animals would be required. With the ALD it is possible to establish a physiological toxic level that does not require death as its end point. Millstone (1989) proposed the maximum tolerated dose (MTD), defined as the highest dose at which the body weight of test animals does not fall more than 10% below that of untreated controls, saying that this weight loss might indicate an undesirable physiological condition. It is possible to do tests that identify dosages that poison without killing.

Almost any of these alternatives are sufficient if the interest is only to allocate the chemical to a rough toxicity class, such as highly toxic, toxic, moderately toxic, and nontoxic, as is done with the LD_{50}. Problems with the LD_{50} are caused by the many factors that influence its determination such as, species, strain, sex, age, ambient conditions, nutrition status, and route of administration (Orlans, 1993)

Another meaningful test is the minimal lethal dose (MLD), the lowest dose that kills any animal. This is the dosage one wants to know to determine the safety of a chemical. The LD_{50} has little to recommend it except tradition, and the MLD is preferable to estimate mortality. The power of regulatory tradition should not be underestimated, however. It took more than ten years for regulatory agencies to accept a fixed-dose procedure to replace the LD_{50} (Botham & Purchase, 1992)

It might be even more preferable (and possible) to have alternatives to animal testing that rely on some level of adverse physiological reactions to obtain safety estimates without killing animals at all. Even this brief review supports the recommendations made by Stephens (1989) that questionable tests such as LD_{50} must be changed, and that scientists should encourage regulatory agencies to support the development and use of alternative tests. Analyses provided by the UK working party indicate that some within the scientific community are proactively taking this responsibility seriously.

The Draize Test   The history of the Draize eye test provides one of the more deplorable tales in toxicology. The test, which involves applying substances to the eye, especially of rabbits, is named after the scientist who developed it. The rabbits usually are restrained in a holding device with only the head protruding, and the treated eye is held closed for a time after a substance is applied. Sometimes a skin sensitivity test is used before the eye test; a small quantity of a test substance is held in place with a gauze pad for about four hours on a patch of shaved skin. The degree of redness and swelling is scaled to classify the degree of skin irritation over a period of time, sometimes for as long as fourteen days.

An in vitro test assesses the corrosive effect of chemicals on slices of rat skin by measuring the change in electrical resistance of the skin. The method predicted 100% of corrosives, and had a false positive rate of about 10% (Botham & Purchase, 1992). This test is formally recognized by the European Organization for Economic Cooperation and Development, which stated that it may not be necessary to test materials in vivo if corrosive properties are predicted on the basis of results from in vitro tests, although they thought it unlikely that in vitro tests would replace the rabbit test totally for at least ten years.

It is presumed that if skin irritation is present, it is not necessary to perform eye tests. In that case the study may be extended for up to twenty-one days to determine if the changes observed are reversible. Tissue damage is rated on a scale to indicate the substance's irritation potential. If skin irritation is minimal; 0.1 ml of the substance is applied to the eye, with the other eye serving as a control, and observations are made at one, twenty-four, fourty-eight, and seventy-two hours. Reducing the volume of the test substance from 0.1 to 0.01 ml increases the predictive value of the test for humans, but regulatory guidelines have not been changed to accommodate this finding.

One of the major criticisms of the Draize tests is that well-conceived alternatives exist that do not involve animal testing. (These alternative are described in the next section.) The other criticism is that the test is often done to screen cosmetics and toiletries that are not necessary to maintain or promote human health, having been developed to compete with, and companies hope, replace commodities already available. Even those who are not particularly sympathetic to beliefs of animal liberationists agree that this use of animals is questionable because the high costs in terms of pain and suffering to animals are not balanced by any particular benefit to humans other than esthetic gains and profits for industry. The threat of consumer boycotts and pressures by animal activists led private industry to conduct in-house research to find alternative test methods not using animals (Stephens, 1989). Industry also has donated research funds to universities to develop alternatives. Several of the largest United States cosmetic companies have ceased using laboratory animals for consumer product safety testing, even while they review plans for alternatives (Singer, 1990a).

Alternatives to Using Animals

Some alternatives that have been developed to replace the LD_{50} test were described. Other alternatives take advantage of a number of different technologies using tissue preparations, bacterial materials, basic chemical reactions, and computer simulations. Many of these techniques were developed in the interest of economies of time, effort, and money as well as to improve the quality of generalizations that can be made from the test preparation to target population. The pace at which these developments occurred undoubtedly was quickened in response to pressures exerted by those in the animal welfare movement on funding agencies, regulatory bodies, and commercial producers.

Singer (1990a) suggested that until satisfactory alternatives to animal testing are available we should do without any new but potentially hazardous substances that are not essential to our lives. I suspect most people would endorse that recommendation, with the problem being to agree on what constitutes a potentially hazardous substance and what benefits are to be considered essential. Regan (1983) insisted his animal rights view is not antiscientific, but is a call for scientists to do science better, rather than relying on the use of traditional models. He maintained, however, that if animals must be used to learn certain things, we cannot learn those things. This means that certain kinds of science cannot be done, and certain kinds of questions cannot be asked whenever they impinge on an animal's welfare, which is contrary to some of what science is about. I now discuss this point further when issues regarding the pursuit of basic scientific research are considered.

It is generally agreed that what is referred to as the three Rs—*replacement* of the use of animals whenever possible; *refinement* of procedures to diminish the amount and degree of pain, suffering, and stress experienced by animals; and *reduction* of the number of animals used in testing—should be dominant in the general guidelines for the development of procedures. The UK working party (Smith & Boyd, 1991) outlined a number of replacement alternatives that can be achieved without great difficulty: There is a need for improved information exchange to avoid unnecessary repetition of animal procedures; physical and chemical techniques should be used that depend on knowledge of physical and chemical properties of molecules; mathematical and computer modeling should be applied to design drugs and other chemicals; bacteria and invertebrate preparations should be used as much as possible; greater emphasis should be placed on research with animal embryos and human fetal tissue; and such in vitro methods as tissue slices, cell suspensions, perfused organs, and tissue cultures, including human tissues, should be developed and used for preliminary screening of potentially toxic materials. In addition to these alternatives that involve experimentation, some call for greater use of human volunteers, surveys of human reactions after products have been marketed, and examination of epidemiological data collected over the years.

In Vitro and In Vivo   Animal liberation activists insist more use should be made of in vitro procedures that either do not involve animals, or require small numbers of animal or human tissues and cells. Smith and Boyd (1991, p. 134) suggested that ". . . many anti-vivisectionists tend to overstate the current availability of replacement alternatives, while scientists tend to overemphasize their limitations."

One of the more promising tests to screen chemicals for carcinogenic potential is the Ames test, which Rollin (1992) endorsed enthusiastically. It is simple, inexpensive, and quick relative to tests using intact animals. It is based on the relationship between somatic mutations and carcinogens, because many carcinogens are mutagens. The Ames test introduces a chemical agent to a growth medium for a special strain of the bacterium *Salmonella*. Changes in growth patterns of the bacteria are used to detect potential carcinogens. The test detected about 80% of mutagenic chemicals, and made false positive identifications of 10% of noncarcinogens (Rollin, 1992). These results suggest the test can be used initially to screen suspect chemicals as part of a battery of short-term assays in mass screening programs. Procedures such as the Ames test reduced the number of animals required for carcinogen tests in the UK; the number fell from 63,000 to 40,000 between 1977 and 1980, even though the demand for carcinogen screening probably increased during that time (Rowan, 1984).

Tissue culture methods could be adopted in many cases where toxicity testing and screening of products are involved. A tissue culture method has been adopted in Canada to replace the mouse inoculation test for rabies, and it is estimated that this spares 30,000 mice a year (Rodd, 1990). In addition, tissue culture alternatives to test diphtheria toxins require fewer animals because more information can be obtained from each individual, and none has to suffer a painful death from the effects of the disease. Exposing tissues of rat embryos to evaluate chemicals for toxicity requires only a few cells for each test culture. Only one embryo would be required for several tests, thereby reducing the number of animals killed and not causing any to suffer. One such test requires only

3 animals for complete screening of a new substance, compared with 300 for a conventional study using intact animals.

A general problem with exclusive reliance on in vitro procedures is that results often cannot be generalized to processes in vivo. For example, studies of individual nerve cell preparations made it possible to understand basic biophysical and biochemical events involved in transmission of nerve impulses. This information, however, does not advance our understanding of the functional outcomes of stimulating a neuron. If the cell exerts an excitatory effect there will be transmission through the system, but if it is an inhibitory cell such transmission will be impeded. Similarly, the functional effect will depend on whether a cell transmits its excitation or inhibition to an excitatory cell or to an inhibitory cell. The only way to understand such events is to study the neural system of interest in its totality. Finally, the function of any system is not produced in isolation from other systems in the intact organism, making it necessary at some point to study intact organisms before an integrated system's functions can be understood. In vitro studies can direct a research program into promising avenues and thereby reduce the number of alternative hypotheses that must be considered (and hence the number of animals required for testing), but they can never completely replace in vivo studies.

Alternatives to the Draize Test   As mentioned, the Draize test has received special criticism, and attention has been directed toward eliminating it. Part of this interest is related to its use in screening what are seen as unnecessary products, such as cosmetics, although the UK working party (Smith & Boyd, 1991, p. 199) wrote: "There is a tendency for such arguments to be based on the tacit assumption that 'What I want is necessary, but what other people want, and I don't want, is unnecessary.'" They concluded that, if society wishes to have certain products, the provider of those products has a moral and legal responsibility to do everything possible to ensure their safety. Animal welfare activists often contend that because the public supports research through taxes, it should be able to control research procedures. If that argument is to be entertained, the desires of the general public for esthetically improved cosmetics should receive consideration.

Several alternatives can replace the Draize test, which is unable to predict many types of human toxicological reactions. The low-volume eye test, in which only 0.01 ml of the test substance is used (rather than the traditional 0.1) has been mentioned. The lower solution volume more accurately predicted toxicity in humans, and that lower volume is now widely used. In vitro methods use isolated rabbit eye, isolated bovine corneas, or isolated sections of rabbit intestines, thereby eliminating days of pain and suffering by test animals. These procedures would not be approved of by antivivisectionists because they require killing animals, although material can be obtained from slaughterhouses where animals are killed for other reason—which also do not meet the approval of radical animal activists.

Another alternative is an assay of the chorioallantoic membrane of developing chick embryo after a small piece of chick egg cell has been removed. This heavily vascularized membrane has no nerve cells, but responds to injury with inflammation. A few drops of a test substance is placed on the exposed membrane and the amount of blood vessel break-down is the measure of toxicity. This test is inexpensive—fertilized eggs cost about $1 for three, much less expensive than to obtain and maintain rabbits for use in the Draize test. It is now used by Colgate Palmolive to screen new formulas and new ingredients (Orlans, 1993).

Physicochemical tests are based on breakdown of proteins in solution. One of them, EYTEX, uses a protein derived from the jack bean. This protein becomes opaque, as measured by a simple spectrophotometer, when a test substance is added. The degree of opacity is proportional to Draize test scores. An artificial skin consisting of skin cells grown on sheets that resemble the human skin tests the safety of household chemicals and has been adopted by several major companies, including Avon and Revlon (Orlans, 1993). Cytotoxicity tests that assess effects of chemicals on cell viability, morphology, adherence or detachment, membrane integrity, and proliferation are being evaluated.

Finally, computers can predict toxicity based on information regarding the structure and properties of new products. These methods compare molecular structure of substances of known toxicity with those of new chemicals. It is possible to screen chemicals and withdraw from further development those predicted to be toxic, thereby making further testing unnecessary. Evidence that alternatives are coming to replace the Draize test is that use of the test was reduced by 50% in 1988, and PETA claimed that more than 350 companies have stopped testing products on animals (Orlans, 1993).

The Draize test story is interesting because it illustrates several realities: Results of the test do not validly predict reactions of humans; the test has remained in place due to tradition and caution on the part of industry and science; public exposure and clamor, along with threats of boycotts, led the public to insist that manufacturers and regulatory bodies clean up their act; in response, industry funded research programs, both in-house and through universities, to find viable alternatives; and these alternative were developed quickly, were even better predictors, and have begun to replace the Draize test. Clearly, this is a success story for the animal welfare movement, and should be taken as a cautionary tale by scientists who resist the idea of alternatives to animal testing.

Some General Alternatives   The classic conception regarding alternatives to animal research embraces the three Rs of repleacement, refinement, and reduction. The replacement alternative was discussed in terms of testing for toxicity. Each of the three Rs is related to the others, so if animal testing can be replaced with a bacterial culture, the aim of reduction also is attained, and the change represents a refinement in terms of method (Orlans, 1993).

It is often suggested by opponents of animal research that computer simulations and mathematical models should be used instead. There is no doubt that simulations can help collate and manipulate data, develop models that reveal general patterns in a set of data, and extrapolate results beyond data parameters that have been studied. The major shortcoming with placing complete reliance on computing techniques is that there must be a data base to input to the computer and its equations. Some data can be obtained from knowledge about basic physicochemical functions that have been obtained in vitro. However, the problem of establishing the range of permissible generalizations regarding in vivo circumstances must still be answered through experiments with living organisms. The computer is able to generate predictive models, thereby refining design, methods, and specific avenues of investigation to be followed in the laboratory, but testing must still be done, and much of it must be done in animals.

Any mathematical model requires some input of factual data to generate predictions regarding physiological processes (Rodd, 1990). If knowledge about how a living system works is extensive, computer programs might be developed to simulate how a variety of treatment regimens could affect patients, and the most promising ones could be subjected to clinical trials.

Computer models probably will be most productive to test toxicity, because information from animal tests of many thousands of compounds of known chemical structure is available and can be used to predict toxicity of closely related compounds that have not been tested (Stephens, 1989). It is doubtful that computers will be effective to investigate questions concerning aspects of basic knowledge about which information is sparse. About all they can do in such new areas of research is generate large numbers of predictions, thereby sharpening theoretical models and pointing the program in directions that might provide critical tests of more promising alternative models.

One implication of the enhanced use of computers would not be comforting to the antiresearch community. The ability to generate models will make it possible to develop more testable alternative models, which might lead to an increase in the number of experiments. Experimental results can be evaluated more quickly, leading to the design of better experiments. Computer simulations and modeling can be important tools to refine animal research, but they are not replacements, and could lead to an increase, rather than reduction in the number of animals used.

Many discussions of ways to improve the quality of research emphasized the need to improve the quality of experimental design and statistical methods used to analyze data. Rollin (1992) considered this one of the simplest ways to achieve refinement and reduction of animals. Adequate preparation of researchers in the niceties of experimental design and statistical analysis is an area in which the scientific community has tended to be irresponsible. Although it is true that there is great sophistication regarding research design and statistical analysis, and the computing hardware and software required are available off the shelf, relatively few researchers are able to use them effectively. This lack is due primarily to poor statistical instruction received by graduate students in many research training programs. Students are introduced to the basics of description, analysis, and statistical inference, but too often their education goes little beyond learning how to plug numbers into standard statistical packages available for computers and how to read printouts. There is a world of complex multivariate statistics with which most researchers in basic biological sciences are not familiar enough to use, or to interpret correctly when they are employed. Methods that involve developing and testing alternative structural theoretical models to understand sets of data could be applied to great advantage, and would improve the quality and precision of experiments.

One of the more important statistical considerations often mentioned in print, but neglected in practice, is the power of a test. This is important because if a preliminary estimate of the size of the score variance and the size of the expected experimental value compared with a control value are available, it is possible to estimate the number of subjects that would be necessary to detect a difference of that size. Being able to make such an estimate would lessen the likelihood that insufficient subjects were included in an experiment to detect a real difference of the expected size, should it exist, or that more subjects than necessary were used. This problem is often acknowledged, but very seldom are the calculations done, mainly because the underlying statistical logic is somewhat difficult, although it has been readily accessible since 1969 (see Cohen, 1988).

Still (1982) examined the experiments published in the journal *Animal Behaviour* in 1979, focusing on methods used to choose the number of animals in studies of behavior. He concluded that refined statistical procedures were not being used effectively. McConway (1992) evaluated the experiments published in the same journal in 1990 and found no evidence of improvements; no clear justification was given for the number of subjects, and no reports of power calculations were included.

One simple and major improvement would be always to include a statistical specialist as a member of peer-review panels. This statistician's tasks would be to review research proposals before experts in the substantive discipline consider the proposals, and to explain the statistical concerns to these experts before they consider the merits of the research. Rodd (1990) even considered it desirable to have a legal requirement that all experiments obtain advice from a statistician—and follow it. A review of statistical considerations should occur at the levels of the IACUC, of funding panels, and of peer review for publication. Experts in a substantive discipline are often focused so heavily on the scientific theoretical merits of proposed research that they either overlook, or are not knowledgeable enough to evaluate, statistical and design aspects. Critics charge that too often methods and analyses are based on traditions within the field, and this can result in unnecessary costs to the progress of the discipline and unnecessary harm to subjects.

Humans could be used more extensively in medical research. According to opponents to the use of animals, if humans are to benefit, it is better that they, rather than animals, pay the cost. Some researchers prefer using available human material because of increased validity of generalizations to the human condition. Early-stage human embryos could be used more (Boyd & Smith, 1991), as could organs from brain dead humans and cadavers (Stephens, 1989), executed criminals, and victims of self-induced substance abuse (Orlans, 1993). Others favor greater reliance on clinical observations of humans (Singer, 1990a), testing of normal human volunteers (Boyd & Smith, 1991; Stephens, 1989) and long-term criminal volunteers in exchange for reduced sentences (Leahy, 1991), as well as increased epidemiological studies (Stephens, 1989; Boyd & Smith, 1991). Although many of these suggestions are sensible, most would produce howls of outrage from various segments of society that would find their moral standards violated.

Research Regulations

Although researchers were considerably reluctant to accept the necessity or wisdom of oversight, a number of laws and regulations were enacted regarding animal care and to improve proposed research at both institutional and federal levels in the United States. These intensive regulations did not meet with the approval of animal activists, such as Singer (1975), who deplores the fact that the regulatory bodies are mainly composed of individuals within the research establishment. He believes such councils should have more representation from the general public, because it provides the money for most research, giving it the right to direct the way its funds are used, a point I disputed. Another complaint of Singer's is that the law has set standards only for transportation, housing, and handling of animals sold as pets, to be exhibited, or intended for use in research. "So far as actual experimentation is concerned . . . it allows researchers to do exactly as they please" (1990a, p. 76). He complains that the law requires no attempts to assess whether research objectives are sufficiently important to justify inflicting pain. Although these procedures are not examined at the level of the Animal Welfare Act (AWA), which was enacted into federal law in 1966 and strengthened in 1976 and 1985, NIH and IACUC guidelines apply whenever pain is present in an experiment. When a series of NIH site visits in 1984 indicated that many committees were failing to meet their responsibilities, the agency defined more precisely the role and duties of animal care committees. Under 1985 amendments, each research facility using animals (a category that, as of 1994, excluded rats, mice, and birds, which are, however, covered by PHS regulations) must establish an IACUC to review all research protocols involving pain, and investigators must consider alternatives to animals and consult with a veterinarian before beginning any experiment involving pain. Other requirements cover presurgical and postsurgical care, prohibition of the use of an animal for more than one major surgical procedure, and approved methods of euthanasia (Orlans, 1993).

Baldwin (1993) and Rollin (1992) presented brief reviews of the 127-page AWA as amended in 1985, that is enforced by the USDA's Animal and Plant Health Inspection Service (APHIS). The act mandates unannounced inspections of animal research facilities by APHIS inspectors whose sole responsibility is to ensure compliance with regulations regarding cage size, feeding schedules, lighting, exercise requirements for dogs, and protection of psychological well-being for nonhuman primates. The AWA also calls for a reduction in painful animal tests and of student exercises that harm animals. In addition, the Secretary of Agriculture was directed to establish an information service at the National Agricultural Library to provide information that would to eliminate duplication of animal experiments.

The AWA set standards for training personnel who work with animals, strengthened reporting and record-keeping standards, and mandated that the IACUC appointed by each research facility must include at least one member not affiliated with the facility to represent better the general community's interest. The amended act excluded regulation of research practices once the general methods had been approved at funding and institutional levels, where appropriateness of experimental procedures are considered in light of overall scientific goals. To protect commercial interests, a penalty was established for any animal care committee member who reveals trade secrets contained in research protocols.

Funding to enforce AWA provisions increased from a mere $300,000 in 1966 to $6.19 million in 1989. In 1990, 1,474 registered research facilities and more than 4,000 other animal dealerships and exhibitors were covered by the regulations (Orlans, 1993). In 1992 there were 1,527 facilities, with 3,205 total sites, with an average of 666 animals per site (Francione, 1995). The USDA reported that, in 1994, there were 1,761 registered facilities.

The basic act is supplemented by NIH policies administered by the Office for the Protection from Research Risks. In addition to mandatory requirements of AWA and NIH, a voluntary mechanism for control of standards is regulated through the agency of a professional accrediting body—the American Association for Accreditation of Laboratory Animal Care (AAALAC). In 1979 the PHS decided that AAALAC accreditation provided the best means to demonstrate conformance with NIH principles, and it was mandated that results of AAALAC reviews be maintained for reference by PHS.

Orlans (1993, chapter 6) summarized review responsibilities of the primary institutional committee—IACUC—whose general charge is to ensure that the minimum number of animals is used to produce valid results, and that pain and distress to laboratory animals are reduced to a necessary minimum. The IACUC is charged to consider the following: A description that is not presented in the scientific jargon of the investigator's field of inquiry; information to make it possible to weigh the expected contribution to knowledge, considered in light of potential harm to animals; and enough information regarding experimental procedures to permit assessment of the justification for the experiment, consideration of alternatives, numbers, and species of animals used, dosages of anesthetics and analgesics, exact experimental procedures, expected reactions of animals, details of possible adverse effects and their severity and duration, steps to alleviate them, and methods of euthanasia.

Animal activists complained that the IACUC is only a rubber stamp established to improve the institutional image, the community is not represented adequately, and an antivivisectionist must be included on the committee. Scientists complained that the added bureaucracy hampers research progress. Another criticism of the decentralized system is presumed inconsistency in decision making from institution to institution. The 1985 revision of AWA required the IACUC to include one community member, a requirement that was opposed by radical antivivisectionists because one is only a token and can be outvoted. Other required persons are a doctor of veterinary medicine and a scientist.

An important review of substantive matters in research plans and financial concerns is done at the level of federal funding agencies, mainly NIH and NSF for biomedical and psychological research. The NIH requires a committee of not less than five persons, including a veterinarian, a practicing scientist experienced in animal research, a nonscientist (e.g., ethicist, lawyer, or member of the clergy), and one person not affiliated with the institution in any way. After adoption of AWA in 1985, NIH immediately started to fund projects to explore environmental enrichment of caged animals, including effects of group housing, optimal cage sizes, modifying the structure of housing, adding objects and apparatus to the environment, feeding enrichment, and foraging boards (Orlans, 1993). Although this move signaled a serious intent by NIH, it did little to assuage doubts of animal welfare activists such as Regan, who want to empty cages rather than improve them. Improvements in animal facilities do not qualify as improvements in the view of activists on the grounds that such changes merely perpetuate the research enterprise (Orlans, 1993).

The 1985 AWA requires IACUCs to ensure that procedures used with animals avoid or minimize discomfort, distress, and pain consistent with sound research design, and that procedures involving animals are designed and performed with consideration of their relevance to human or animal health, the advancement of knowledge, or the good of society. Another requirement is that a minimum number of animals be used to give valid results, and that alternatives should be considered.

Animal welfare groups complained that IACUC meetings are not open to the public. They claim that the presence of members of the public at meetings would influence researchers to pay more attention to ethical implications of research. Research institutions express worries about security if the public is allowed to inspect research facilities, fears that researchers would be harassed, and that confidentiality of continuing projects would be compromised. Some universities opened ethics meetings to the public, and in at least one (University of Florida in Gainesville) this has worked well (Orlans, 1993).

Another level of review exists at the level of professional societies and their scientific journals (e.g., American Ornithologists' Union, American Physiological Society, American Psychological Association, Animal Behavior Society, British Psychological Society; see Orlans, 1993, p. 225 for a more complete list). Most biological, medical, and behavioral journals require those submitting research articles to assert the work was reviewed by appropriate institutional committees, and that procedures conformed to guidelines published by the learned society publishing the journals. In addition, those who review manuscripts for publication are asked directly if they detect or suspect any violations of animal care and experimentation guidelines. If there are violations, reviewers are asked to spell them out to the journal editor, and if the research is in violation it will not be published and institutional authorities can be alerted.

Poll results reveal solid support for the use of animals in research, which can be attributed to public acceptance of a need for animal research, and confidence that safeguards guarantee institutional accountability and maintain adequate standards of animal welfare (Newcomer, 1990). In spite of the large number of regulations that have been adopted, Singer (1990a, p. 77) concluded that there is a ". . . complete absence of effective regulation in the United States . . . in sharp contrast to the situation in many other developed nations." This view is based on what he characterizes as a lack of assessment of the justification to inflict pain to achieve research objectives. The fact that assessing the justification of pain is one of the primary charges of IACUC review process does not satisfy him because he considers the composition of the committee to be inadequate. He insists it is necessary (p. 79) to give appropriately constituted institutional committees control over what happens during an experiment. I suspect he means a committee approved by animal welfare activists, not the presently constituted institutional committees.

In his less political comments Singer (1996, p. 229) stated: ". . . science should properly be regarded as subordinate to ethics, and the protection of both human and animal subjects of research should take priority over the desires of scientists to perform particular kinds of research." An effective way to achieve a balance between science and ethics would be to instruct scientists in ethical issues, and to raise the consciousness of scientists, ethicists, and animal welfare activists regarding the complexity of the issues that must be considered to evaluate relative benefits and costs. For example, discussions of animal issues could be introduced into university undergraduate curricula, academic chairs established in animal welfare, courses on ethical concerns included in veterinary schools, and academic centers established to consider alternatives to animal research (Orlans, 1993). I agree, and add that, to appreciate problems involved in determining the importance of similarities and differences among animal species, instruction in the principles of evolutionary biology should be provided to researchers, philosophers, and policy makers.

Morton (1989, p. 190) concluded his discussion of possible refinements of research procedures with a sensible suggestion: "It should be remembered that, regardless of laws, animal welfare is best served and protected by the individual. It is up to each research worker to consider the ethical issues involved and to choose techniques that will not only answer the scientific question but cause least distress to the animal. Serious consideration should be given to whether the knowledge is worth gaining—at the end of the day that is a personal decision." Similar sentiments were expressed by Rowan (1984), who suggested that the ultimate protection for laboratory animals depends on the conscience of the scientific researcher, whose level of awareness must be raised through educational programs. In other words, the most important control point for laboratory animal welfare in the United States is the local institution. Rollin (1992, p. 191) considers the major benefit of AWA to be generation of dialogue among scientists on morally problematic aspects of animal research, ". . . thereby eroding the indefensible ideology that in the past served to allow animal research to be seen as a value-free activity." He believes this goal has been approached because more papers on animal pain and its control have been published since the passage of AWA than during the previous hundred years.

A number of bad practices have been tolerated by the scientific community for much too long. However, serious attention has been devoted to eliminating many of those practices, and adequate regulatory mechanisms have been developed and are being improved with experience. The goals represented by the 3 Rs are being realized, although none of these changes will result in the abolition of research in animals, short of forbidding science to ask certain questions.

11

Setting Research and Educational Policy

Scientists and Basic Research

In chapter 10 I suggested care should be taken to distinguish between different activities falling under the rubric "animal research." Rodd (1990) grouped purely technological uses of animals at one end of the spectrum of animal use and pure science at the other, with intermediate categories clearly delineated, and that scheme is used here. An instance of unhelpful overgeneralization is an analogy made by Rollin (1995, p. 109) when discussing the welfare of farm animals: "White veal production is to animal agriculture as the Draize test . . . is to animal research. Both are perceived by the public as examples of these activities at their worst." Appropriateness aside, the analogy does not involves basic scientific research—the first half is an analogy from one product-oriented activity to another, and the second half from product to science. It only confuses matters to blur distinctions that demarcate different uses of animals by humans.

Views regarding the intentions and processes of basic science range all over the map. Large numbers of negative views regarding scientists and science have been noted throughout this book, and if those expressing them believe what they write, there is little hope of any rapprochement between them and the scientific community. Finsen (1988) considered animal research to be so exploitive that she wrote that the current institution must be abolished. Collard (1989) believed all funds used to support laboratory research should be redirected to the study of pollution and to promote the banning of polluting products. One beneficial outcome of such redirection would be to force scientists to think of alternative methods or careers. Sperling's (1988) animal rights activist informants viewed scientists as driven by profit motive and career concerns that suppressed ethical and spiritual goals, and supported materialistic ones in the interest of dominating nature. Collard characterized the researcher's drive for power to lie at the core of experimentation, and scientists were intellectually dishonest about the real goal of their research—their personal welfare—as well as insensitive sadists. In the *LA Times* Alice Kahn (1990) propounded: "Those who can, do, those who can't, teach. And those who can do absolutely nothing, do research." For those having such negative beliefs there is no reason they should do anything more than attempt to abolish animal science and force scientists into occupations that do no harm. Scientists have no reason to attempt to engage in positive dialogue with people voicing those views; the appropriate response is to adopt a bunker mentality in order to mount strong political counterattacks.

Less vituperative but still negative characterizations of scientifici research have been directed at what is called the exercise of idle curiosity and irresponsible duplication of experiments. Fox (1990) considered much research to be repetitive and nonproductive, and Hazard (1989) proposed legislative action to prevent duplication of experiments, claiming that this would save money by rejecting grant applications for duplicative projects.

Hazard seems not to accept the fact that one major purpose of peer review is to impanel experts in a substantive research area to detect and reject duplicative studies. A review of previous findings is required in all federal grant applications, and a common reason to reject proposals is that the principal investigator has not demonstrated mastery of the literature. It is critical to decide what duplication means. If a finding is of great practical or theoretical importance, many in both the lay and scientific communities insist it be replicated independently, especially if the finding has strong economic or public health implications. It is also desirable to determine the limits of application of findings and establish their robustness when the particular background variables are varied. The issue becomes one of insisting that necessary, but not unnecessary, duplication is done, and it is difficult to determine where to locate that line. If the consensus of members of society is that moral implications of a research finding are great enough (assuming the results are successfully applied or increase understanding of critical theoretical matters), scientific peer review probably is the best way to locate the line where it is necessary to replicate and beyond which unnecessary duplication lies. Such determinations should be made in terms of the scientific merit of performing what might appear to the general public to be duplicative experiments. Rather than mindless copying, repetition of critical experiments is often necessary to evaluate the validity and generality of critical theoretical points.

The antiresearch faction claims that scientists routinely approve of anything using traditional methods, insisting that scientists support what they know best how to do. The old saw is "give a child a hammer and things will be found that need pounding." No doubt a great deal of the research involved in toxicology testing, for example, relied on traditional methods too often and for too long. Individual workers in toxicology laboratories have little influence on the methods used because some standard tests are demanded by government regulations.

It is true that science has strong and often unexamined traditions. Standard methods and the research literature describing them are communicated to students during training. This conservative aspect of science was characterized by Kuhn (1962) as a research paradigm. However, conservative methodological traditions are challenged continually, usually without success; but these unorthodox challenges sometimes produce enough anomalous results that a prevailing scientific program is abandoned in favor of one that is simpler, explains more, and has greater heuristic value (Lakatos, 1970).

A second major goal of peer review is to question the appropriateness of experimental procedures to address theoretical issues. Resolution of this question presupposes that by peer review it can be maintained that the theoretical issue is important, and the need to address the theoretical issue at all has been considered. Morton (1989) emphasized the importance of not causing animal suffering unless it is strictly necessary to pursue the scientific objective, which presupposes that the objective is of sufficient importance. Francione (1995, p. 141) objected to letting scientific experts determine the necessity of experiments because these experts ". . . routinely and slavishly defend virtually any use of animals.

Indeed, the complete lack of critical analysis of the notion of necessity is remarkable." I believe this charge is without basis, and stated in chapter 10 that peer review and institutional committees provide adequate levels of critical analysis.

On the issue of necessity, Smith and Boyd (1991, p. 37) took the view that if certain conditions are satisfied, crucial judgments are of a scientific rather than moral nature. In general, a scientist must satisfy at least four conditions: (1) The goal is worthwhile; (2) it has a high moral claim to be achieved (arguments involving cost-benefit analyses regarding the welfare of society); (3) there is no less drastic method to achieve the goal (questions regarding alternatives); and (4) a reasonable possibility exists that the project can achieve the goal. The first two conditions involve the moral level, and the last two evaluate the likelihood of achieving the moral ends with available scientific methods.

Current research-funding structures receive strong input from both the executive and legislative branches of government, which not only set funding levels, but establish areas of research priorities when specific budgets are established for various agencies, and these agencies usually are charged with specific responsibilities in terms of objectives. Following input regarding conditions (1) and (2) above, responsibility rests with agency heads, who rely primarily on peer reviews done by panels that channel their reports through a scientific executive council established for each branch of each agency. All of these safeguards and levels of review will not satisfy the objections of those who view scientists to be beyond the limits of acceptable standards of morality and honesty. Scientists will claim they have attempted to address the concerns, but the antiresearch faction will consider these attempts to be nothing more than window-dressing to allow cruel, wasteful, and unnecessary research to continue.

Basic Nonapplied Research
Strong disagreements surround the permissibility of causing suffering for the sole purpose of developing basic scientific theory. Arguments in favor of such research assume that advancement of knowledge is an absolute good (Hollands, 1989). Regan (1983, p. 383) challenged the idea that scientific experiments should be done to increase understanding of basic principles. Much research is a waste of time when viewed in retrospect,

and we can never say in advance whether a given experiment has been done ". . . by an incompetent researcher who doesn't know what he is looking for and wouldn't recognize it if he found it." Peer review would not be able to detect such cases, and it might be ". . . just as well to draw straws instead."

Rollin (1992, p. 170) insisted that ". . . it is immoral to close the door to the advancement of knowledge; it is a rejection of our very humanity," but then (p. 195) wanted to ". . . exclude invasive research which produces no benefit, but simply advances knowledge or careers." He wrestled with the question of the importance of serendipity—that it may not appear that a particular piece of research will produce a benefit, but such a result might arise adventitiously. It is a contradiction to assume it is possible to plan for serendipity. Because granting agencies reject research that is poorly designed or considered to be of slight importance, he rejected positions based on serendipity, because if serendipity was so important, one would logically be compelled to fund everything!

Rollin was unable to resolve the dilemma, concluding that the law should allow local committees that have greater representation from the citizenry at large to pass on the value of a piece of animal research; society pays for the research, and scientists should have to defend expenditures of public money to hurt animals. Earlier, however, he (p. 135) observed that ". . . opponents of animal experimentation know little about research and often discredit themselves by offering wholly implausible 'alternatives' to the use of animals." How can people who know so little about research make wise decisions regarding what investigations should and should not be done? It is questionable that either the general public or many of those opposed would be able to evaluate the adequacy of experimental and statistical designs to improve the quality of research and arrive at more powerful tests of theoretical questions.

I stated in chapter 10 that it is important for members of the scientific community to improve their knowledge of design and statistical issues beyond the basics. Can it be that people who know little of the substantive methodological and theoretical aspects of a science, let alone the complexities of statistical measurement, design, analysis, and inference, would be able to make wise decisions? I think the possibility is nil, and behave that the dialogue among committee members from the nonscientific community would not concern intricacies of design and analysis or logic relating data to theory, but would revolve around political and ideological differences. The public should have input regarding the merit of practical and scientific goals and the moral costs and values in their achievement, but technicalities of procedure are beyond their competence. Societal and economic concerns establish the research missions that receive priority funding, and these are the proper (and adequate) inputs from the general public.

Wall (1992) raised an important point when he noted that most often justifications for animal research are stated in terms of usefulness to produce cures for disease and to ease suffering. These justifications are based on acceptance of an unfortunate spirit of the times that defines value only in terms of the marketplace, and such terms do not reflect the nature of science as it exists for most scientists. No place would be left for some of the greatest intellectual and practical achievements and challenges of our times, ones that were produced by those solely interested in the pursuit of pure knowledge.

Laypeople sometimes consider animal research pointless merely because they do not understand it. They understand the rationale of trying a new compound on an animal before testing it in humans, but have greater difficulty understanding why investments should be made in what looks like mindless basic research that takes funding away from important applied research questions, or from dealing with environmental issues that affect public health. Rodd (1990, pp. 153–154) asked how likely is that lay people would understand ". . . how basic research . . . looking at the diffraction patterns of chemicals extracted from a plant virus, the development patterns of sea urchins, the pigmentation of snapdragons, or the genetics of maize could have medical importance." However, studies of each of these problems won Nobel prizes for physiology and medicine, and they were of fundamental importance for the development of modern biotechnology. She (p. 154) concluded: ". . . there will be a tendency for non-scientists who are involved in the control of research funds to favour the more obviously relevant higher-animal work at the expense of projects which use organisms less closely related to humans but which share the characteristic which is of interest for the particular study in question." The dilemma is that animal research activists will object to using those "higher animals" for research at all. So, what's a good scientist over to do?

The burden of proof is on the shoulders of those who claim that a panel of citizens would be able to perform a useful function other than obstructing research progress. One bit of evidence suggests the kinds of difficulties those outside the research discipline have when evaluating technical matters. Orlans (1993) surveyed sixteen members of the community who were animal advocates serving as members of IACUCs. They tended to be well educated (doctoral, master's, or baccalaureate degrees) and were at middle or top managerial levels of humane societies. Those most satisfied with their service expressed appreciation of science, were able to withstand role ambiguity, and could deal with group pressure. Although few proposals were disapproved, investigators often would be limited to performing pilot studies in a minimal number of animals under strict veterinarian supervision. One of the most effective committees developed a series of written policies covering problematic procedures and circulated them to investigators, with the result that projects following those procedures were no longer submitted.

Among the impressions of different members were the following: Impressed with the overall concern for animal welfare on the committee; lacked scientific background and had considerable difficulty in understanding protocols; protocols were not comprehensible to a nonscientist, but the committee chair permitted her to seek help from scientists she knew; discussions of the social merits of some animal experiments were disallowed; although a veterinarian, could not understand the science in some protocols; although a "lay abstract" was provided with all protocols, did not understand what was going on and felt intimidated due to a nonacademic background, although the committee members provided help; kept the committee "honest" because his presence forced them to look at things more carefully.

Often the protocol information given to committee members was deficient, making meaningful review impossible, although the institutions continually revised their standard protocol forms to improve the quality of information provided. The consensus was frustration because it was very rare for any animal experiment to be disallowed completely, often with the community member being the only negative vote. Some animal advocates experienced rejection by other animal advocates as well as by other committee members. Orlans believed that community members performed a valuable role by providing a constant reminder of the outside world, often bringing up social and ethical issues. She recommended that the numerical representation of nonscientists and students be increased, a nonscientist be appointed chair or cochair, and instruction regarding ethical issues required for investigators who would use animals as subjects. These recommendations seem reasonable, and would move committees closer to performing a needed function.

Ten chairpersons of IACUCs, all scientists, were also interviewed by Orlans, and all thought community members served an important function, the intent of Congress was being fulfilled, and no changes in committee membership were necessary (although one thought having a community member was "primarily a PR move"). They thought an antivivisectionist would be unacceptable as a committee member. Most agreed that an outsider's presence made investigators explain what they were doing and why, and that it made them more introspective about their work. Orlans concluded the chairs were more satisfied with the role of community members than were the members themselves, especially those from the animal rights movement. She recommended that a national commission on animal experimentation be established with respresentation that "reasonably reflects" current social attitudes. This commission should make policy recommendations on specific functions of IACUCs (which still are not clear), and clarify the role of community committee members (which is still poorly defined).

The permissibility of using animals for basic research in which the aim is to develop theory rather than to produce direct applied benefits remains a major concern of many animal welfare activists. I have noted remarks by those who characterize such research as an exercise in "idle curiosity," "mindless animal testing," and "pain for trivial purposes," and who conclude that "harm done to animals in pursuit of scientific purposes is wrong."

Gallistel (1981), a research psychologist who is an expert in the history of the study of adaptive specializations, discussed one of the most important discoveries in the history of biology—that the spinal cord dorsal roots are sensory in function and the ventral roots are motor. No rational physiology of the nervous system was possible before these separate functions were discovered, and the information made it possible to establish current concepts of the physiology of the central nervous system. The experiments were performed by Magendie in 1822, twenty-five years before the discovery of anesthetics. Gallistel proposed that the ethical problems involved in this research were placed in sharp relief. The results were of utmost importance, puppies were used in the experiments, and the pain of the surgical procedure was both intense and unalleviated. The experiments incurred widespread moral censure and helped fuel the anti-vivisection movement in nineteenth-century England.

Gallistel admitted that science and medicine cannot progress without such experiments, even though they cause pain to animals. He acknowledged that most animals that suffer in the course of neurobehavioral research do so in vain because many experiments do not yield data that are decisive or meaningful. The discovery of the Bell-Magendie law, however, produced scientific knowledge of immense importance from which flowed many human and humane benefits. The dilemma is that it is never possible to know before the study is performed whether a proposed line of inquiry will be in vain or will provide immensely important knowledge. All that can be assured is that the research team is competent, the questions are important, and the study is designed adequately. Gallistel (1981, p. 360) found it impossible to comprehend ". . . how it can be right to use animals to provide food for our bodies but wrong to use them to provide food for thought."

Francione (1995) disagrees strongly with Gallistel's position, and does not believe that scientific knowledge should outweigh animal suffering. Rather, the acquisition of knowledge can count as a benefit entitling a researcher to inflict pain or death on an animal, virtually any use of animals can be justified. This is a sticky point, especially when the history of science is examined, especially if the intent is to understand how scientific progress occurs. Examination reveals the power of serendipity, as well as advancements that were made possible by a number of small increments in the knowledge of how the world goes 'round.

Rollin (1992, p. 169) acknowledged: ". . . one never knows what applications a piece of research may have, however far removed from reality it may seem to be." Not only is it impossible to know before an experiment is performed whether it will or will not produce valuable information, but one cannot even be sure that the results will be interpretable. The research plan might appear to be justified in terms of the significance of the theoretical question, and the procedures might be adequate to lead to a potential answer. The research can be planned carefully, but especially when exploring a new area, it is often only after the fact that flaws in the design can be appreciated. If those flaws can be corrected, an improved experiment can be done; if they cannot be corrected, the entire approach might have to be abandoned and attention directed toward what appear to be more promising avenues.

In Rodd's (1990) view, a person who believes animals possess rights is not in any way committed to general opposition to scientific inquiry. The proper concern regards the extent to which these rights ought to limit the kinds of experiments that are ethically justifiable. She believes scientists have almost universally accepted a cautious position in the case of experiments involving the human animal, and I think evidence is increasing that they are willing to accept this position regarding nonhuman animals and to engage in dialogue regarding the extent of limits that should be established.

The wisdom of scientists who adopt ethical systems that see knowledge as supreme can be questioned. Rodd held that it is crucial to decide the extent to which animals should be allowed to suffer, and it is incumbent on experimenters to attempt to decrease that suffering. If it is not possible to avoid causing extreme suffering, we might be better off in blissful ignorance regarding the answers to some questions. It might be possible to assess whether an experiment or line of research is justifiable by considering what would be done if we had to deal with a new disease for which there was no animal model, and she posed several alternatives: We could content ourselves with letting nature take its course; we could conscript humans to the research effort; we could conscript volunteers; we could decide how destructive the new disease would have to be before any of the above alternatives would be used; and we could estimate how much risk to experimental subjects would be justifiable to combat the new disease.

She entertained an example where such a test might be possible (pp. 147–149). Chimpanzees are used to produce and test vaccines against one strain of hepatitis virus that causes a serious disease in humans but only a mild one in chimps. At first glance, the experiments seem justified because of the higher level of suffering by humans compared with that of chimps. When the situation is examined more closely, however, the cost to chimps is higher than it at first appears. Many chimps used for the research are captured from the wild (which often is done by shooting mother chimps to capture their young), mortality during transport is high, young chimps are generally kept in isolation in tiny cages in the laboratory, and those who become hepatitis carriers are usually killed because of a risk of infecting humans.

When these facts are laid out they could indicate how the research might be modified so it does not involve such gross costs to chimpanzees. If a program was established that eliminated or severely reduced all of those costs, it might be justifiable. If we are convinced of the importance of medical investigation in such instances, there could be a duty on the part of humans to volunteer to serve as subjects, at least in experiments that do not involve lasting harm. Rodd (1990, p. 149–150) suggested that members of animal rights movements should be prepared to volunteer to replace animals in particular experiments, which ". . . would spare animals and allow the human subjects direct experience of scientific work, giving them a more realistic ability to understand, while there is much wrong with scientific use of animals, random cruelty or sadism is rarely the problem." Her proposal requires decisions to be based on the applied application of research findings, and is moot regarding the pursuit of research that concerns only theoretical objectives.

Bateson's Decision Model

Bateson (1992) developed a promising conceptual scheme that could drive the process by which research projects can be evaluated. He believed the pain, distress, and anxiety generated by scientific research on animals is the issue that most exercises the public, and proposed a "decision cube" that could be constructed to conceptualize the relevant factors to decide whether a project should be conducted. On one dimension of the cube is degree of animal suffering, scaled from low to high. A second dimension is quality of the research design, and on a third is the likelihood the benefit will be realized, both also scaled from low to high. Although

Bateson framed the model in terms of medical benefit, Emlen (1993) said it would be better to characterize it as scientific value. This value could be considered in terms of the conceptual importance of the question being asked and the likelihood that interpretable results would be obtained and be generalized to other species. He considered this latter point important, because fewer experiments ultimately would have to be done using different species if the generalizability of studies were greater.

Bateson proposed that high levels of animal suffering should be tolerated only when both research quality and likelihood of benefit (either in terms of improving welfare or enhancing scientific understanding) were high. Very high levels of animal suffering could well be unacceptable regardless of the high quality of the research and a likelihood the benefit would be realized.

The decision rule would permit any high-quality research that involved little or no animal suffering, even if the research had no obvious potential benefit but was intended only to enable scientists to understand phenomena. Bateson was emphatic that the decision cube is not an exercise in crass utilitarianism, because the consideration of costs and benefits does not depend on a common currency or on balancing incommensurable properties. Rather, it is a set of rules used to decide whether a research project should go ahead, with the boundaries for making a positive or negative decision not always remaining fixed. The aim of the process is to encourage the pursuit of research with maximum benefit and minimum cost, and he expressed the belief that fair-minded people, even though they start from completely different moral positions, can find ways to reach agreement. He concluded, "For this reason, I believe that the dark age of intolerance will not last for ever" (p. 33).

I strongly endorse his belief that fair-minded people can use rational methods to reach agreements and thereby enhance the likelihood of attaining benefits while minimizing costs, even though those with different moral positions might not be completely satisfied with all of the decisions. The value of the exercise is that it highlights difficulties to be faced. An important problem is that those with different moral positions might have strong disagreements over what constitute high and low degrees of suffering by animals. However, it still would be possible to engage in dialogue to seek ways to reduce costs without diminishing benefits, even though a level of disagreement regarding many basics might remain.

The UK Working Party (Smith & Boyd, 1991), of which Bateson was a member, spelled out factors that could be involved in conceptualizing degree of suffering: The animal's capacity to experience events that might damage it or shorten its life; an estimate of how damaging the proposed procedures are likely to be; the adequacy of care facilities; the response of the animal to being kept in laboratory conditions; the adequacy of veterinary care; the use of a minimum number of animals; the response of animals taken from the wild to procedures involved in capture, transport, quarantine, and acclimatization; and the effect of removal of animals on the welfare of the wild population.

The benefits of research could be weighed in terms of the project's likely contribution in several areas: Improvement of the health and welfare of humans and other animals; likely contribution in terms of originality, timeliness, and effect on scientific understanding; contribution to the general education and training of specialists; effects on employment and the economy; and effects on the conservation of natural resources and on the reduction of the environmental impact humans produce.

These concerns address most of the important issues involved when costs and benefits are considered, and they are stated broadly enough that specifics can be treated differently as situations and conditions change. Because some of the concerns are quite specialized, it might be helpful to have experts from a variety of disciplines who can evaluate them. These experts would provide the panel with more valid information than would be possible if total reliance had to be placed on the knowledge of only those who were members of the panel.

The Working Party developed a qualitative assessment scheme (Smith & Boyd, pp. 141–146) to evaluate potential costs and benefits, and to arrive at an overall assessment of the potential likelihood benefits will be realized using the proposed scientific approach. This represents an attempt to spell out morally relevant factors and interests in enough detail to make it possible to develop weighting procedures by examining specific case studies. To understand how the scheme might be employed and even quantified, they applied is to seven case studies (pp. 146–181), analysis of which indicated that the approach has merit. Research protocols were examined, and they were able to arrive at general recommendations, both in terms of overall merit of proposed research and specific suggestions for improvement of projects that had merit. Although this approach will not satisfy everyone, it could provide guidelines that IACUCs might find helpful and that focus their activities. As mentioned above, it might be possible for individuals with different conceptual and technical abilities to contribute to at least one portion of the evaluation, and for everyone to contribute something of value to the final decision, even though they are not competent to decide in all areas.

Psychological Research

As mentioned in chapter 8, animal welfarists are especially critical of behavioral and psychological research using animals. Most of the public, and some in the animal welfare community, accept the necessity to conduct certain types of biomedical research because potential applied benefits easily can be understood and appreciated. Most accept the permissibility of animal testing to determine possible toxicological effects of pharmaceuticals, although they believe alternatives should be found. Fewer agree to such testing if the product is for cosmetic use or represents merely an improvement over some existing product adequate to the tasks for which it is intended (although the extent of such animal testing has decreased). Many find it more difficult to approve of animal research aimed at testing ideas that are of theoretical significance, with no immediate benefits intended other than the acquisition of knowledge about basic physiological processes. Even stronger objections and doubts have been expressed regarding the permissibility and usefulness of psychological research. These objections have been strenuous, and equally strenuous defenses have been made by behavioral and psychological researchers.

I discussed Rollin (1992) in chapter 8, where I aired his complaints regarding procedures used in experimental and comparative psychology, noting that much of his attack concerns not present-day psychology but the school of Behaviorism that was dominant in previous generations of theory and research, and which was represented by psychologists of the first half of the twentieth century, such as Watson, Thorndike, Guthrie, Hull, and Skinner. This ideological school is no longer is ascendancy (and none of those mentioned above are alive), and many of its formal principles have been rejected in favor of avowedly cognitive approaches to the study of behavior. These newer approaches do not deny that animals have cognitive processes, and they accept the fact that animals can experience pain and have interests. Questions regarding animals that cognitively oriented psychologists address were raised in chapter 6, and one of the central concerns is how cognitive processes differ from animal to animal and species to species.

Many indictments of bad experimentation consist of lists of "stupid and useless" psychological experiments (see Rollin, 1992, chapter 3; Singer, 1990a, chapter 2) accompanied by descriptions of procedures considered to be offensive. Although some of the procedures are extreme, it is the importance of the theoretical issues that should be the central focus, not procedures used to manipulate variables. Midgley (1989) questioned some of Harlow's research on the basis of procedures, stating that such things as the "steel wells" in which monkeys were housed have little relevance, because these things do not happen to humans. Research should be judged, however, on the importance of theoretical issues; the way variables are manipulated should be examined, but appropriateness should be judged within the context of theoretical issues. A related issue was raised by Russell and Nicoll (1996); many of the complaints of animal welfare advocates are based on a confusion between conclusions and results. The results of an experiment may well be valid, while the conclusions drawn from them are not; whereas results may remain constant, conclusions are subject to change without necessarily repeating the experiment, especially if the experiment was designed to evaluate alternative hypotheses.

Rollin (1992) held that psychological researchers should be forced to justify their research on a utilitarian basis—possible benefits that might accrue to humans should balance animal suffering—and justify their investigations according to basic canons of scientific methodology and logic. He suspected that in many cases this cannot be done, and that research should be evaluated in light of the theory being tested and the truths being unearthed. If investigators are unable to meet this test of adequacy, they should not be funded, on both moral and economic grounds. These are sensible proposals, yet when he cited examples of impermissible research, they all highlighted procedural matters rather than the theoretical issues those procedures were intended to illuminate.

Rollin (1992, p. 183) insisted that the National Institute of Mental Health (NIMH), which funds a great deal of psychological research, should have research projects examined in the "cold light of day" by people "outside the circle of mental masturbation." He suggested an appropriate group would be the Friends of Animals, an animal welfare organization. I suggest it might be better to use Bateson's (1992) decision model to approach the question of the permissibility of research; this model evaluates research in terms that balance degree of suffering, benefit produced and the likelihood the benefit will be realized, and is endorsed widely by people in many fields of animal research. Experimental psychologists are neither worse nor better than other research workers in their desire to proceed ethically, to avoid causing unnecessary pain, and to investigate theoretically meaningful issues.

The strident objections to psychological research seem disproportionate, given the small proportion of animals involved. Gallup and Suarez (1985) surveyed the number of animals housed for research in graduate departments of psychology in the United States. Of a total 252,687 animals, rats and mice constituted 90%, birds (mainly pigeons) 5.7%, and dogs, cats, and primates combined only 1.2%. The British Psychological Society stated that psychological research accounted for about 8% of the annual British use of laboratory animals (Rowan, 1984). Over 80% of those 43,000 animals were rats, with mice and pigeons making up most of the remainder. Small numbers of monkeys were used, about 50% in observational studies, 15% in drug studies, 15% in relatively severe deprivation protocols, and 10% surgery; 10% received electric shock. The pattern of usage in the UK appears comparable with that in the United States. The number of animals used by psychologists is small, and the number of these that are members of cherished companion animal species or primates is minuscule.

It seems that issues in psychological research with animals are emphasized because they compel popular interest and stir the public's imagination, invoking anthropomorphic sentiments to which most people are sensitive. Mother love, learned helplessness, neurosis, and behavioral dysfunction evoke strong intuitive responses in most people, and it is easy to have empathy for a young monkey deprived of its mother. These appeals attract supporters and make it easy to attract financial support, especially when attention is directed toward the welfare of nonhuman primates and companion animals.

Miller's Defense of Psychological Research

One of the most vehement supporters of psychological research is the eminent experimental psychologist Neal Miller, who defended the value of psychological research in several publications. Coile and Miller (1984) surveyed all 608 articles appearing from 1979 through 1983 in the four APA journals that report animal research. They challenged six accusations made at the 1984 APA meetings by the group Mobilization for Animals. The group stated that the tools of experimental psychologists are mutilation, castration, agony, starvation, and insanity. The specific accusations were that animals are given intense repeated electric shocks that they cannot escape, until they lose the ability even to scream in pain any longer; they are deprived of food and water to suffer and die slowly from hunger and thirst; they are put in total isolation until they are driven insane or even die from despair and terror; they are subjected to crushing forces that smash their bones and rupture their internal organs; their limbs are mutilated or amputated to produce behavioral changes; and they are victims of extreme pain and stress inflicted on them out of idle curiosity in nightmarish experiments designed to make healthy animals psychotic. The survey found not one article during those five years that supported those accusations, and it was concluded that such studies were perhaps published somewhere, but not in APA journals. They concluded it is misleading to imply that such procedures typify experimental psychology.

Singer (1990a) claimed that one of the most common practices in experimental psychology is to apply shock to animals, and Rowan (1984, p. 143) stated that electric shock is a widely used aversive stimulus in psychological research. Coile and Miller found that only 10% of the studies surveyed used shock (only 0.5% involving monkeys, dogs, or cats), and none of the shock levels was strong when considered in terms of their effect on humans. No periods of food deprivation were longer than forty-eight hours, and only 0.6% were longer than twenty-four hours (they noted that most peoples' pets are usually fed once a day), only 0.7% used water deprivation of over twenty-four hours and none for more than forty-eight hours, and no animals died of thirst. Early studies performing limb removal and limb deafferentation did involve intense inescapable shock and social isolation, but studies of some of the types described in the litany of horrors were done years ago, many of them by physiologists, not psychologists. No such studies were reported in psychology journals between 1979 and 1983, and they now would be subjected to stringent review by granting agencies and IACUCs, and probably not be permitted. Current research review requires extraordinary theoretical justification to allow such drastic procedures, and they would have to be evaluated along the lines of the Bateson decision model before they would be permitted.

Coile and Miller noted that the annual cost of behavior research on animals supported by NIMH and NSF was only about 0.0002 of the cost for the care of mental illness, which fact they used to suggest that the economic impact on the funds available for care is nil. Singer's (1990a) reference to this study is based on a report to the Office of Technology Assessment, he does not reference Coile and Miller at all, and he says that studies using electric shock still appear in other journals not associated with APA, even suggesting that many are not published at all. The point made by Coile and Miller stands—only 10% of the 608 studies reported in experimental psychology journals over five years used shock, a percentage that hardly supports the charge that that is a major source of abuse and suffering caused by experimental psychologists.

Miller (1985) defended the value of behavioral research on animals by citing benefits to humans that resulted. Among these benefits were treatments for human urinary and fecal incontinence, behavior therapy to treat eating disorders, behavioral treatment of scoliosis, rehabilitation of neuromuscular disorders, understanding and relieving stress and pain, discovery and testing drugs to treat anxiety, psychosis, and Parkinson's disease, understanding mechanims involved in deficits of memory that occur with aging, and development of biofeedback procedures to treat a host of behavioral and physiological disorders.

Baldwin (1993, p. 128) added to this list: ". . . rehabilitation of persons suffering from stroke, head injury, spinal cord injury, and Alzheimer's disease; improved communication with severely retarded children; methods for the early detection of eye disorders in children . . . ; control of chronic anxiety without the use of drugs; and improved treatments for alcoholism, obesity, substance abuse, hypertension, chronic migraine headaches, lower back pain, and insomnia." The evidence is strong enough to refute assertions that psychological research using animals represents "mental masturbation" by "insensitive sadists" serving the interest of "idle curiosity."

Spinal Cord Regeneration

A particularly compelling defense of animal research was presented by Feeney (1987), a paraplegic physiological psychologist who studied rats' recovery of function from hemiplegia that he induced by damaging their cerebral cortex. He found ways to enhance the rate and extent of recovery in rats, and is extending this potential therapy to humans with stroke. Feeney noted that after World War I almost all paraplegics died within a year; only following World War II did they survive, and currently it is possible for them to live active and useful lives because of changes brought about by the Americans with Disabilities Act.

Psychologists studying animal behavior made important contributions to both rehabilitation and cures of brain and spinal cord injuries. Rehabilitation frequently involves biofeedback, a technique developed through research with animals. In early experiments rats were conditioned to control heart rate and blood pressure, and the techniques are now being extended to enable human paraplegics to maximize the use of what little voluntary muscle control they may have. It is hoped that in the future surgical procedures might heal the effects of spinal cord damage. An indication that this hope is not far fetched was provided by the research of Cheng, Cao, and Olson (1996). The spinal cords of adult rats were severed, leaving a gap, and a bridge of nerve cells obtained from the animals' chests was sewn microsurgically across the gap to guide the severed nerves in their effort to regenerate. The animals dragged their hind legs behind them like dead weights for three weeks, after which time they started to flex their legs, and their ability to move continued to improve. Some animals were followed for a year, and were able partly to support their weight and move their legs, although they could not walk normally. Anatomical studies found that nerves had regrown from both ends of the injury, downward into corticospinal tracts and upward into subcortical regions.

Young (1996), professor of neurosurgery, physiology, and neuroscience, wrote an enthusiastic commentary on this study; it suggests that spinal cord regeneration is possible in adult animals, and that the task of inducing it might be easier than anticipated. He noted that very few axons crossed the gap, probably no more than 10%, and concluded that repairing spinal cord injury is no longer a speculation but a realistic goal. Cheng et al. (1996, p. 512) cautiously suggested: "It remains to be seen to what extent our technique is applicable to the chronic paraplegic state and to humans." The technique was based on knowledge regarding the function of nerve growth inhibitors, and on the idea that growth factors can be used to stimulate neural proliferation and growth. Understanding these processes was made possible by basic research with rats and cats.

Some general comments regarding this progress are in order. The original psychological research with animals was done to develop procedures to alleviate symptoms and permit recovery of function in the face of organic damage, and to alleviate psychological and neurological disorders. Basic research, such as that conducted by Feeney, led to techniques that speed recovery of function after severe nervous system damage in rats. With sophisticated techniques of microsurgery, accompanied by better understanding of principles of nerve cell growth and function, it was possible to achieve spinal cord repair hitherto considered impossible.

It should be emphasized that the experiments reported by Cheng et al. subjected animals to great suffering, some for as long as a year after surgery, culminating in death to conduct anatomical studies. The costs to the animals were severe; the potential benefits to what Feeney estimated to be as many as 300,000 trauma victims who are permanently disabled each year are very great. Not only were the costs to rats involved in that particular study great, but the costs to the many more animals required to obtain basic knowledge regarding physiology and biochemistry of the nervous system and to develop the microsurgical techniques also were severe. These costs and benefits have to be weighed, but the relevant facts are available, and perhaps the optimism expressed by Feeney (1987, p. 599) is justified: "By working together, scientists, animal welfare advocates, and we incurables may be able to reach a compromise to reduce human suffering and keep the concern for animal welfare at a balance in favor of humanity."

APA Guidelines

Rowan (1984) attacked the general guidelines for ethical conduct in the care and use of animals adopted by APA in 1979 (they were revised in 1985, and are available in published form; American Psychological Association, 1986) on grounds that they are little more than platitudinous endorsements of avoiding suffering where possible. A concrete objection concerned permissible levels of food deprivation, whether it is appropriate to maintain animals at 80% of their free-fed weight by restricting food intake; he suggested the lower limit might well be set at 85%. He maintained that such questions must be addressed before it can be claimed guidelines for animal research are adequate. I agree, but believe the question should be considered in terms of the appropriateness of procedures to address theoretical issues, rather than in terms of establishing some universally applied standard that would be considered appropriate in all cases.

The revised APA guidelines were established for field research and the educational use of animals. Eleven major sections address matters such as those involved in training personnel, establishing and maintaining facilities, justifying research goals, and specific questions regarding experimental design and procedures such as surgery and issues in suffering.

In addition, the guidelines specifically address aversive or appetitive procedures. When appetitive procedures are equivalent for the purposes of the research, the appetitive procedures should be done. The strength of aversive stimulus levels should be minimal, although compatible with the aims of the research, and psychologists are encouraged to test painful stimuli on themselves. Extensive food or water deprivation should be allowed only when minimal deprivation is inappropriate to the design and purpose of the study, with convenience to the psychologist not acceptable as a justification for prolonged restriction of intake.

The guidelines are based on the assumption that an animal's immediate protection depends on a scientist's conscience. This represents an inevitable reality, but it will provide little comfort to animal welfare advocates who view all scientists, and especially psychologists, as being beyond the pale of decency.

Individuals publishing in an APA journal have to attest to the fact that animal research was conducted in accordance with the guidelines, which are to be posted conspicuously in every laboratory, teaching facility, and setting where animals are maintained and used by psychologists and their students. Violation of the guidelines are to be reported to the facility supervisor, and if not resolved at the local level, allegations of violations are referred to the APA Committee on Ethics, which is empowered to impose sanctions. This empowerment by APA is exceptional because few scientific organizations take positions on enforcement (Dresser, 1988). It is also mandated that psychologists be aware of all federal, state, and institutional laws, especially NIH guidelines, and that housing conform to those guidelines. All procedures must be reviewed by the IACUC to ensure that they are appropriate and humane.

The guidelines cover a range of care, design, and procedural matters and seem to be about as inclusive and specific as a set of voluntary guidelines can be. Federal and institutional reviews, supplemented by peer review of grants and publications, are the major mechanisms of enforcement. Little more can be done short of posting monitors or police in every facility to observe every procedure and all aspects of care and maintenance. Again, if one insists that members of the research community are morally bankrupt, policing would be the only satisfactory solution, short of abolishing all research using animals. It might be useful to heed Leahy's (1991, p. 210) reminder that, "A practice may be abused without its necessarily being a bad one. We would not wish to outlaw parenthood on the grounds that some children are abused, even murdered, in the home."

Orlans (1993) discussed an instructive review by an IACUC of an experimental protocol involving prolonged water deprivation to induce rhesus monkeys to perform a visual discrimination task. The task was chosen to investigate the development and alleviation of strabismus in children. The IACUC considered the task appropriate, but questioned the period of water deprivation. Monkeys were deprived of water for twenty-two out of every twenty-four hours. Each monkey was placed in a restraint chair and tested for an hour to an hour and a quarter, being given one drop of water as a reward each time it performed the required response. During the remaining forty-five to sixty minutes of the twenty-four hours the animals were allowed to drink as much water as they wanted, and were allowed free access to water on the sixth and seventh days of the week (when the experimenter rested, presumably).

The investigator was not allowed to proceed, and he expressed anger at the suspension of the experiment, claiming that the twenty-two-hour deprivation was common practice, and that any change in the protocol would make useless the baseline data he had collected for more than six years. He also argued the monkeys seemed to be in tolerable condition, that they maintained satisfactory body weight, and none had ever died from water deprivation. The IACUC responded that because a procedure was standard practice did not necessarily indicate it was justifiable, and the fact that no animal had died was an unacceptable justification—life can be sustained under many intolerable conditions. They also noted that the claimed interference with baseline data was an untested assumption, because at that point alternatives had not been tested. I also question the robustness of any generalization that depends on a narrow range of background conditions; the investigator should be confronted with the suggestion that it would be better to study the phenomenon under a more variable and representative set of conditions if generalizations are to be made to conditions not identical to those used in the experiment.

The IACUC disapproved the water deprivation because thirst had no relevance to the subject of investigation—vision—but was used merely as an inducement to perform a task. Reasonable alternatives existed that would induce monkeys to perform the tasks, such as high-preference foods or drinks that could be provided as a reward, as rhesus monkeys will work well for mandarin oranges, yogurt, Gatorade, and malted milk. To reach these conclusions the IACUC solicited expert opinions from primatologists, psychologists, physiologists, and relevant professional scientific associations. A literature search was done to little avail, and the investigator could provide no published research articles that bore on the question of whether or not the deprivation procedure had an effect on animal welfare.

The IACUC examined the APA guidelines, which call twenty-two hours of water deprivation into question. The investigator requested a test period of one hour or more to collect a satisfactory volume of data each day. Orlans concluded that the investigator's decisions obviously were based on convenience to himself to accumulate data more quickly, and did not concern welfare of the monkeys. The APA guidelines specifically reject grounds of convenience to the investigator as a justification of prolonged restraint, and the decision arrived at regarding the convenience of water deprivation violates the spirit of that guideline.

The point of pursuing this case in detail is that it represents an instance in which the regulatory controls worked as they should: Animals were protected, and the investigator could proceed if he adopted procedural changes. Cases such as this support the conclusion that the rules and regulations in place are appropriate to protect animal welfare if they are followed. If the IACUC performs its functions, investigators will find it to their advantage to design experiments that comply with regulations in order to avoid delays, they will become educated regarding the necessity to consider animal welfare, and they will stop suggesting controversial procedures.

None of this should be construed to mean that psychological researchers have carte blanche to do whatever studies they wish, nor would it be possible for them to do so, given the effective regulatory mechanisms that now exist at many levels. It does mean, however, that the strongly negative characterization of research they do should be seen as political statements by those who want all animal research stopped, no matter the loss of benefits. It is hard to believe that many of the rhetorical slogans are more than calls to inspire conflict, to overthrow the research institution, and to solicit funds.

Harlow's Monkey Research
An interesting case history is provided by the research of Harry Harlow and his associates. Their early work stressed curiosity as an important driving element of monkey behavior. They developed a conception of learning that emphasized the development of learning sets (a cognitive construct), and expanded those ideas into an error factor theory to account for the process by which learning takes place. I consider the question of whether this early research was worth doing at the time, whether it made a contribution to science, or was just another exercise in

idle curiosity to prove what my grandmother already knew. First, however, I examine Harlow's later and most controversial work.

The research that received extensive publicity was begun in the 1950s and investigated maternal deprivation—removing infant monkeys from their mothers and raising them under a variety of abnormal conditions. This work was the target of derisive attacks from animal welfare activists, but it was defended by the research community. The aims were to establish the extent to which early social experiences affect subsequent behavior, and to determine the permanence of such affects. Hinde (1974) and Alcock (1989) presented succinct summaries of the basic findings, and they should be consulted for primary references. Rhesus monkeys were raised under severe conditions of social isolation shortly after birth. Some were placed in a cage with a surrogate mother, which might be a bare wire cylinder or one covered with terrycloth, but which had a bottle from which the infants could nurse. Although the young monkeys showed normal physical development, they began to crouch in a corner, rocked back and forth, and frequently bit themselves. If presented with a strange object or another monkey, they withdrew in terror. When other infants were raised in the presence of only their mother they appeared more normal, but developed neither normal play nor aggressive or sexual behavior, tending to react to other monkeys with excessive fear or inappropriate violence.

To develop normally, it was found that infants must interact with peers early in life. Totally isolated monkeys would display normal behavior when they were introduced into a cage with three peers for just fifteen minutes each day. Isolated monkeys raised on a mobile mother (a plastic pony with a rug saddle) that was moved several times a day in the infant's cage showed relatively normal adult social behavior, with several able to copulate successfully with new social companions, a behavior that never took place by those raised in total isolation or with stationary surrogate mothers.

Total isolation for only three months produced abnormal behavior, but no permanent effects, whereas isolation for six months produced permanent deleterious effects and isolation for one year destroyed all social abilities, with the most sensitive period occurring between three and nine months of age. One of the most important findings was that the most effective therapeutic tactic was to place a three- to four-month-old isolate with one-month-old monkeys who had been reared normally.

This research was condemned in the strongest possible terms by many animal welfare activists for two main reasons (Rowan, 1984). One was Harlow's unfortunate tendency to use deliberately provocative and sexist language that many found highly offensive, and to make flippant remarks, the intent of which was clearly to annoy as many people as possible, a personal tendency that typified his behavior in many aspects of his life. The second and more important complaint concerned the extent of mental suffering endured by the monkeys, accompanied by statements that it was not necessary to use such extreme procedures. I would add as a third reason that the research dealt with issues that arouse the strongest evolved responses in humans—those concerning the affection toward and nurturing of an infant by its mother. Strong empathy is evoked by the attendant suffering of the deprived and helpless infant that physically resembles young of our own species. Midgley (1989) expressed such a view when discussing the Harlow research. She suggested that a baby monkey placed in a stainless steel well probably does feel something like the same kind of misery and fear that a human baby might be expected to feel in the same situation. These empathic responses are understandable and certainly should neither be dismissed nor ignored; they are evidence of a high moral sensibility.

This third point also relates to a dilemma Rachels (1990) posed when considering Harlow's research. The work was justified on the grounds that animals are models for humans. One horn of the dilemma is that if the animals are not sufficiently like us to provide a model, the entire experimental program is questionable. If this position is accepted, insurmountable differences indicate that nothing of human value can be learned by depriving infant monkeys of maternal care. The other horn is that if the animals are enough like us to provide a good model, it may be morally impermissible to justify treating them in ways we would not treat humans. Rachels (1990, p. 220) remarked, "The problem is that one cannot have it both ways." Once again, we are faced with the problem of how much similarity makes a treatment impermissible, and where one crosses the line that represents that adequate degree of dissimilarity. Chimpanzees and humans share about 98% of their genetic material

(Orlans, 1993). Is that enough to consider them too similar to use in ways we would not use humans? The 2% that is not shared represents a lot of differences in physical and psychological characteristics, and this fact can be used to maintain an insurmountable difference exists between the species. The issue of how one should consider such similarities and differences is treated more extensively in chapter 1.

Some of the procedures developed using young "therapists" with older deprived monkeys were successful in promoting the rehabilitation of human children who had been reared under conditions of social deprivation (Hinde, 1982). A reasonable assessment is that Harlow's findings helped us understand the course of psychological trauma in human infants, as well as develop therapeutic techniques. If this assessment is accepted, although the procedures were extreme and costly to the monkeys, they produced benefits to both monkeys through the establishment of better laboratory-rearing conditions and human infants through the development of better therapeutic methods.

Harlow's earlier primate research referred to at the start of this section was innovative. He (1949) developed the Wisconsin general test apparatus (WGTA) that did not require restraining the animal. The monkey sat facing a tray containing two stimuli, one of which, when chosen, would have food hidden under it. The experimenter recorded behavior while observing through a one-way screen. Monkeys learned these discriminations rapidly, but not in a routine, mechanical fashion, as was expected on the basis of classic learning theory. They developed learning sets, indicating they had acquired a general learning strategy. When exposed to 100 problems, by the end of training, the first choice would result in a 50% chance of being correct (there being no way to tell which of the two stimuli was the correct one on first presentation), but performance on the second presentation would be 80%, rising to 95% by the sixth presentation. Thus with experience, a general strategy had developed: If you win on the first trial, stay with that choice; if you lose, shift to the other.

Harlow (1953) found it was neither necessary to deprive monkeys of food or water or give them extrinsic rewards, nor punish them to test their learning abilities. They would work just to take apart mechanical puzzles, so that over a course of twelve days, the number of errors made in manipulating puzzles dropped to nearly zero, and the manipulation behavior was highly resistant to extinction. Making monkeys hungry disrupted their puzzle-manipulating behavior, rather than improving their performance. Harlow interpreted these findings to mean that monkeys have a curiosity that is strong enough for them to work for nothing more than the incentive of performing an activity.

One might still say, so what, so monkeys are curious and they can figure out how to do puzzles better and better. The point of describing this research is not to extol Harlow, but to appreciate the difficulties involved in evaluating the contribution of research done many years ago, without also appreciating the dominant conceptual context of that time. In the 1950s the dominant learning theory was the stimulus-response reinforcement theory of C. L. Hull (1943), a hypothetico-deductive theory based on a postulate that learning occurs as a result of need reduction. A basic underlying assumption was that the learning of complex tasks can be understood as the formation of strings of simple associations, and the processes involved in forming these simple associations are the same for all species with a synaptic nervous system. It was assumed that this basic mechanism of learning was uniform across species, and increased associative abilities between species were due to the ability to construct more and more complex compounds of associations.

Theories such as Hull's can be considered as the experimental translation of those propounded within the philosophical tradition of British associationists (e.g., John Locke, and James and John Stuart Mill), by way of John Watson and Edward Thorndike (see Petrinovich, 1973, for a discussion of and references to this literature). These reinforcement models held sway for the first half of the century, and were extended to develop complex models to explain psychotherapy and language acquisition (none too successfully). Hull's initial intent, as expressed in his 1943 book, was to extend the theory to include all of human social psychology.

Given the tenor of the times, Harlow's research was highly important, because it led to recognition that external causative psychological factors could be important determiners of behavior, as well as those internal physiological ones emphasized by many Behaviorists. Now that the point is recognized and accepted by most, it seems obvious. At the time, however, it represented not only a new way of thinking about the formal mechanisms causing and the principles regulating behavior, but helped overthrow the dominant theoretical paradigm that had grown within philosophy, physiology, and psychology for many decades.

The fact that a theory now seems obvious does not mean that building strong empirical support to establish it was a trivial matter involving endless and meaningless repetition of experiments. Whenever entrenched theories and ideas are to be overthrown, it is necessary to replicate experimental findings in a variety of contexts to establish their generality and to argue for the inclusion of new ideas. The first reaction by the establishment to an anomalous finding is usually to insist that it is a special case falling outside the boundaries of the general theory. Only after a number of such exceptions have been observed do theorists begin to search for alternative theories that will explain more of the known phenomena in a more parsimonious fashion, meaning that it is necessary to make fewer ad hoc assumptions.

The idea that animals have learning sets was important because it made it difficult to characterize skills and complex habits as merely composed of an assemblage of simple compounded elements. Animals—rats (Krechevsky, 1932) as well as monkeys—approach tasks with active, dynamic hypotheses, which meant they should not be considered to be simple associative mechanisms on which the hand of experience works its automatic ways.

Harlow was one of the prime movers who helped establish the idea of strong similarities among mammalian species in terms of mental mechanisms. He created the WGTA and used it to test animals without subjecting them to deprivation of food or water or punishing them. He (1953, p. 46) expressed ". . . hope of finding and analyzing in subhuman animals motivational mechanisms which parallel the important characteristics of human motivation . . . ; the extreme persistence of motivation, motivation toward nonmaterial goals, and motivation independent of basic drives or intense affective states."

To achieve that end he began the maternal deprivation experiments to understand the processes, their timing, and permanence, and to develop therapeutic techniques to undo the traumas he had caused. The value of the research should be judged in the terms Rodd (1990, p. 9) suggested as appropriate: ". . . to find out what constitutes a good model of the diseased state and how this relates to the pragmatic search for successful treatments." It is ironic that, although Harlow advanced methods to enable the humane study of primate behavior and elevated the terms in which their problem-solving capacities should be considered, he also conducted some of the most reviled research that continues to be a major target of animal welfare activists.

Education and Animals

Issues closely related to using animals for research concern their use in education. Traditionally, animals have been used in high school biology classes and undergraduate classes in several disciplines in colleges and universities to train graduate students in methods of research and veterinary medicine, and to train medical practitioners in the principles and techniques of their craft. Two major levels must be considered: One is in formal classroom and laboratory education, in whatever setting; the other is to develop skills and knowledge required to do research and apply the results in treatment settings.

The key to Regan's (1983) discussion of the use of animals in educational settings is his belief that, although acquisition of knowledge is a good thing, the value of knowledge does not by itself justify harming others, especially when this knowledge is obtainable by other means. There should be no quarrel with this guideline, especially in high school and college laboratories. Usually these laboratories teach anatomy and physiology, with the traditional practice being to have each student or team of students, perform dissections on dead animals, or conduct routine physiological exercises on anesthetized living specimens.

Given the technology now available, there is little reason to continue these practices. Anatomical information can be communicated more effectively through a videotaped dissection performed by an expert. Time in the laboratory can be better spent observing and learning biological principles, rather than learning skills necessary to perform laboratory exercises, especially when they will never be put to use beyond the classroom. Excellent computer-driven programs are available that instruct students in principles of anatomy and physiology, especially the mammalian nervous system.

One technique uses computers, along with computerized tomographic and magnetic resonance imaging (MRI) scans, to construct three-dimensional images of human bodies. These virtual images can be rotated and flipped, and taken apart and put back together using a computer scan (Grady, 1996). The technology has advantages over traditional methods. It is necessary to destroy a specimen as it is dissected in a laboratory, but here it is possible to go back and forth to visualize structures. As mentioned, the dissections are done by experts who have a level of skill far beyond that of students. These images are stored in a computer at the National Library of Medicine in Bethesda, Maryland, and are accessible over the Internet, making it possible to apply them in any number of teaching and research settings. Although the technologies required to produce the original materials are costly and difficult, they could eliminate the need for bodies of members of any species to teach anatomy, and the initial costs can be amortized over the years.

Orlans (1993) searched the literature and found little evidence to support the belief that hands-on experience in dissection yields more benefits than using models, charts, or textbooks. Despite the paucity of evidence, she marveled at the widespread performance and long history of dissection, and wondered why so little educational evaluation has been done.

Animal experiments are also done by teenage students in the United States for projects in high school science fairs. Having judged such projects I am convinced students should be encouraged to participate. Most of the projects entered in competition in the area of psychology involve relative noninvasive testing of humans, often using computer displays, and most are replications or slight modifications of published research. In my experience, the outstanding projects were surprisingly innovative and those students were moving toward productive scientific careers. All projects should be under strict regulatory control and close supervision by qualified professionals who have experience beyond that of the typical high school biology or psychology teacher. Except for unusual circumstances, student projects with animals should not be invasive, but should rely on observations of normal functions in natural habitats, zoological parks, or aquaria. Many of the methods and procedures of science can be learned in such noninvasive ways more effectively than using primitive apparatus to shock animals, or subjecting them to severe deprivations or deleterious substances.

The UK working party suggested that vertebrate animals should be used in education in ways not likely to cause them pain, suffering, or lasting harm. Animals should be kept as pets in the classroom, and rather than engaging in invasive manipulations, observational, behavioral, or breeding experiments should be done. It is desirable to conduct animal projects at some level in schools to raise ethical issues surrounding animal research in a context that will be meaningful to students. Informed and sensitive discussions might result in a balanced and accurate perspective, and they should involve arguments both for and against the use of animals in a variety of settings and for a range of purposes.

Nicoll and Russell (1990) suggested that scientists take a proactive role and teach students at all levels that science involves acquiring new knowledge and transferring it to new generations, and that immense benefits have been derived from these activities. These authors (1991) also worried that organizations such as PETA provide information packets to school libraries and individual teachers and students to indoctrinate them with the animal welfare activist agenda. Their concern was that animals activists are succeeding in winning over the young to their cause thanks to widespread ignorance about benefits that have accrued as a result of animal research. They blamed scientists and members of the biomedical community for this public ignorance, and called on them to go into the community and schools to explain why animals are used for research, how research is conducted, and how it is regulated.

The APA guidelines recommend that consideration should always be given to the possibility of nonanimal alternatives for educational purposes, and that justification should be stronger if animals are to be used for education than for research. Animals should be used for educational purposes only after review by a departmental committee or an IACUC. The guidelines encourage psychologists to include instruction and discussion of the ethics and values of animal research in both introductory and advanced courses. In addition, students should be taught to ask and answer questions regarding the value of experiments in terms of what is already known about phenomena under consideration (Hollands, 1989).

They should consider whether a scientific problem could be better answered using a nonanimal model, if the choice of animal is appropriate, and if the procedures were selected with a consideration to minimize suffering.

The only instances in which it is necessary to teach students dissection and physiological procedures are when they must acquire skills in these areas. It is necessary to train scientists who will use these skills and methods, and surgeons must learn the manual skills and other niceties involved in their craft. Such skills can be acquired only by hands-on experience. Because advanced training in research is best taught by apprenticeship, the science professor should introduce graduate students to techniques in the course of performing research that has been approved by appropriate regulatory agencies. If operative and physiological skills are acquired in this way, it will result in almost no waste of effort or animals in training research specialists.

To train surgeons, both human and veterinarian, it is necessary to practice on live animals to acquire experience with technique, and to encounter problems that arise in postoperative care. Once again, this learning can be done most effectively if under the careful supervision of expert surgeons, physiologists, and medical specialists. Plastic bones are now being used in some schools to teach veterinary students to drill, pin, and wire, instead of actual dog bones (Orlans, 1993). The University of Illinois uses thawed frozen chickens in beginning surgery, which cuts costs and saves about 100 dogs a year—a case of the institution doing well while doing good.

In the UK it is not permissible to use live animals to gain manual skills other than in microsurgery, and it is not permissible to harm animals in experiments conducted in elementary and secondary schools. In the United States the policy states only that surgical or other painful procedures should not be performed on unanesthetized animals paralyzed by chemical agents (e.g., the neuromuscular blocking agent curare), and certain methods of euthanasia are absolutely condemned (e.g., agents such as the convulsant strychnine). It seems progress has been made in terms of enhancing animal welfare in educational settings, probably because the issues are more clear cut, and fewer complex conceptual issues are involved there than in research settings.

12

Eating the Other: Human and Nonhuman

I have considered issues concerning the use of animals in research at length because they are central to many arguments on one topic, and issues regarding the nature and progress of science are central to my areas of professional competence and interest. An even more critical set of issues concerns the permissibility of consuming animals for food, which leads to the question of whether procedures used to raise and slaughter animals for consumption meet acceptable ethical standards. These practices are more critical than those involved in research because of the immense number of animals consumed throughout the world, and the fact that humans (with additional nutritional supplements to a strictly vegetarian diet) can survive and prosper without animal protein. Even if vegetarianism is not regarded as the solution for everyone, a major concern exists regarding the practices of "factory farming" that were developed solely for economic reasons. The conditions in which animals are raised jeopardize their welfare so greatly that serious moral questions arise.

Eating Humans

Before dealing with issues involved in eating nonhumans I cast the net more broadly and consider under what conditions it is permissible to eat the other when that other is human.

Cannibalism, the eating of humans, is one of those activities that occasions strong revulsion among most who consider themselves members of civilized society. The taboo is strong in most Western societies, similar to those regarding incest, infanticide, murder, and torture. Cannibalism has taken place frequently in many parts of the world, and it is not uncommon under circumstances of chronic famine or extreme acute starvation. Ritual cannibalism, which has no direct relationship to obtaining protein, has been practiced in many societies throughout history.

Without going into the reasons for cannibalism or the reasons why most societies abandoned the practice, it is reasonable to conclude that a fair number of societies at some time or another have practiced it, and for several reasons. A major biological reason is to provide essential protein in marginal habitats or in time of famine. Among ritual functions are those intended to enhance or maintain human fertility by consuming reproductively significant parts of others, to appease hungry, vengeful gods, to celebrate the achievement of advanced warrior status, to demonstrate to others the ferocity of the society, to activate and affirm social exchanges between families or societies, and to deal with the grief attendant on the loss of loved ones, especially those lost in warfare. Sanday (1986) maintained that it is reasonable to consider cannibalism as an integral part of the cultural logic of life, death, and reproduction. In fact she said that one way to deal with a conquered people is to take the "raw wives" for breeding and the "cooked men" for food, both of which could increase the reproductive potential of the winning community.

In several instances cannibalism was a response to famine: Among the Windigo of the Algonkin Indians of northeastern North America and the Huron of Canada (Sanday, 1986), the Aztecs of Mexico (Harner, 1977; Harris, 1979), and the Anasazi pueblo in southwestern Colorado (White, 1992). In two major incidents, a group of citizens, separated from society at large, faced incredible hardship and disaster and resorted to cannibalism to avoid starvation. In addition, a large number of incidents involved so-called lifeboat cannibalism. The first was the Donner party, which, in an attempt to cross from Wyoming to California in 1846 to 1847, was stranded in the high Sierras during one of the harshest winters on record (Stewart, 1960). A second involved an amateur rugby team from Uruguay whose plane crashed in the high Andes in the winter of 1972 (Read, 1974). They reveal a similar pattern: An initial reluctance to eat human flesh, but once this was overcome, both groups consumed people in a pattern consistent with evolutionary expectations. These cases suggest that underlying evolutionary biases come directly into play when the rules that regulate normal society are no longer operable.

The events that occurred with the Donner party make sense in terms of evolutionary expectations. No one ended his or her own life voluntarily; animals were consumed in a reasonable order—first those brought for food, then work animals, and finally pets; when animals had all been eaten, parts usually considered inedible, such as hides, were boiled and consumed. When all of these food resources were exhausted, cannibalism began, but the people were always unwilling to eat dead members of their own family. This might be expected in terms of proximate mechanisms that would increase ultimate reproductive success: eat foodstuffs, then animals who normally are not food, then pet animals with which you have a social bond, then usually inedible protein, then human strangers, then friends, and last of all, kin.

A similar pattern was found with the Andean plane crash. When the possibility of eating human flesh was first raised, it was proposed first to consume those who were not members of the community—the dead pilots. When it was decided to eat the flesh of those who had died, those who cut up the bodies did not distribute it to the others, adding to the depersonalization of the process, and no one knowingly ate their relatives. Another interesting aspect of both instances is that cannibalism was accepted as an understandable act that was required for survival. It was held explicitly that not to have eaten human flesh would have constituted suicide, an act that would not be accepted morally. The patterns of behavior in these situations support the belief that dimensions revealed by examining moral intuitions using hypothetical dilemmas are indeed what are important when real social dilemmas are resolved.

The order of survival in lifeboat crises is for the crew to be favored over passengers (to handle the boat to enable any to survive), women and children favored over male passengers, men with family favored over boys, foreigners being in jeopardy, and slaves and animals going first. There has never been any legal or moral question regarding the practice of seafaring killing of anyone for consumption when lots are drawn among voluntary participants (Simpson, 1984).

Cannibalism as practiced in modern China (Zheng Yi, 1996) was done in the name of striking terror, exacting revenge, for reasons of acquisitive greed, or to enforce political dogma. Such practices are repugnant to the point that moral condemnation was directed at the entire society for having permitted them. These motivations strike at the heart of cherished beliefs regarding those things that establish and maintain social bonds that permit communities to exist, and they threaten the moral stability of all societies.

Eating Nonhumans

Throughout human history wild animals have been hunted for food, and in later periods they were domesticated, bred, and herds grown to provide renewable food resources. Animals have been used to draw wagons and sleds, to transport people and goods, and to perform tasks such as plowing and grinding grain. Many species have been raised, slaughtered, and eaten, and in recent years the meat industry has moved from what was primarily a family farm system to what now are called factory farms, using modern biological technology and large programs of selective breeding to increase production of meat, eggs, and milk at reduced cost.

Most cultures approve of eating meat, and for many societies throughout history that was the only way to obtain certain essential amino acids humans cannot synthesize from other foods. There have always been vegetarians who, for a variety of reasons, object to killing animals for food. It is possible to obtain a nutritional diet from nonmeat sources (plants and vitamin supplements) and to maintain a kitchen from which nutritious and palatable meals can be served. Many vegetarian cookbooks have been published, and most cities have a range of excellent vegetarian restaurants. As Benson (1978) remarked, however, we were meat eaters before we were moralists.

Vegetarians usually draw a line beyond which they consider it impermissible to eat an organism. For some the line is four-footed mammals, but they eat fowl and fish. Others do not eat fowl, because birds definitely have pain receptors. Some eat only fish, shrimp, oysters, and other shellfish, although it should be pointed out those creatures, too, have pain receptors. The most extreme position is that of vegans, who do not consume any animal products—no milk, no eggs, no animal flesh.

Many animal activists contend that factory farms producing meat, eggs, milk, and by-products such as leather should be abolished. Others believe all consumption of animal products should be considered morally impermissible, no matter how animals are raised.

The Questions

In chapter 9 it was documented that the numbers of animals used for research and education are not large relative to those expended for other purposes, and that many regulations have been established and are being followed to enhance living conditions and welfare of those animals. Far less attention has been directed toward regulating practices involved in raising and preparing animals for their meat and dairy products, although billions are killed each year for such purposes.

An interesting aspect of the proposals offered by animal welfarists is their relative lack of acrimony and willingness to advocate incremental steps to improve conditions and reduce the amount of meat and meat products consumed, tolerance that is not often extended when considering animal research. I suspect there are several reasons for such a benign attitude. It is easy to demonize research scientists, and to search the extensive biomedical and psychological literature to find procedures that alarm the public. This is especially the case when research investigates abstract theoretical principles that are difficult for the public to understand and whose possible importance is hard to appreciate. Attacks on academia can be successful because academics are by the nature of their calling argumentative, and it is not difficult to arrange forums for active debate among them. Educational institutions are predicated on the permissibility of exchange of opinions. Much of their research is supported by public funds and performed in public facilities, which opens matters to discussion by the public and politicians.

Another reason is that many who are sympathetic to the animal welfare movement consume meat, and it would not be wise politically to mount a direct assault questioning their morality. Vegetarians have express tolerance for social customs and traditions that support consumption of meat and dairy products, and educational campaigns to promote vegetarianism tend to be characterized by understanding.

Yet another reason is the immense economic implications of shutting down the huge agribusiness interests. The dislocation that would occur for workers whose economic welfare is jeopardized, as well as the political might of agribusiness, would arouse violent opposition to attempts to eliminate or seriously regulate those industries. Educational campaigns to restrict agribusiness have been marked by tolerance, accompanied by appeals to principles of morality and compassion.

A practice that enrages the animal welfare community, and occasions spirited defense, is hunting animals for sport and food. The defense of hunting is centered on traditional cultural values that make wild animals "fair game" and represent the deep biological nature of "man the hunter." Appeals to tradition lack force; if traditions arose in response to conditions other than those that now prevail—that is, hunting animals to provide food necessary to survive—they might well be changed in light of new realities of contemporary society. The biological-urge stand commits the naturalistic fallacy; because there are biological propensities in a given direction does not mean that a system of morality should use those propensities to derive the *ought*.

Another position cites the rights, and even duties, of gun owners to practice their skill and to use guns as they wish under the protection of the Second Amendment to the Constitution. This defense often stresses the importance of having a gun-skilled citizenry that can act as a militia to defend the country against some or another "them." Even if one accepts statements regarding the necessity of maintaining a high level of skill at shooting, it is not necessary to use live animals as targets.

We do not have to use animal hides for clothing because satisfactory alternative fabrics are available from plant fibers, wool, plastics, and even artificial furs if the peculiar qualities of fur are desired. Some contend that raising animals for fur is no different from raising them for meat. It is much more difficult to adjust diets to avoid eating meat, but little problem to avoid wearing fur (or leather for that matter). The strongest justifications for wearing fur and leather in contemporary urban society are esthetic ones, and border on questionable bases that are similar to those used to justify toxicological tests to establish the safety of frivolous cosmetic products. However, as Varner (1994b) suggested, relying on renewable animal resources might cause less harm to the environment than relying on nonrenewable resources such as petroleum products.

It is seldom morally permissible, under anyone's rules, arbitrarily to kill another person to survive (ignoring problems of ritual cannibalism and all kinds of nationalistic rituals such as war). Such actions violate what have variously been termed a person's interests, rights, agency, freedom from harm, and sanctity of life. No matter how the issue is phrased, the action is impermissible. It generally is permissible, when the situation resembles that of the lifeboat dilemma (as in the Donner, Andean, and shipwreck cases), for a fair lottery to be held if all involved agree, with the loser killed and eaten. This permissibility is based on an assumption that social contracts, freely entered into and with each person having an equal chance of survival, quite properly are involved in regulating most of society's comings and goings, and that interests of community cohesiveness are of paramount importance to survival. If a person does not want to be part of the lottery, that person should not participate in the benefits for which the rest of the community take a risk; nor should that individual be used as "fair game."

There is little question about the moral permissibility for people to eat animals whenever it is necessary to survive. I imagine most people, no matter what their belief system would agree. A problem arises when eating animals is not essential to human survival, given that it is possible to have an adequate and balanced diet without doing so.

I maintain that factory farming generally should be considered morally impermissible, because the conditions are not satisfactory to allow animals to live a minimal life that respects their welfare, and practices used in transport and killing are often cruel. A gray area involves cases in which animals are bred for food, are raised in a manner that respects their welfare while living, and are killed painlessly. Part of my equivocation is based on respect for the power of generations of social tradition and culinary habits and preference. Perhaps educational campaigns should be launched more forcefully to induce people to forego meat in their diet, to inform them of acceptable alternatives, and to describe benefits that can be secured by consuming those items. Such campaigns have been used to combat generations of other social customs, such as slavery, the use of alcohol and tobacco, driving while substance impaired, and overweight. All of these behaviors were, and some still are, customary and permissible among "good" folks, but now encounter various degrees of condemnation.

Philosophical Arguments Regarding Eating Meat

It has generally been considered permissible to eat human flesh to avoid starvation and to use human skin for protection from the cold. If one is to consider the moral permissibility of eating nonhuman animals, it is appropriate to understand the positions of Singer and Regan because, once again, they established the two dominant moral positions against consuming animals and for vegetarianism.

Singer's Utilitarianism

Singer (1975) believed that because all animals, human and nonhuman, have an equal capacity to suffer they are equal morally. He applied this philosophy of preference utilitarianism to issues of both conducting research and eating animals. In general, people eat meat for taste pleasure and to have a varied diet. Singer rejected this stance on the basis that a trivial interest, such as peoples' taste preference, should not prevail over the more important one of animals' survival. A large portion of his comments was directed against the intolerable conditions involved in factory farming, a practice that exists solely for the economic reason of producing cheaper meat to increase consumption and hence profits.

One of Singer's key intents regarding vegetarianism is to refute the notion of replaceability. It states that, although meat eaters are responsible for the death and loss of pleasure by the animals they eat, they are also responsible for the creation of more animals; if no one ate meat, those animals would not be bred at all. Singer (1993) challenged this view on two grounds: (1) Even if replaceability is valid, it would not justify eating animals that were reared in factory farms where they are so crowded and restricted in their movements that their lives are more of a burden than a benefit to them; they could be maintained under conditions that allow them to have a pleasant life; and (2) if it is good to create a happy life, then it is good for there to be as many happy beings as the planet will hold, supporting the conclusion that human beings should be eliminated to accommodate larger numbers of smaller happy animals. He admits these points do not go to the heart of the matter, but does not believe a more satisfactory alternative has been suggested.

He concluded: ". . . it would be better to reject altogether the killing of animals for food, unless one must do so to survive. Killing animals for food makes us think of them as objects that we can use as we please. Their lives then count for little when weighed against our mere wants" (p. 134) He allows interests of humans to prevail over those of other animals in circumstances of survival, which means that in some conditions humans count more than other animals. This is another instance in which species membership is a critical consideration, and it also means that the status of animals is being evaluated relative to the needs of humans.

Singer contended that plants should be rejected as holders of preferences and interests, and wrestled with what should be considered an animal "person." He believed our near relatives—chimpanzees, gorillas, and orangutans—should be extended all protections we extend to human beings, and suggested that a case also can be made, with varying degrees of confidence, on behalf of whales, dolphins, monkeys, dogs, cats, pigs, seals, bears, cattle, sheep, "and so on", perhaps even to the point of including all mammals. He decided fish might be conscious, but are not persons because they are not conscious of self, and also rejected self-consciousness for shrimp and oysters, although he was not so sure about the octopus. He worried that oysters might have the capacity to experience pain, and decided the line should be drawn between a shrimp and an oyster, noting that he occasionally ate oysters, scallops, and mussels, but avoided eating even them because they might well have a capacity for pain. Singer (1990a) changed his views regarding fish because they have a nervous system that is centrally organized and show most of the pain behavior that mammals exhibit. He concluded we should avoid eating fish, and felt that those who continue to eat fish while refusing to eat other animals have taken a major step, but that those who eat neither have gone one step farther.

His ideas in favor of becoming a vegetarian are based on the belief that the one thing we should take responsibility for in our lives is to be as free of cruelty as we can, and one step toward that end is to stop eating animals. The first step should be to stop buying the products of modern factory farming, which means one should not buy chicken, turkey, rabbit, veal, beef, and eggs, although it is less objectionable to do so if the products are produced by free-range methods. Lamb has a degree of permissibility because it tends not to be intensively produced, the lambs lead a relatively normal life, and their welfare is respected, even though they are killed while young.

He suggested a reasonable and practical strategy, even if he does not consider it to be ideal: Replace animal flesh with plant foods; replace factory farm eggs with free-range eggs, otherwise avoid eggs; and replace milk and cheese with soy milk, tofu, or other plant foods, but do not feel obliged to go to great lengths to avoid all food containing milk products. Although it would be admirable to give up all animal products including milk, he offered these suggestions so that people would not be deterred from doing anything at all, a course that would allow the exploitation of animals to continue. Finally, the only necessary nutrient not normally available from plant sources is vitamin B_{12}, which is present in eggs and milk, but can be obtained from seaweeds such as kelp, a soy sauce made by traditional Japanese fermentation methods, and a fermented soybean product.

Fox (1990) similarly stated, that an enlightened person should eat conscientiously, including only animal products from animals treated more humanely than when intensive methods are used. By this he meant products available from free-range dairy cows over intensively maintained ones, meat from beef that are humanely slaughtered, broiler chickens (preferably free-range) rather than intensively raised ones, and eggs from free-range chickens over battery-caged laying hens. He also recommended eating less or better yet no farm animal produce, which would mean no veal and probably no pork. As long as people consume farm animals and their produce, research to improve farm animal health and well-being is ethically acceptable.

Regan's Rights Views

Regan (1983) considered it permissible to eat meat if circumstances are such that required nutrients could not be obtained from other sources, just as did Singer. When humans (such as Eskimos) live in a subsistence economy, it is morally permissible to kill and eat animals to avoid starvation and to provide clothing and shelter. I believe this is another bit of Singerian utilitarianism lurking in Regan's arguments whenever difficult moral choices must be made.

Regan (1983, p. 240) used the word "animal" to refer to all (terrestrial, at least) moral agents and patients. Later (p. 349) he suggested that chickens and turkeys should be included, but (p. 417) that birds and fish are not subjects-of-a-life; he excluded sponges and oysters (p. 10) on the grounds that they probably are not conscious. If the subject-of-a-life stipulation is accepted it could remove fowl, fish, sponges, and oysters from the protected animal list. As discussed in chapter 7, he is not clear and consistent regarding what should be included as an animal.

I am not compelled by viewpoints that rely on the fact that animals can experience pain, because there is strong evidence that fish, lobster, crab, oysters, clams, mussels, worms, and insects have pain receptors of the types that could signal distress. One could claim that plants, although not having nervous systems, react positively and negatively to stimuli; they are constructed to respond protectively when traumatic stimuli are applied and positively to benign stimuli. Most do not include plants in the morally protected category, but relying on criteria that emphasize patterns of reaction to noxious stimuli walks a fine line.

DeGrazia (1996) made a sensible distinction between nociception and pain. Nociception refers to pain receptors (the necessary machinery and plumbing), which are present in all mammals and birds, indeed, all vertebrates and possibly some invertebrates. He used the term pain to refer to an unpleasant mental state, which implies that an affective state exists, which in turn implies a state of consciousness, which is probably not true of invertebrates and maybe not poultry.

Regan (1983) listed eight reasons that have been used to justify eating meat, to each of which he offered a rebuttal:

1. Animal flesh is tasty.
2. It is rewarding to prepare good-tasting dishes.
3. It is convenient and our habit to eat meat.
4. Meat is nutritious, and it could ruin one's health to stop eating it.
5. Many people have strong economic interests in raising food animals, and eliminating the market would lower their quality of life.
6. The nation has an economic interest in the maintenance and growth of the meat industry.
7. Farm animals are legal property, and farmers should be able to treat them as they wish to maximize the use of that property.

8. Some farm animals, e.g., chickens and turkeys, are not covered by the principles prescribed by the rights view.

Regan challenged the first two point on grounds similar to those Singer used: Such trivial reasons do not give one a right to violate important consequences when an animal is killed and eaten. If one loved the taste of ghetto children, it does not follow one had a right to kill and cook them in the interest of culinary adventure, a less than compelling analogy if the species barrier is accepted to make a moral difference, as held here.

His rejection of point 3 is based on the idea that custom does not justify morality. It was a custom to keep slaves, and we still are in the habit of discounting the equal moral standing of women and minorities, but most agree those practices are not moral. In addition, because something is convenient does not mean it justifies overriding rights. All of these seem to be sensible views.

Point 4 is that meat is a nutritious food, containing essential nutrients more difficult to obtain from other foods, with which Regan agrees. However, it is possible to take the modest trouble to obtain an adequate vegetarian diet, providing sufficient grounds against this point. The fact that consumers will neither take the time nor be intelligent enough to learn how to obtain the essentials is "patronizing in the extreme." It should be remembered, however, that people are well aware of the consequences of consuming too many fats and carbohydrates on their weight and consequent health, yet the problem of overweight individuals persists (let alone the continuation of smoking in spite of the strong likelihood of health problems). Even though arguments regarding the difficulty of maintaining an adequate vegetarian diet might be patronizing, they might still be correct.

Regan invoked the worse-off principle (see chapter 7) to counter the economic considerations involved in points 5 to 8. Regarding 5, he examined the idea that the farmer and his relatives would be worse off than the animals they raise because they would be financially ruined. His rights view does not permit aggregation (in chapter 7 I contested this claim in terms of its correctness, as well as his use of it), which makes it necessary to consider the case animal by animal. He observed that the farmer is engaged in a risky business venture and has voluntarily chosen to compete, which suspends the worse-off principle, and the farmer

should understand that fact. A response is that when the farmer voluntarily chose to compete he was not under the threat of vegetarian practices. If he had known the risks perhaps he would not have entered the
competition. An apt analogy might be that I could agree to a fencing
match provided we use guards on the tips of the foils. If, in the middle of
the match, you decide to remove the guards, that ain't right. Regan
suggested it is the responsibility of the farmer, meat packer, and butcher,
rather than the consumer, to take action to prevent their kith and kin
from being made worse off. If this idea is accepted it could also justify
militant counteractions to the vegetarian movement on the part of those
affected by any change in rules.

Carruthers (1992) sided with factory farmers when he balanced their
economic loss against what he called the admirable sensibilities of animal
lovers. He considered earning a living and maintaining a viable business
to be morally significant interests that should take priority over feelings,
and interests of humans override whatever harm is done to animals. In
respect for the feelings of animal lovers, society should be altered so that
it has no need for practices causing suffering to animals on a regular
basis, including compensation for those who might lose employment or
income. He regarded (p. xi) "the present popular concern with animal
rights in our culture as a reflection of moral decadence," which diverts
our attention from the immense human suffering that exists in the world.
Our response to animal lovers should not be (p. 168), ". . . 'If it upsets
you, don't think about it', but rather 'If it upsets you, think about
something more important.'" I find it difficult to believe many will agree
with his relative weighting of utilitarian values, which equates animal
rights with moral decadence, or his rather cavalier treatment of differences of opinion.

Another antiwelfarist, Leahy (1991), attributes welfarists' view that
using animals for food is a cardinal vice to the fact that disproportionate
numbers of animals are killed for food. He sides with Midgley, who
proposed that what animals need most urgently is a campaign for treating
them better before they are eaten, moving gradually toward consumption
of less meat. As usual, I agree with Midgley. However, I cannot agree
with Leahy's conclusion that those who regard eating meat as an evil
invasion of animal rights are "promulgating a sham"—their positions

may be disputed, but they are respectable ones. He conceded that it is possible to defend vegetarianism because the cruelty involved in raising and killing animals for food is unacceptable.

Regan held that farmers assume a moral burden when they breed or acquire animals, and that these moral duties are analogous to those they acquire when they have or adopt children. I suggest the analogy is bad: One's biological children reflect the output of the reproductive game that humans are evolutionarily set up to play, and adopted children receive the enhanced consideration due human moral patients by the human moral community, as well as being the beneficiaries of a social contract.

According to Regan, individual animals have inherent value and should not be treated as renewable resources (discussed in chapter 7). If the principles of equal inherent value and nonreplaceability are accepted, termination of an animal's life before it has run its natural course cannot be justified by saying that when it is killed its place will be filled by another. This violates the respect principle and treats an animal as a renewable resource based on its utility relative to the interests of others, rather than as an individual with inherent value.

Regarding the treatment of poultry (point 8), he changed his ground from when he placed chickens and turkeys outside the scope of principles prescribed by the rights view. The change reflects the difficulty in drawing the line between animals that do and do not satisfy the subject-of-a-life criterion, and we should not tolerate treatment of any farm animal as a renewable resource; therefore, chickens and turkeys should be included as rights holders. These are difficult views to accept on such a flimsy basis because it is critical to draw a clear line—permissible treatment depends on which side of the line an organism falls.

Regan's (1983, p. 345) conclusion regarding the meat industry is similar to that regarding scientific research in animals: "The rights view will not be satisfied with anything less than the total dissolution of the animal industry as we know it." He maintained (1975) that it should not be the vegetarian who is on the defensive to demonstrate how his "eccentric" way of life can be rationally defended, but the nonvegetarian who must justify the pain and suffering produced by his carnivorous way of life. The meat eater cannot escape the issue by the simple expedient of buying from farms where animals are not raised intensively because the animals are still killed, whether "humanely" or not. Such treatment only eliminates the further wrong of harming the individual before and while it is killed; it is less wrong, but that does not remove the fundamental injustice. He conceded that buying animals from farms that do not use intensive rearing methods would at least be a first step in the proper direction.

Positions based on national economic interests are denied because basic injustice still exists, and it is wrong no matter at what level the injustice occurs. He acknowledged that it is unlikely everyone will have an overnight conversion to vegetarianism, resulting in an instantaneous collapse of the meat industry. Rather, dissolution of the meat industry will be incremental, and the world will have time to adjust to the change in dietary lifestyle, as well as to absorb the economic impact.

Singer (1990a) agreed that dissolution of the meat industry will be gradual, and soon raising animals for food will become less profitable. Loss of profitability will induce farmers to turn to other types of farming, and giant corporations will invest their capital elsewhere. The result will be that the number of animals in factory farms will decline, because those killed will not be replaced. In a similar vein, Rollin (1995) discussed the advisability of having farmers raise pigs in the open rather than in confinement stalls. Then they will be able to get out of the pork business because they will have less capital investment in their facilities, and can put the land to other uses when the pork market becomes problematic. The factory farmer who uses confinement stalls must continue to make huge payments on expensive buildings and equipment, and is likely to fail unless the operation is part of a large corporate structure.

Laws that regulate the legal status of and set standards for treatment of animals are inconsistent, illogical, and badly in need of revision. As discussed in chapter 7, they do not consider animal welfare directly, but are based on the intended use, of the animal, and many laws regulating animal welfare apply only to those used in research. The USDA regulations implementing AWA are not abolitionist, but simply intended to guarantee that animal suffering is controlled (Rollin, 1995). Animals used in agriculture or raised for food have no legal protection other than the laws and regulations regarding the treatment of property, along with appeals to prevailing standards in the industry. Revision of such laws would be a major step toward reducing cruelty to animals, and it is a relatively simple and noncontroversial one to take.

Although animals are property under the law, Regan maintained that property rights are not absolute. The law should be reformed to impose strict constraints on what a farmer can do to an animal in the name of exercising his property rights. More fundamentally, animals should be recognized as legal persons, a point I dispute on the grounds that the status of personhood is a biological and social event attained only by humans at birth. It should be remembered that, under the law (discussed in chapter 7) many human persons are treated as property in contemporary society, including children, the elderly, and, to some extent, women.

Regan and Singer agreed that killing animals for meat should not be permitted, but the way they reached that conclusion differed. Regan characterizes Singer's utilitarian position as one that derives the right to equal consideration from the capacity for suffering and enjoyment. Singer believes animals' interests ought to be given equal consideration with the like interests of humans. Regan holds that Singer's preference utilitarianism must count the interests of humans involved in the industries of meat production when utilitarian calculations are made. Because these human interests involve considerable economic realities in support of the welfare, health, and education of vast numbers of people, they will weigh heavily in the balance, especially if matters are considered globally, thereby diminishing the value of animals in the calculations. He believes Singer trivializes the pleasures of taste because many go to great trouble and expense to prepare and consume tasty food.

The point of these reservations is to cast doubt on the adequacy of the utilitarian position as a challenge to meat eating and factory farming, especially if aggregation of interests is allowed. Regan notes that calculations that support Singer's position do not exist, and believes Singer must demonstrate that the consequences for all concerned would be better if all were vegetarians than if not, a challenge Singer cannot meet because he cannot produce the necessary empirical details. For these reasons, the rights view is more satisfactory. Because necessary empirical details have not been developed does not mean they cannot be. A serious attempt to scale costs and benefits should be attempted before the utilitarian position is rejected out of hand. Regan seems to have begun with an a priori conclusion and rejected out of hand any argument that weakens it.

Judgments of the degree of animal and human suffering have to be anthropocentric (Devine, 1978). All such judgments are made by rational human beings and thus filtered through their personalities and affected by social institutions, even though no particular bias may be universally shared. Morality is a human phenomenon, and all moral words are words in human language. In addition, all morality is egocentric, always involving questions of what I should do, with the root of morality being my conception of myself as a moral agent.

For example, unease is expressed about boiling lobsters for food, partly because of their violent reaction to being placed in boiling water, which evokes strong empathic reactions by humans. Less concern is expressed regarding fish, probably because they do not respond as vividly and have no appendages to flail about with, although they do have exquisite pain receptors. Few object to eating shrimp, and even fewer oysters and other bivalves, although they, too, are placed in boiling water while alive. Part of the basis for these beliefs depends on how much people identify with the animals' reactions, and party on a construal of the degree of suffering involved in the methods of killing them.

Devine (1978) rejected the premise that it is wrong to benefit from another's wrong-doing. If we live in the United States, the land on which we live and on which our bread is grown is land that was unjustly taken from the Native Americans. Yet, he finds it difficult to propose that we have an obligation to leave the country or abstain from all products grown here. A person might have an obligation to protest against injustices, but has no obligation to refuse to consume the products of injustice. He concluded (p. 483), "There has been so much injustice in human history that untainted merchandise is not available."

Factory Farming

One of the most questionable practices affecting animal welfare is the use of intensive methods to raise large numbers of animals with minimal regard for their quality of life. Singer dubbed this practice factory farming, and it has become the dominant method to raise and maintain livestock for meat, hens for eggs, and cows for milk products. The advantage of factory farming is its immense economy. Only a few technicians are required to maintain large numbers of animals, and they do not have to be highly skilled in the art of animal care. In 1940, each farm worker supplied food for eleven persons in the general population, and by 1990 each supplied for eighty persons (Rollin, 1995). The economies realized are sizable: In 1950, 30% of disposable income was spent on food, and in 1990 the figure dropped to only 11.8%. These economies are obtained by increasing productivity while decreasing feed costs For example, during the last half-century in the United States the number of eggs a hen lays doubled annually, but the amount of feed consumed for each egg decreased by 50%. At the same time, the cost of eggs to the consumer rose by only 40%, considerably less than increases in the cost of most other consumer goods (Mench & Tienhoven, 1986).

Another economic reality is that the mechanization required for factory farming requires construction of capitalized facilities, which means that agribusiness has become very large and most ordinary family farmers have been driven out of business. Recently, trends by concerned consumers to prefer and be willing to pay more for free-range turkeys, chickens, and eggs have made it possible for small ranchers to compete in that small market.

High technology makes it unnecessary (and impossible) to pay attention to individual animals (especially poultry, given that each bird has little economic worth), with the total emphasis on increased productivity at the lowest cost possible. It is axiomatic that welfare of the animals is given low priority. In previous times farmers had small numbers of animals raised under conditions more similar to those in which the animals evolved, thereby respecting them as a bundle of evolved characteristics. In earlier times, as Rollin (1995, p. 7) stated: "Producers did well if and only if animals did well, and . . . 'did well' for the animal meant playing out its biological nature in an environment for which those powers had been selected by both natural and artificial selection." Rollin characterized the western rancher's dictum as, "We take care of the animals; the animals take care of us."

Singer (1975) devoted considerable attention to the methods used in factory farms, and spurred the liberation and vegetarian movements through his stark portrayal of the conditions produced by such methods. One startling fact is the extremely large number of animals involved in these operations. In addition to billions of chickens, millions of turkeys, cattle, and pigs, about 10.7 million sheep are raised for wool and food (Conway, 1995). Sheep have received little discussion because almost all are raised and kept in free-range conditions, and lambs are not subjected to the tortuous experiences that veal calves (who also are killed at an early age) undergo. Methods of maintaining sheep are similar to those that have prevailed for many generations. I consider factory farm practices for three animals, poultry, cattle, and swine.

Poultry

Singer (1990a) cited estimates that 5.3 billion chickens are killed annually in the United States, with eight corporations responsible for 50% of them. Of these, 102 million broilers are killed each week when they are about seven weeks old (the normal life span of a free-range chicken is about seven years), and they weigh four to five pounds at slaughter. The Center for Science in the Public Interest reported that, by 1996, the United States produced 7 billion chickens (DeWaal, 1996). Most are raised in highly automated plants to which they are brought at one day of age, and placed in dim lighting with about half a square foot of space each. A typical cage holds three to five hens, and has wire floors that slope to the front of the cage so the eggs will roll down and be collected mechanically; wastes fall through the floor. To reduce the amount of feather-pecking and cannibalism that occur under such confined conditions the hens are debeaked. The beak has a highly sensitive soft tissue that resembles the "quick" of the human nail. About fifteen birds a minute are debeaked by burning away the upper beak with a hot blade, a procedure that probably causes severe pain.

In addition to birds raised for meat United States has millions of laying hens, with many producers having more than 500,000 and the largest over 10 million (Singer, 1990a). In 1990, 90% of laying hens in the United States were caged, $2.5 million is required to set up a 300,000-layer operation, and only one laborer is required per 100,000 birds (Varner, 1994a). The whole flock of layers is replaced every twelve to fifteen months, a less costly procedure than routinely culling hens that are not producing. To maintain 300,000 layers it is necessary to have about 600,000 births per year; given that half the chicks will be male, it is necessary to slaughter twice as many birds as there are layers.

In 1933 the average annual yield per hen was 70 eggs a year, and now it is 275 per year (Rollin, 1995), a much higher increase than Mench and Tienhoven reported in 1986. This immense increase is due to improvements in nutrition, disease control, intensive confinement systems, and breeding programs to select for egg-laying efficiency.

Another large segment of the poultry business is the $2 billion turkey industry. In 1985, 207 million turkeys were raised, with 20 large corporations producing 80% of them. DeWaal (1996) reported that 277 million turkeys were produced a year by 1996. The birds spend thirteen to twenty-four weeks in intensive conditions before they are slaughtered. There is no doubt that these intensive procedures are economically successful; the consumer is able to buy cheaper products and producers realize greater profits, although most small producers no longer are in business. Switzerland, The Netherlands, and Sweden have phased out the use of battery cages, and Britain is considering doing so (Singer, 1990a). Swedish laws passed in 1988 disallow confinement agriculture based on efficiency alone, mandating that the animal rearing be suited to the animals' natures (Rollin, 1995). Sweden has almost eradicated *Salmonella* contamination in chickens, and in the United States about 25% of broiler chickens are *Salmonella* contaminated (DeWaal, 1996).

Factory farming forces chickens to endure conditions that are below the acceptable minimal standards of life. The implication extends beyond that regarding the welfare of chickens. Intensive slaughtering and the preparation methods used to process the hundreds of thousands of chickens produced each day pose severe dangers to public health. Several procedures contribute to high contamination rates in poultry. First is the method used to kill them. They are shipped in cages crowded with other birds, and often arrive at the abattoir with feces on the feathers and skin; then they are hung by their feet and stunned. At this point they are brain dead, but other physiological processes continue, often resulting in defecation, with fecal matter remaining on the skin and feathers. Then they go through machines that have small rubber fingers to loosen and remove feathers, which can be another source of contamination. Machines are not cleaned between birds, making it possible for contamination of the dirtiest bird to be distributed to clean ones. Birds are then placed in a hot water bath to loosen any remaining feathers, followed by chilling in large vats of cold water. These baths allow carcasses contaminated with the two most frequent bacteria, *Salmonella* and *Campylobacter* and *E. coli* to infect clean carcasses. During the time in the baths carcasses gain up to 8% additional weight from the water, which often has chlorine added to it to minimize levels of bacterial contamination. Finally, contamination can be spread when birds go through automatic evisceration machines, and it is not possible to prevent intestinal contents from spilling into the cavity.

Under the Poultry Products Inspection Act, federal inspections are required to examine birds prior to slaughter, inspect each carcass after slaughter and before processing, inspect plant facilities and all slaughter and processing practices to ensure sanitary conditions, and verify the truthfulness and accuracy of product labeling. Birds are inspected while they are on a conveyor line, and the NAS observed that inspectors have only two to three seconds to examine each bird to decide on its suitability (DeWaal, 1996).

These methods are quite different from those used with beef and pork. When a poultry carcass is contaminated with fecal matter or stomach contents it is reprocessed by washing with chlorinated water. Beef and pork must be trimmed to remove contamination. Poultry are chilled by total immersion in cold water (often chlorinated), whereas beef and pork are chilled using cold air along with spray chilling. Many European and Canadian producers use air rather than water chilling. One study was reported to have found that the prevalence of *Salmonella* on carcasses increased by as much as 28% from the prechill to postchill sampling points. DeWaal (1996) estimated that *Salmonella* and *Campylobacter* contamination of meat and poultry products is responsible for as many as 4 million illnesses and up to 3,000 deaths per year in the United States, and the USDA estimated that health costs are as much as $3.4 billion a year.

Cattle

The United States cattle herd is estimated to be 98 million (Conway, 1995), and 34 million cattle were slaughtered in 1987 (Singer, 1990a).

Most beef cattle spend much of their early life in range conditions, and the feedlots to which they are sent before slaughter are considered to be the least problematic of all intensive production units (Rollin, 1995). Rollin noted that many of the questionable procedures involved in cattle ranching are not due to industrialization, but are holdovers from early traditions. Some of these procedures are castration done under field conditions with no anesthetic or asepsis, branding with a hot iron (which lowers the hide value for leather by about $7 a head), dehorning, and rough handling ("cowboying"), especially while transporting the animals. Simple alternatives to these practices are available, and Rollin believes ranchers are more open to correcting them than are those involved in other aspects of the meat industry, especially because the improvements would be to the economic advantage of ranchers in terms of better health and quality of animals. Although beef consumption has dropped over the years, the total number of animals killed, when both beef and poultry are counted, has increased 300% due to a concomitant increase in poultry consumption (Varner, 1994a).

Another aspect of the cattle industry is the dairy business, which has become increasingly dependent on large, intensive operations, with as many as 3,000 cows maintained in a relatively small acreage. It was estimated that there were about 10 million active milk cows in the United States in 1990 (Varner, 1994a). The calf mortality rate is about 20% in dairy farms, and a milk cow is slaughtered after about three years of production.

Intensive methods make it possible to devote closer attention to the welfare of the cows, which is important because of the high economic worth of each individual. A cow can produce 10,000 to 36,000 pounds of milk per year, thereby making it worth the dairy owner's time to protect that valuable capital asset.

Because of these economic interests, much attention has been devoted to research aimed to improve the welfare of both cows and calves. Outside hutches reduce calf mortality compared with inside ones. Separating a calf from its mother right after birth causes less stress to the pair than does the usual procedure of separating them after three days, and separated calves seem content when they can see calves. It appears that calves raised under the stress of isolation produce more milk as adults, although the research is not extensive.

An aspect of the cattle industry that has received widespread criticism is the production of white veal. Veal is the flesh of a young calf, and traditionally the calf was killed before weaning. This flesh is tender and pale because the calf has not yet begun to eat grass, living only on mother's milk. The preference for pale veal led ranchers to raise calves in confinement, feeding them high-protein food and not letting them have iron in their diet, practices that enhance the light color of the meat produced by the sedentary, anemic calves. Veal of this type is highly preferred, especially in expensive restaurants and upscale markets, where it commands a high price.

The veal calf is confined in a wooden stall 1 foot 10 inches wide by 4 feet 6 inches long, with a slotted wooden floor raised above a concrete shed floor. The calf is tethered so it cannot turn around and it has no straw or bedding. It is fed a totally liquid diet based on nonfat milk powder with vitamins, minerals, and growth promoters sixteen weeks, at which time is weighs as much as 400 pounds, as compared with 90 pounds at birth (Singer, 1990a).

Even cattlemen find the procedures used to produce white veal offensive (Rollin, 1995), especially because a calf could be killed while young without subjecting it to the torture of confinement. However, the difference between the 400-pound calf and the 90-pound newborn represents a sizable monetary difference. The veal industry is not large, and its practices could be modified or restricted to slaughter of newborn calves without any great loss to society or agribusiness. The British government requires that the calf be able to turn around and fed a diet containing sufficient iron to maintain it in full health; similar laws exist in Sweden.

Swine

All things considered, pigs appear to have one of the worst deals in the meat industry. Authorities consider pigs to be the most intelligent of farm animals, to have a high level of curiosity, high learning ability, and a complex behavioral repertoire. Over 90% of the estimated 56 million pigs in the United States are raised in some kind of confinement (Conway, 1995; Rollin, 1995). The typical practice is to keep sows in gestation stalls while pregnant, which is most of their three to five-year life. These stalls are 2 feet wide, 7 feet long, and 3.3 feet high, and are in environmentally controlled facilities. The pigs are fed and cared for by unskilled labor. It is possible to maintain them with a minimal amount of food because they do not expend energy on thermoregulation or movement. They show the strong stereotypical behavior indicative of abnormality, such as bar chewing, chain chewing, and vacuum chewing at nothing. Merely providing straw in the stall reduces or eliminates these stereotypies, but it is usually not provided because it interferes with the common procedures for waste disposal—concrete slatted floors for manure to fall through into an automatic manure-handling system that cannot handle straw easily (Rollin, 1995).

European studies led to the abolition of confinement in Sweden, and to the development of alternative housing systems in a number of other countries (Rollin, 1995). These studies varied degrees and types of confinement and rearing conditions. One involved 1,600 sows in a 40-acre facility. No gestation stalls were used, and the sows were placed in farrowing crates for about four weeks to avoid crushing piglets. The rest of the time about sixteen sows were kept in group pens that had both a concrete and a sand portion. They could dig, root, and play in the sand, and displayed almost no stereotypical behavior or fighting. When the weather was bad they could move to the concrete portion. Some of the animals were housed in outdoor pens to finish them before slaughter. The bottom line indicated that the cost per pound of pork was two cents higher than when the pigs were finished indoors. The down side is that the labor force must be knowledgeable about the animals.

Another study compared the conventional system with an alternative one that included pen gestation, straw bedding, pen farrowing, free feeding during lactation, an area for piglets to creep in, and weaning at four to six weeks of age. The average cost of facilities per sow was 50% higher with the conventional system, suggesting that alternative methods might result in more profits for the owners, as well as improved life for the pigs. Rollin noted that little research has been done, and with a commitment to research, vast improvements could be realized in the industry. He suggested that the USDA should hire a full-time swine behaviorist to develop an understanding of the animals, and to make it possible to put that knowledge to practical use.

Rollin (1995) surveyed the farm animal industry and concluded that alternative approaches to many of the problematic aspects of current systems already exist. Relatively small expenditures of research money could produce noticeable results fairly quickly, improve economic gains for producers, offer a higher quality of life for animals, and mean a safer product for consumers. Callicott (1980) concluded that rather than eating vegetables in preference to meat, it is important to resist factory farming, especially with its liberal application of pesticides, and herbicides. He also objected to the use of chemical fertilizers to maximize production of vegetable crops.

Attempts to label products that are genetically engineered, or where hormones have been administered to the animals or the product, are strongly approved by the dairy and meat industries. Fox suggested the poor should be educated regarding less costly substitutes in their diets should they not be able to afford meat products, a suggestion that might well be met with storms of protest among many who would see it as patronizing and elitist.

Most vegetarians (estimated to be between less than 1% to 4% of the United States population) are working toward the abolition of meat eating by degrees, although as soon as possible. Fox (1990) suggested the effective first step is to become a "conscientious omnivore" know "whom" you eat, how it was raised, transported, and slaughtered. It is hard to disagree with this suggestion, unless one adamantly holds the position that meat eating is a human right, or is an inherent part of our carnivorous beginnings. The first position is difficult to defend on philosophical grounds, and the latter smacks of the naturalistic fallacy. Fox suggested that all should endeavor to eat "low on the food chain" to reduce inefficiencies, waste, animal exploitation, and the environmental costs that excessive meat consumption produces. Again, this is a difficult position to contest. Francione (1995) expressed pessimism because conservationists express concern only for animals mistreated in modern agriculture, but not to the extent of agreeing to pay for alternatives.

Fox (1990) proposed that farm animal produce be graded in terms of how the animals were raised, so that informed consumers could select products from humanely raised animals. This is done to some extent in the poultry industry in the United States, with consumers able to buy free-range chickens and turkeys, free-range eggs, and poultry and eggs from animals that are grain fed and are hormone free. Of course, these products are more expensive than those produced by intensive methods, making it likely that only the economically advantaged and informed citizenry will be free to make those choices.

Vegan Diets

The extreme position is taken by those who simply refuse to eat meat or use meat products, who consume only plant products and eschew all animal and dairy products, a group estimated to represent about 2% to 9% of vegetarians. The vegan position is without doubt the most consistent one, but it also means that those who accept and practice it experience the most disruption of usual customs and traditions of human society.

The adequacy of a vegan diet that excludes consumption of all animal products has been debated. The issue is whether an animal-free diet would place humans at serious risk compared with the usual omnivorous diet or a semivegetarian diet including milk and eggs. The question of adequacy should be examined for different classes of people who have different nutritional requirements: Adult men, infants and children, adolescents, pregnant and lactating women, the elderly, poor, and undereducated.

Such a debate was engaged in the *Journal of Agricultural and Environmental Ethics* in 1993 and 1994. Part of it was represented by Pluhar (1993, 1994) and Varner (1994a, 1994b) upholding the adequacy of a vegan diet; George (1994a, 1994b) questioning its adequacy; and nutrition experts Mangels and Havala (1994) and Dwyer and Loew (1994) weighing in with moderate commentaries. The disputants raised economic, moral, and nutritional issues, but I concentrate on the last, with only an aside regarding the first two, these having been discussed at length throughout this book.

Pluhar (1993) insisted that it is not necessary to supplement vegan diets as long as the skills and knowledge of a registered dietitian are used to obtain unconventional food sources (especially high-calcium vegetable greens, such as kale). She distinguished between planned and unplanned vegan diets, noting that the former can be adequate in all respects, except for Vitamin D; that, however, can be obtained through adequate exposure to sunlight. It may be difficult to obtain adequate amounts of vitamin B_{12} unless one eats cereals that are fortified with the vitamin. In fact, nonvegetarian diets can be unhealthy due to overconsumption of meat and calories, which can lead to health problems, especially those related to obesity. She concluded that both vegetarians and nonvegetarians should have their diets monitored and receive information and education regarding nutrition. Most problems would be avoided if milk and eggs were consumed, with a strong moral caveat that they not be obtained from sources involving factory farming.

George (1994a) maintained that a vegan diet favors middle-class adults in high-technological societies, especially men because their dietary needs are less stringent than those of women, children, and the elderly. Also, a vegan diet is too high in bulk if it is adequate in nutrition. She (1994b) agreed with Pluhar that vegetarian and vegan diets can be safe if they are monitored carefully, and if individuals live in a society (such as ours) where a wide variety and quantity of foods, education, and medicine are available.

It is harder for women and children to achieve an adequate diet than for adult men. Adult males rarely suffer from anemia, do not lose iron through menstruation, and do not carry fetuses in their bodies or nurse infants. For these reasons George rejected Varner's (1994b) comment that all diets have risks and that inequalities can be corrected by taking supplements; she considered this viewpoint based on the principle of separate but equal.

George (1994b) compared the nutritional aspects of hamburger and green leafy vegetables in terms of the quantity of each a fourteen-year-old girl would have to eat to get the same nutritional benefit. A three-ounce lean hamburger patty has the same amount of iron as four cups of lettuce, two and one half cups of green beans, and three-fourth cup of spinach. In terms of calories the hamburger provides 190 kcal, the lettuce 40, green beans 75, and spinach 30. Because the teenager is still growing and requires more energy than adults, and also has a smaller stomach capacity, the amounts necessary to maintain adequate levels of energy, protein, and nutrients may be excessive. The same picture emerges for iron: 20% of iron from lean beef is absorbable, 18% from chicken, 7% from soybeans, 1.6% from black beans, 1.4% from spinach, and 4.4% from lettuce (George, 1994b). The adolescent would have to eat twelve times the three-fourth cup of spinach, or four point five times the four cups of lettuce to get the same amount of iron as contained in the beef patty.

A semivegetarian diet might be preferable, especially a lacto-ovo-vegetarian one, which is a hyphenated way to say one that excludes meat but includes milk and eggs (Mangels & Havala, 1994). In addition, lactating women, infants, children, and adolescents on a Vegan diet are at greater risk of nutritional deficits than men, and pregnant women require supplements especially of vitamin B_{12}, calcium, and iron. Iron needs of pregnant women rise so much after the second trimester that supplements are usually required, especially since a lesser proportion of iron from plant sources is absorbed by the gut (Dwyer & Loew, 1994). High doses of iron should be avoided, however, because zinc intakes tend to be low in vegans, and too much iron may depress serum zinc levels even lower. The authors also recommended calcium supplements for all pregnant women, especially vegans.

Vegan children should eat foods with high caloric density, have B_{12} supplements, and vitamin D if they are not exposed to enough sun, and they should consume nondairy calcium by eating dark green, leafy vegetables (Mangels & Havala, 1994). Care should be taken to avoid hypervitaminosis due to extreme supplementation. The authors (p. 118) concluded: "Health professionals need to be more tolerant of vegans. They follow their diets for strongly held beliefs and deserve the same respect afforded to other groups that have dietary restrictions, such as Jews, Muslims, and Hindus." This admirable sentiment could be endorsed, while remembering that some religious sects have unusual diets and eschew health care (e.g., yogic groups).

A study of vegan children discussed by Varner (1994b) reported that between 37% and 52% of weaned children fell below the twenty fifth percentile in weight and length for their age. This might not be due to diet as much as to the fact that 49% of children followed a macrobiotic diet and another 24% were members of yogic groups. Still, caution is in order whenever dietary regimens are out of the ordinary.

Where people do not have access to a variety of nonanimal foods, eschewing meat all but ensures malnutrition, and strict vegetarianism has several economic impacts (Varner, 1994b): It might be more detrimental

to the environment to fashion clothing and other products out of nonrenewable sources such as petroleum products than to continue exploiting
renewable animal resources; if laying hens were not kept in factory farms,
eggs would be less uniform in quality, higher in price, and less widely
available; if dairy cattle were not kept in factory farms, milk would be
more expensive and less available; and health care costs would be greater
due to inadequate nutrition status of the underprivileged, who would be
affected more because they could not afford the high cost products. The
principle of equal consideration of interests requires us to accommodate
similarly situated individuals, while at the same time recognizing differences among cultures. Respect for equal treatment might result in a
different view of human's moral relationship with animals, depending on
the circumstances a culture faces.

A similar thesis was mounted by Pluhar (1993), to the extent that
moral agents who are unaware that sentient animals, as well as humans,
are rights holders hardly qualify as immoral when they kill and eat
sentient nonhumans. Pluhar extended this to include moral agents who
"sincerely and non-culpably" reject this rights view, or are poor, uneducated, or disadvantaged omnivores. I find this view unsettling; it
could be extended to justify human cannibalism if it was decided that
those outside the community did not hold rights, an intuitively unacceptable conclusion. It could justify the view that rational adults, who must
abide by principles of moral right and wrong, could be excluded if they
were ignorant. This argument is insufficient because it could be used to
excuse a murderer who "in good faith" rejected a moral rule against
killing innocent persons (George, 1994b). Pluhar's view of morality
could be used to excuse almost everyone in the world except those in
Western societies, which George took to mean something is wrong with
that view.

Conclusions

The emphasis throughout this discussion of methods used to produce
meat, dairy, and poultry products focused on the welfare of animals and
on the economic realities facing producers and consumers. Major concerns also arise regarding the safety of products for consumers, especially
methods of processing chickens. Another important problem is the effect

meat industry practices have on broader conservation issues. Maintaining large herds of sheep and cattle can have disastrous environmental consequences. In many instances ranges are overgrazed, rivers polluted, and native environments devastated by too many animals in herds maintained on the land. The resource input (in the form of feed grain) required to produce beef could better be used to feed starving populations of humans. Beef cattle may be so high on the food chain, that they must have a negative impact on environmental resources, and thus it is impossible to harvest enough resources to feed starving populations throughout the world. Therefore, efforts should be directed toward making more effective use of natural resources.

Callicott (1980) challenged the idea that it would ecologically be better for us all to become vegetarians, that the trophic niche of humans should be shifted from those of an omnivore with carnivorous preferences to an herbivore. This shift would shorten the food chains that terminate at humans, and represent increasing efficiency in the conversion of solar energy from plant to human biomass. If food resources are increased, the human population would be expected to expand as a result, there would be fewer nonhumans, and more humans, who have far more elaborate requirements than do domestic animals. These requirements would tax natural resources (such as trees for shelter and products, minerals that are mined at the expense of topsoil and vegetation, and overuse of agricultural lands) more than at present. Thus a vegetarian human population would be more likely to be ecologically catastrophic than result in an ecological godsend.

13

Species Preservation, Zoos, and Pets

Major threats to animals and the habitats on which they depend resulted from actions by human agents. Rampant human destruction of ecosystems on which many species of plants and animals depend produced radical environmental changes and caused an almost unprecedented rate of extinction of species in recent years. These extinctions raised strong concerns regarding issues in biodiversity (e.g., Wilson, 1992) that led to the development of a land ethic (Leopold, 1949, Callicott, 1980). Some maintain that species preservation is of major importance, and the world's zoos responded. The importance of preserving ecosystems to support living beings at all levels was stressed. E. O. Wilson (1994, p. 362) phrased the matter clearly: ". . . the most important implication of an innate biophilia is the foundation it lays for an enduring conservation ethic. If a concern for the rest of life is part of human nature, if part of our culture flows from wild nature, then on that basis alone it is fundamentally wrong to extinguish other life forms. Nature is part of us, as we are part of Nature." Many animal rightists and liberationists consider efforts to preserve species misguided, preferring that the major effort be directed toward preserving habitats rather than capturing and removing animals from the wild.

In this chapter I sketch issues concerning species preservation, and consider the importance of maintaining biodiversity. I assess the role of zoos and how the zoo community responded to the challenge of saving endangered species with the intent of reintroducing them into the wild. The general purposes of zoos, as well as the status of pets, is addressed in light of objections made by animal welfarists regarding the permissibility of keeping animals in captivity for any reason. Although many animals are kept in captivity in zoos, many more are kept as pets in human households. Another large captive population of animals is used as companions to assist humans in their everyday activities; for example, working dogs, draught animals, tools for falconers, guide dogs for the blind, and companions for the lonely.

Problems of the Ecosystem

Statistics indicate that species are becoming extinct at an alarming rate, and that most of these extinctions are caused by human exploitation and misuse of the environment (Wilson, 1993). About 1.4 million species have been named to date, with the actual number likely to be between 10 and 100 million. About 1.6 million are fungi, 8 to 10 million arthropod species found in tropical rain forests, millions of invertebrate species on the floor of the deep seas, and untold numbers of species of bacteria.

Wilson estimated that the number of species on earth is being reduced by a rate that is 1,000 to 10,000 times higher than was estimated to have occurred throughout prehuman times. Much of this increase is attributed to removal of tropical rain forest at a rate of about 1.8% of the cover each year, which at present logging levels would leave about 10% standing in twenty years (Conway, 1995). Humans also are destroying other species-rich habitats, such as coral reefs, river systems, lakes, and heathlands, the loss of which decimates resident populations of organisms. Wilson's widely cited estimate is that 20% or more of the earth's species will disappear or undergo early extinction during the next thirty years.

There is a sense of urgency that immediate action must be taken to save many animal species or it will be forever too late (Norton, Hutchins, Stevens, & Maple, 1995). Extinction is forever, and rare species should be the focus of conservation biology (Wilson, 1993, p. 228). Wilson likened the sense of immediacy held by conservation biologists to that of doctors in an emergency ward: "They look for quick diagnoses and procedures that can prolong the life of species until more leisurely remedial work is possible." In Norton's (1987) analogy, the extinction of a species was like the burning of all copies of a book.

It is agreed that humans largely are responsible for losses in biodiversity, and this culpability creates a moral obligation to respond to impacts of the expansion of human populations on wild habitats. Disagreements exist regarding what should be done, whether the effects on the ecosystem and evolutionary processes are all negative, and at what level the impact of extinctions should be evaluated. Norton (1995) advised care regarding the level at which preservation priorities should be set: To preserve genes, individuals, populations, species, communities, ecosystems, all of the above, or none of the above.

It is important to understand the science of ecology to have proper respect for the complexity and interrelatedness of ecosystems. Norton, professor of philosophy at the Georgia Institute of Technology, in his book *Why preserve natural variety?* (1987), wrote that an ethic founded on ecology is essential because it is built on values embedded in observations of the world that are influenced by cognitive values. Because ethical statements are not derived abstractly from relations between statements, there is no naturalistic fallacy: The *ought* is not deduced from the *is*—they are separated by reflection regarding the complexity, interrelatedness, and fragility of biotic systems, and this places humanity in a position that reflects the importance of the integrity of ecosystems.

Individualism

Concerns over the level of analysis are examined first because they sharply demarcate the philosophical differences between animal welfarists and environmentalists. An exclusive focus on individuals constrains one from considering animal welfare in terms of general aspects of evolution and ecology. Part of this constraint is produced by sheer ignorance. For example, DeGrazia (1996) does not find it plausible that the discontinuation of a single species out of the innumerable species on earth can inflict terrible damage on the ecosystem, a statement that flies in the face of abundant ecological data. A snowball effect is often seen whereby elimination of one key species causes the collapse of an entire ecosystem and extinction of all species within it. According to one estimate, for every plant species that becomes extinct, fifteen animal species can be expected to follow (Norton, 1987).

Advocates of animal welfare positions, such as the rights views of Regan, constrain analysis to the level of moral rights of individual animals, denying the permissibility of aggregation across individuals or consideration of attributes of larger "superorganisms." Regan (1995) spoke against any holistic position that emphasizes monitoring the harmony of the larger community of life: It is the interests of particular animals that are of paramount importance. The holistic view represents what he considers an inadmissible utilitarianism, regarding individuals as meaningful only in the instrumental sense of promoting the welfare of the biotic community. In terms of the survival of endangered species, Regan (1983) concluded that if a choice is to be made between saving the last two members of an endangered species or saving another individual who belonged to a plentiful species, but whose death would be a greater harm to that individual than the harm of death to the two, the individual from the plentiful species should be saved. In his view, numbers make no difference; it does not matter whether the choice is between saving the last 2,000 or million members of a species rather than only 2. Aggregating over numbers of individuals is impermissible: The proper test must involve the greater harm done to each individual. I find this not only a counter-intuitive conclusion, but one that is incompatible with much of what is known about general processes in biological sciences concerned with organism and environment interactions.

Singer (1993) rejected the idea that species have interests above and beyond those of their individual members. Because species are not conscious entities, they cannot have preferences and interests that should be respected. He confined his notions to the interests of sentient creatures. DeGrazia (1996) maintained that there is no being corresponding to the words "nature," "biosphere," or "the environment" who would benefit, thereby making the interests of individuals primary. Both Regan and Singer contended that because one organism is a member of an endangered species, the rare individual is not intrinsically more important. Whenever species preservation and animal welfare conflict, DeGrazia (1996) did not see any justification to sacrifice an individual's interests, especially if the individual is going to be kept in captivity and forced to mate.

Sober (1986) considered this point of view to represent a major difference between welfarists and those environmentalists for whom the endangered status makes all the difference. The animal welfare ethic is based on the life situation of an individual, whereas that of the environmentalist is based on stability and diversity of populations of individuals.

Some hold (e.g., Jamieson, 1995a, 1995b; Loftin, 1995) that efforts would better be expended to save habitats than to capture, breed, and reintroduce animals, because no habitats will be available to introduce animals into. Jamieson's view (1995a) is that if the last few remaining animals are removed from a habitat and the habitat is saved, nothing will be left to inhabit it except the few captives, and they will be unlikely to survive and reproduce upon reintroduction. For this reason, most zoo breeding programs are a "cruel hoax." Most zoo animals are not going back to the wild, because the wild no longer exists for them, which led Maple (1995) to justify the existence of zoos primarily for reasons of public education. Regan (1983, p. 361) concluded that the best policy regarding animals is to "*let them be!*"

Environmentalism

Environmentalists reject the idea that basic analyses should be at the individual level. The broadest view is the land ethics approach (e.g., Leopold, 1949; Callicott, 1980) that considers the good of the biotic community to be the ultimate measure of moral value. Leopold (1949) is the pioneer of the land ethics movement, and it is appropriate to begin with a brief quotation from *A Sand County almanac* (p. 204): "A land ethic of course cannot prevent the alteration, management, and use of the 'resources,' but it does affirm their right to continued existence, and, at least in spots, their continued existence in a natural state. In short, a land ethic changes the role of *Homo sapiens* from conqueror of the land-community to plain member and citizen of it. It implies respect for his fellow-members and also respect for the community as such."

The land ethic generally assigns more value to an animal of an endangered species than to one of a common species, no matter what the level of cognitive or sensory development. In this view, an endangered plant could be valued more than an introduced rabbit that eats it, even though the rabbit has more qualities that would confer on it a higher moral value. Each species has a role to play within the ecological system, and the important factor is the relationship among them. The land ethic extends moral consideration to plants, microorganisms, and insects, not for their own sake, but for that of the entire system (Loftin, 1995).

The land ethic accepts captive breeding if and only if the goal is restoration, but not if the goal is to keep the species in captivity forever. If there is no alternative to allowing the extinction of a species, animals should be taken from the wild for captive breeding programs, but only as a last-ditch, desperation effort. When species are endangered, captive propagation is the only alternative to condemning species and ecosystems willfully to certain and very cruel death (Geist, 1995). Such beliefs were upheld by Leopold (1949) and E. O. Wilson (1984) using the first rule of the tinkerer: Keep all the pieces.

According to Norton (1995), it is permissible to sacrifice a member of one species for the well-being of another whenever that sacrifice can be justified as necessary to protect natural communities and habitats to perpetuate large numbers of species. Natural evolutionary processes are more basic than the interests of individuals because they direct the creation and sustenance of individuals in the long run.

With natural selection at work, each assemblage of successive species modifies the environment to make it unfavorable to themselves, favoring the path for a new assemblage that can exploit those changed conditions more efficiently (Vrijenhoek, 1995). Or, the members of a species might adapt in ways that make them able to exploit the new conditions more effectively and continue as the same species, with a few modifications here and there. Vrijenhoek (1995, p. 78) described evolutionary processes in a compelling manner: "What really evolves is a cloud of genes. New mutations arise in the cloud, many are lost, and some replace ancestral genes. Sometimes, a cloud splits (cladogenesis) and gives rise to independent lineages, or even new species (speciation). Together, cladogenesis and anagenesis are responsible for the diversification that we associate with the evolutionary process. In contrast, discrete clouds sometimes hybridize and fuse (reticulate) into one."

Rolston (1992) discussed the values and disvalues involved when examining nature. He proposed a series of natural occurrences that may be considered to be disvalues that, at one level would be considered bad, but when viewed at other levels could be seen to have strong positive values. One was predation: Certainly if you are a prey animal it is bad to be eaten. However, predators have a positive value when considered systemically because the death of the prey means life to the predators. The most fundamental fact of life in the biotic community is to be eating—and be eaten. Whatever moral entitlements a being may have as a member of the biotic community, right to life is not among them.

Matters are not quite so simple, however. Although the individual prey is killed and loses its life, the population of which it is a member might gain, because there is selection for better skills at avoiding predation, and more prey will become more sentient and cognizant of the danger, allowing them to reproduce more successfully. As Rolston (1992, p. 254) stated it: "Being eaten is not always a bad thing, even from the perspective of the prey species. The predator depends on a continuing prey population; they have entwined destinies." He goes on: "A world without blood would be poorer, but a world without bloodshed would be poorer too. Among other things, it would be a world without humans—not that humans now cannot be vegetarians but that the evolution of humans would never have taken place." Cost or benefit to any individual is not the relevant consideration; it is the effect on biological systems that plays an important role to tune the players to act in the theater of life being played on the evolutionary stage. Callicott (1989) added that the humane eradication of predators could destroy a biotic community because it could destroy the very species that are intended beneficiaries of this misplaced morality; prey species often depend on predators to optimize levels of their populations.

Another example of seeming disvalue is parasitism. Surely, one must consider a parasite evil—it often sucks nutrients out of the host, cripples it, and takes a tremendous toll on life. Considered in a broader perspective, however, what is found is coevolution of vertebrate hosts and parasites; infections caused by common parasites tend to be of low virulence. Such coevolution is necessary if the parasite itself is to survive. If it becomes too effective it exterminates the individuals of the host species to a level that the species may face extinction. A parasite can also increase its chances of surviving by increasing the host's chance of survival by developing a symbiotic relationship that is to the benefit of both—you scratch my back and I'll scratch yours. A good strategy for a parasite is to benefit the host a bit. The advantage to the host might be the parasite's ability to eliminate other disease vectors, leading the host to develop general immune responses to the effects of those vectors. This process of give and take can regulate animal populations at many levels.

Another idea is that natural processes entail great waste. Many species of plants and animals produce immense numbers of propagules, only a few of which mature and enter the breeding population; they are said to be r-selected. Does this mean these surplus expendables represent profligate waste in nature? Not in the least. As something dies, something else makes a living by scavenging it. "One organism's waste is another organism's treasure" (Rolston, 1992, p. 269). There is not much waste in natural systems, although there are exuberance and fecundity.

A distinct difference exists between naturally directed extinctions and those inflicted by humans. Naturally directed selection always works with existing gene assemblages within the context of the environment that imposes the selection pressures that induce change. Aspects of the environment change when species succession occurs, along with characteristics of such elements as vegetation and soil. A pioneer species starting a new process of exploiting the environment is expected to disappear during the course of various phases of succession (Brennan, 1986). When natural extinctions occur, a transformation accompanies the losses that affects related and competing lines of organisms.

Because extinction is natural in evolutionary reality, it may be better to let things be and hope that life on earth is completely extinguished (Hargrove, 1995). Then speciation will begin again, and sooner or later massive biodiversity will reappear. Under current policies, zoos can be considered the arks that will eventually land and discharge their passengers into reconstructed habitats. Some doubt, however, that the boat ride will ever end, and if so zoo breeding programs are less justifiable. Perhaps efforts should be directed toward docking the ark at miniature natural habitats [construed by Maple (1995) as *naturalistic* environments], bringing the journey of some species to the natural conclusion of extinction. Although these suggestions have merit, the idea that we should let existing species be extinguished and hope for a better roll of the dice next time does not excite me. I would opt for any number of sunnier possibilities.

In contrast to the gradual natural processes involved in species and habitat succession, human activities produce more devastating and rapid effects through massive habitat destruction and fragmentation, environmental pollution, and excessive harvesting and hunting. Artificial extinction occurs without issue. Doors are not opened—only closed. Humans generate and regenerate nothing when they induce extinction, they only dead-end the extinguished lines.

For any species population, freedom is the absence of human intervention of any kind in the natural processes by which it preserves itself (Taylor, 1986). However, a problem concerns what should be done when the processes of natural selection already are relaxed due to human intervention. From an evolutionary perspective, the struggle for survival is important to the continued viability of a breeding population of organisms. If the genetic composition of individuals in the population is variable, if this variability has produced some individuals that can cope with a change in selection pressure, and if that coping adaptation is heritable, humans should not interfere with natural processes. However, if humans have domesticated or otherwise restricted the free patterns of animals, and the same selection pressure (for example, a disease vector) appears, it would be appropriate for humans to intervene, treat the animals, and nurture them to survival. Even though this might result in a population that is less resistant to disease, humans have placed them under the protective custody of captivity, and having interfered with the natural struggles for life, they must nurture those whose full freedoms they curtailed.

Concern for the protection of each individual animal does not begin until the pool of animals representing the species becomes so small that the death of any individual may lead to extinction of the species (Hargrove, 1995). When such an endangered status no longer exists and the species has been restored to acceptable levels, concern for individual animals disappears and the emphasis once again is to preserve the species. With this emphasis a primary task is to preserve those aspects of the environment essential to the survival of the species. The focus on species rather than on individuals is one of the stumbling blocks that makes it difficult for welfarists and environmentalist to agree.

It might not be possible to avoid conflicts inherent in the positions held by those endorsing different philosophical premises, and it might be necessary, especially for zoo professionals, to take steps to understand, coexist, and manage within a contentious social context (Wuichel & Norton, 1995). As with many differences in the moral sphere, it may not be possible to reach agreement, given different initial premises. It might be possible, however, for welfarists and environmentalists to make some coordinated efforts to deal with the preservation of endangered species at least as far as rescuing the remaining individual animals and restoring crucial habitats are involved.

It is possible that even this expectation is too optimistic, given the views of some welfarists that it is never permissible to hold any animal captive because the animal's freedom is compromised (Regan, 1995). Regan believes the only permissible reason to capture an animal is to remove it temporarily from the threat of human predation, with a caveat that when this threat has abated the animal is reintroduced into the wild. This rights view does not consider it permissible to confine animals in zoos for educational or recreational purposes, to provide models for scientific research, to benefit the local region economically, to protect rare or endangered species, to ensure a genetic stock, or for any other reason that forwards the interests of other individuals, humans or nonhumans. It will be difficult for any environmentalist to work within the confines of such proscriptions.

Many positions adopted by those who espouse the individualistic liberationist and rightist philosophies can be construed to be antihuman. Regan insists it is permissible to capture animals under threat of human predation, but not if the predator is a nonhuman animal, even if the natural threat might eliminate all individuals of a species. Again, his suggestion is, "let it be." Jamieson (1995b) believes the essential conflict involved in killing or confining an animal to preserve a species is between the interest of the animal and the human desire to preserve the species. We have little evidence that animals other than humans care about the preservation of other species, a point with which I readily agree. I would add, nor do they care about moral philosophy, duties, or obligations. These matters worry only us, and not them.

Here is a basic paradox: The individualistic ethic begins by emphasizing similarities between human and nonhuman individuals, but ends with greater willingness to sacrifice human individuals than nonhuman ones because humans have the ability to deliberate and choose heroism. Other animals, lacking this capacity, do not have an obligation to help even their own kind. Because humans are able to establish moral values and recognize rights, individualists consider them to be in a less favorable position to enhance their own species' well-being than are individuals of other species. This paradox strikes me as "curioser and curioser," and it appears that the rational anthropocentrism of which humans are capable is being turned to the disadvantage of the welfare and interests of many human individuals (often the deserving needy).

Some animal conservationists contend that it is wise to permit controlled hunts to regulate populations, and that shooting is a more humane death than starvation. Regan (1983, p. 354) finds the idea that death by trapping or shooting is better than starving, "is far from credible," because not all hunters are expert shots and not all trappers tend their traps responsibly, and use leg-hold traps that cause intense suffering. I believe it not credible that dying from starvation is necessarily better and think that animal populations could be controlled by allowing only expert shooters to participate and regulating the types of traps used.

Trapping animals for fur is another practice that meets with almost universal disapproval by animal welfarists for a number of reasons. The most compelling reason is that many animals lie maimed and injured for long periods after they have been trapped, which can be said to constitute intense torture. This objection could partially be met by adopting padded offset traps that do not injure animals severely. Rollin (1995) cited a court case that established the precedent that procedures such as trapping fulfill a legal human purpose, and should not be regulated by anticruelty laws; such regulations require legislative action to be extended.

Lacy (1995) adopted a utilitarian position to justify the need to maintain the lives of some animals at the expense of sacrificing others, noting that the decision is not whether animals should be killed, but which will be killed. Animal rights activists consider this view environmental fascism because it is based on anthropocentric values of humans regarding the relative importance of biosystems over individuals.

All animals born will die, most will experience pain when dying, and death from disease, starvation, or aging usually occurs slowly and with suffering (Lacy, 1995). Culling surplus animals from the natural population kills them, but frees resources that would benefit other animals in the wild population. However, hunting and trapping done in the name of wildlife management should be reoriented toward benefiting wildlife rather than serving the interests of hunter, trapper, and wildlife consumers (Callicott, 1985), a point that is well taken.

When surplus zoo animals are culled, cage space is freed so that animals of greater value to enhance biodiversity can be housed. Using extra resources to protect favored but surplus animals could mean that even more species will become extinct. Welfarists insist that the value is a human value, and they deplore this because it is anthropocentric.

Zoos

Now that general issues regarding biodiversity and species preservation have been considered, the role of zoos can be discussed in terms of their responsibilities toward the public, the animals, and the environment. About 1,700 exhibitor permits have been issued by the USDA. These animal collections range from shopping mall petting zoos to nonprofit public institutions with large scientific and teaching staffs and extensive collections of live animals. There are 164 zoos and aquaria accredited by the American Zoo and Aquarium Association (AZA), a body that considers conservation its highest priority (Conway, 1995). Those accredited zoos have annual operating expenses of nearly $800 million a year and a work force of about 16,500 people. They have survival programs for 117 species of animals, two-thirds of which are mammals (Hancocks, 1995; Koontz, 1995). More than 3,000 vertebrate species are being bred in zoos and other captive facilities, with about 93% of all mammals and 75% of all birds added to AZA collections in recent years having been bred in zoos (Koontz, 1995).

Beck (1995) identified 145 projects that released captive-bred animals in this century. The goal of these releases was to reestablish or reinforce wild populations to promote conservation. About 128 endangered species breeding programs are now active, about one-half of them in zoos. He noted that only about 12% of the programs can be documented as successful, a topic that is addressed below.

The goal of AZA is to institute survival programs for at least 200 species by the year 2000, hoping to slow the rate of extinctions until humans are better able to manage negative environmental impacts and stabilize populations. Vrijenhoek (1995) asserted that the real problem facing the globe is that it contains too many people, and he urged political and religious leaders to recognize population control as the essential problem causing ecosystem collapse.

A major role of zoos is to educate the public regarding the natural behaviors and lifestyles of well cared for and well-exhibited animals. The current emphasis is to present animals in naturalistic rather than caged settings, and to bring people into closer contact with animals. About 100 million people went to zoos in 1991, and 14 million participated in zoo education programs—about 10 million children and 35,000 teachers. These figures indicate that zoos play an extensive educational role.

Another role is supporting research. About 70% of the 120 North American zoos and aquaria were conducting research of some kind in 1983, 46% indicated an intent to expand their research programs, and it appears that even more are engaged in such activities since that time. In 1992 and 1993 AZA-accredited institutions supported nearly 1,100 scientific and conservation projects in more than 60 countries, and between 1990 and 1993 produced more than 1,300 technical articles on wildlife biology, conservation, and management of captive animals (Hutchins, Dresser, & Wemmer, 1995).

As might be expected, animal welfarists object to most of these educational and research activities. From Regan's (1995) rights view, zoos are morally not defensible because the freedom of animals is compromised by conditions of captivity. Others object to educational justification of zoos. Jamieson (1995a, 1995b) characterized the profound message communicated by zoos to be that it is permissible for humans to dominate animals, observing that the entire experience of a zoo is framed by the fact of captivity. He believes zoos are for us, rather than for animals, and said they are in the business of entertainment rather than species preservation. DeGrazia (1996) agreed; however, he allowed that animals may be kept in zoos if their basic physical and psychological needs are assured, and they have a good life compared with what they would likely have in the wild; Such treatment is just as reasonable as restricting human children's liberty to protect their basic needs and interests. The problem with this position is that the life of many animals in the wild is difficult, and they have to cope with physical and psychological hardships they would never encounter in a good zoo. Yet, one would not prefer that as many wild animals as possible be removed from harsh wild circumstances and placed in zoo rest homes.

It is no surprise that few zoo biologists subscribe to the principles of the rights or liberation movement. Their global biological interests generally are centered on the health of entire populations, species, and ecosystems rather than on individuals. One point of general agreement among almost everyone—pro and anti-zoo—is that humans have a moral responsibility for individual captive animals, and this poses difficulties when the issue of what should be done with surplus animals arises.

Some maintain that surplus animals should be culled to free cage space for those from more endangered species, or to avoid genetic problems produced by inbreeding the same animals year after year. Many such surplus animals can be transferred to other zoos that need them, either as exhibits or to enrich their own breeding population. Lacy (1995) expressed concern that decisions regarding the culling of animals in zoos often are based on maximizing the human pleasure derived from exhibits featuring attractive species and individuals, rather than concerns regarding moral imperatives of animal welfare. It would be nice if Ehrenfeld (1995) was correct when he suggested that both sides are right, and the only thing to do is to search for common ground that will lead to a mutually acceptable path, although that path might not be one entirely acceptable to all parties. I doubt such a solution is possible, but perhaps a few points of agreement can be exploited to everyone's satisfaction.

Zoo advocates say educational programs are especially useful because they have naturalistic displays that attract public attention to animals' habitats, and to the interrelationships between all components of those habitats and residents. Such a focus could lead to better public acceptance of the importance of habitat preservation, and shape attitudes regarding the need for species preservation. Hancocks (1995) extolled this virtue, but suggested that each zoo should sharpen its particular focus, giving more attention to regional elements and avoiding duplication with other zoos. It seems to be generally agreed that the classic concept of having as large a number of species as possible for exhibit should no longer prevail, and that the emphasis should be not on how many animals there are, but on how they live.

Species Preservation

One of the primary missions assumed by zoos is to breed individuals from endangered species in order to release them into the wild and establish stable breeding populations. Some charge that capture programs of zoos are a major factor in reducing many species to endangered status because excessive numbers of the wild population have been removed for purposes of exhibition and to stock breeding programs. Data do not support this charge; Conway (1995) could find no instance where zoo collecting was among the significant causes of endangerment of any species.

Beck (1995) compiled a data base to study the effectiveness of reintroduction. There are 145 documented projects that have released captive-bred animals in this century to reestablish or reinforce a wild population. More than 13 million captive-bred animals have been reintroduced, mostly fish, toads, and salamanders, but more than 70,000 mammals, birds, and reptiles of 100 different species. Zoo-born animals were involved in 76 (59%) of 129 reintroductions in which the source of animals could be determined, with about 10,000 of the more than 20,000 animals involved in these projects being birds and mammals.

Only 16 (11%) of the 145 reintroduction projects contributed to the establishment of a self-sustaining wild population: the criterion of success being a stable or growing population of at least 500 individuals that are independent from provisioning or other human support, or otherwise considered self-sustaining. Beck unfortunately found no overwhelming evidence reintroduction is successful. The remaining 89% of the projects were not all failures, however, because progress has been made toward producing self-sustaining wild populations. Indirect benefits also accrued in terms of increased public awareness and support for conservation, professional training of wildlife experts, enhanced habitat protection, and increased scientific knowledge.

One of the major reasons reintroduction has not been successful is that captive-bred animals are not able to cope with the stresses they encounter in the wild. Although they have the necessary biological heritage, they have no practiced survival skills. In addition, whenever endangered species are reintroduced, a new life is given to poaching, which drove some exotic species, such as the golden lion tamarin monkey, to extinction in the first place. This factor, combined with decades of habitat destruction, doomed many attempts at reintroduction. Major efforts now are being directed toward preparing animals to cope with predators, hunger, parasitism, climatic extremes, locomotor and orientation challenges, and the social competition they will encounter after reintroduction. To serve these ends, life in zoos has been made more naturalistic, although these changes might drastically decrease the welfare of individual animals. This fact will not please welfarists who oppose capture in the first place, and who are adamant that if animals lose their wild freedom, human captors must assume a social contract to enhance their welfare.

Studies indicate that reintroduction programs are twice as likely to be successful when wild animals are translocated in the wild. He suggested that a mixed strategy might be appropriate wherein excess or doomed individuals are translocated to suitable, unoccupied habitat and integrated with captive-born animals. This policy, accompanied by a long period of postrelease support in terms of provisioning, veterinary care, and rescue of distressed or lost animals, might improve success rates.

Loftin (1995, p. 170) objected to captive breeding programs, expressing a general concern that they encourage a "man-manipulates-nature" attitude that might give "corporate culture an excuse to continue its rapacious way." In addition, the programs are a waste because they put animals back into the same situation that brought them to extinction in the first place. His other concerns were that taking animals from the wild hastens the demise of the threatened remnant population, resources are shifted from field to laboratory studies, captive breeding sacrifices the interests of individual animals to those of the species, and captive rearing lowers fitness so that the process of natural selection is disrupted, therefore making reintroduced individuals less able to survive in the wild.

Some of these objections should be considered seriously, but others seem to have little merit. There is considerable merit regarding alterations of the fitness of released animals, including decreased survival with increased inbreeding. However, concerted efforts have been made to deal with these problems, and they do not appear insurmountable. Problems involved in habitat preservation are most serious. It might be necessary to abandon some habitats because they have been so devastated that they can no longer support a population of animals. However, efforts should be made to restore critical aspects of habitats, to prevent further destruction, and to reintroduce animals only into healthy, restored habitats.

The game is not zero-sum whereby a gain in any one activity produces a corresponding loss in another. No either-or choice has to be made between habitat preservation and captive-breeding programs because we are not dealing with a unitary source of finite funding. Different people and agencies are willing to support one or the other, and competition is not for a single pot of gold.

It is true that captive breeding programs emphasize the welfare of species and ecosystems rather than that of individuals. As discussed in the preceding section, differences in holistic and individualistic philosophies represent an unbridgeable gap between environmentalists and animal welfarists, and progress is going to have to be made with the understanding that the two sides are working from different basic premises, making it unlikely they will ever agree completely.

There is no reason that laboratory and field studies should be viewed in an either-or manner either; we need more and better studies of both kinds, and environmentalists, ethologists, and ecologists strongly support both types to develop the best procedures for species preservation and to enhance the welfare of individual animals in the wild. DeGrazia (1996) proposed that zoos engage in species preservation only if the program stressed family preservation, and if a great deal of space were available to provide enriched environments that afford ample opportunities for climbing, exploring, problem solving, and playing, especially in the case of apes. I believe most of these goals are accepted by zoo professionals, with the possible exception of what he might mean by family preservation. If that means using only intact, natural families in breeding programs, they will not agree.

Zoo and aquarium research is aimed primarily at issues in conservation biology that are broader in scope than many studies in the biological sciences. It tends to be opportunistic and noninvasive, and usually does not involve large numbers of animals, often being done with members of endangered species that have been removed from the wild. Specific research topics include ecology, reproductive biology, genetics, nutrition, behavior, disease, anatomy, physiology, and clinical veterinary medicine; the research is done in both captivity and in nature (Hutchins et al.,

1995). One of the primary aims of zoo biologists is to develop and refine technological advances that potentially can make contributions to wildlife conservation, with studies of birth, parental care, and various social interactions particularly valuable.

It is reasonable to agree with Hancocks (1995) that zoos are not the best places for sustained captive breeding programs, which could be conducted better in facilities dedicated to that purpose. Zoos can probably make their greatest contribution to conservation through education, especially by emphasizing the importance of saving habitats. A trend has developed to move away from the traditional zoo concept to one of naturalistic wildlife conservation parks. This process should be accelerated by increasing the emphasis on the functioning of animals within their ecosystem, and representing more adequately the importance of smaller life forms that are essential to maintain biodiversity and preserve the complexity of biosystems. Hancocks, director of the Arizona-Sonora Desert Museum in Tucson, Arizona, appealed for more regional specialization to bring home the full message of conservation to local audiences. Most of these suggestions should please critics such as Jamieson, who do not like the entertainment and exhibition quality of the classic zoo, but who seem more comfortable when zoos educate the public regarding the value of preserving habitats and species.

Pets

Immense numbers of captive animals are used by humans as pets and companions. Much of the fire generated by animal welfare activists is stimulated by perceived mistreatment of favorite pets and attractive mammals. Rollin (1992) estimated that between 6 and 14 million healthy dogs and close to that many cats are killed each year; about 12% of the total number of dogs born in the United States are killed by animal control staff. Conway (1995) estimated that of the nearly 118 million dogs and cats in the United States, 13 million are killed each year. For 1989, Francione (1995) claimed there were 125 million dogs, cats, horses, and birds living in American homes, and revenues in the veterinary field are about $5 billion per year. Such figures led Rollin to recommend stronger constraints on pet ownership and harsh punitive measures for those who violate their responsibilities, because acquiring an animal morally is more like adopting a child than buying a wheelbarrow. He recommended incentives to sterilize pet animals, and Feeney (1987) proposed that laws should be passed to mandate neutering in order to stop the slaughter of millions of dogs and cats each year, noting that this degree of harm far exceeded that produced by animal research.

Few would dispute that any human who acquires a pet enters into a social contract with that animal and assumes duties and responsibilities to maintain its welfare. It must be demonstrated the animal is not made worse off by becoming a pet (DeGrazia, 1996). Cats and dogs are accorded the highest concern by the public, as are most nonhuman primates, and horses are favored by many individuals. Rollin (1992) claimed that many people would probably choose to have the interests of their family dog supersede the interests of the life of a nomad in central Asia, although he allowed it is difficult to consider such a decision morally correct. However, we have data that this is not the choice people make: When a hypothetical dilemma was posed, pitting a favorite pet against a person from China, the person was favored by almost all respondents. Laws regarding cruelty to animals afford special protection to dogs and cats, and strong objections are expressed about using animals that are common pets as research subjects because that is seen as betrayal of a social contract (Smith & Boyd, 1991).

There is also a Bambi effect—humans tend to find animals attractive that have characteristics similar to those provided by human babies, such as a short face in relation to a large forehead, protruding cheeks, and maladjusted limb movements. Lorenz (1943) suggested these characteristics serve as sign stimuli to release the "parental instinct" in humans.

The animal liberation movement has relatively little to say about keeping pets, even though this involves captivity, thwarts many of the natural behavior tendencies of animals, could be construed to be involuntary servitude, values animals for their human entertainment value, and consumes vast food resources—exactly the reasons they consider the existence of zoos to be impermissible. Regan (1983) does not include an entry for pets or companion animals in the index to his book, and Singer's entries (1990a) refer to the theft of pets to be used in research, and a notation that vegetarian diets are available for dogs and cats. As Rodman (1977) observed, Singer proposed radical changes to diminish the suffering of domesticated animals, but stopped short of challenging domestication itself.

Leahy (1991) cited Jamieson's moral presumption against keeping wild animals in captivity and used it to maintain that zoos are detrimental to animals. Fox (1990) thought it justified to keep pets because they are given affection, understanding, and satisfaction of their basic needs in reciprocation for their companionship and devotion. Some animal rightists contend that animals should not be kept as pets or bred to become pets, but Fox placed such exploitation in an "essential" category when their needs are provided for and they are treated with respect and understanding. DeGrazia (1996) accepted as a basic principle that sentient animals should not be confined unnecessarily, but denied that this implies we should not have pets. He based this denial on the fact that having pets does not confine animals in the relevant sense that it precludes their having a good life, whereas zoos confine animals unnecessarily, which is impermissible. Considerable arbitrariness surrounds what is considered essential and permissible: Captive animals kept as pets and companions are essential and okay, but keeping animals in zoos is not because the animals are captive. Fox believed it would be better to use resources to conserve animals in the wild than to maintain and breed them in zoos. One can ask whether the extraordinary expense of keeping pets might not be better used as well. One should also remember that animals kept as pets consume tremendous resources of foodstuff, both animal and plant, and arguments that oppose raising animals high on the food chain for human consumption seem even more applicable here.

Dogs engage in many natural behaviors, such as urinating on handy upright objects and rolling in excrement, which are not permitted. Humans housebreak dogs by procedures that could well be described as cruel to the dog and contrary to its *telos*, forcing it to behave in an unnatural fashion for the rest of its life. And this behavior is founded on fear of punishment. In the interest of consistency, one could object to this practice and argue against keeping pets. On the other hand, as Leahy concluded, most well-fed, well-cared-for, and well-trained dogs give no indication of wanting to escape the family home. Anyone who has seen a trained dog, such as a border collie, herding sheep would be hard pressed to conclude the animal is working contrary to its nature and that it is not experiencing pleasure. It is highly tempting to conclude that the dog enjoys herding and is delighted by the shepherd's approval. It is difficult to conclude the animal is working under threat of punishment and should be released to do whatever it might, unconstrained by a human master. It appeared to me a partnership existed between shepherd and dog—which did work against the natural tendencies of the sheep, however.

Conclusions

Many other uses of animals could be discussed, and the general principles developed in this book can be applied to them, such as having animals assist disabled humans in their day-to-day activity (e.g., guide dogs), for entertainment, as companions for the elderly, and in therapy for the depressed. I will not discuss these uses because there is no new ethical ground to be covered, and the conclusions are apparent from consideration of the principles developed in this book.

With this comment I conclude the long journey into the Darwinian dominion of evolution that was begun in the preceding two books dealing with the permissible use of humans by humans, and ending with this book considering the permissible use of animals by humans. I believe evolutionary principles provide an adequate grounding for moral decisions. When the basic tendencies that constitute human nature are understood, it can be realized that to attain a just society, a principle must be added that guarantees freedom from harm and assurance of respect.

Utilitarianism views costs and benefits in an avowedly anthropocentric light, but leaves room to honor social contracts that arise because of human actions, such as domestication of animals and destruction of habitat. Actions to fulfill these duties and responsibilities should be undertaken with a sense of compassion and concern for the welfare of all individuals, but should recognize that concerns transcend individuals and respect existence at higher levels of the biosystem. The holism accepted by environmentalists establishes an unbridgeable gap between animal welfarists and land ethic environmentalists.

I recast the essentials of the arguments contained in this book in the next chapter, a brief epilogue, where I reflect on the issues that have been dealt with in this and my earlier two books. I hope that these views contribute to the understanding of difficult problems in applied ethics that confront citizens in modern society. They were developed from a deep concern with principles of evolutionary biology, and are offered in the spirit of demonstrating the principle enunciated in the preface—and evolution shall have dominion.

14

Epilogue

Evolved Morality

At least three levels of theory run throughout the three books that comprise my theories regarding morality. One deals with the evolutionary biology of reproduction, which I maintain is the fundamental grounding, the "glue" if you will, of much of our social cooperation and communication. As we move from realities at the level of evolutionary biology we come to a second level—characteristics that differentiate moral agents from moral patients. A decision must be made to determine when a developing human should be accorded moral standing, which I believe begins at birth. It is at this point the neonate is a public entity, entitled to the respect that all human moral patients should have.

A distinction was made between human and nonhuman moral patients. When a recognizable human neonate appears it is accorded respect as a member of our species who will, under normal circumstances, represent and perpetuate the genes of its parents and kin. For this reason the human neonate has greater ultimate value to caregivers than neonates of other species or those outside the social community. The ultimate biological contribution the neonate represents is established, cemented, and enhanced by behavioral interactions between it and caregivers that create emotional bonds and channel continuing development.

Moral agents in the social community must honor the obligations and duties that constitute what I refer to as a social contract. This social contract is biologically mandated, exists among members of social species, and is forged by experiences during development. Its function is to mold members of the community into a cooperating, self-perpetuating entity. Critical aspects of the contract involve both emotional bonding and development of communicative networks that will permit the development of cognitive functions on which the status of moral agency is forged. The ultimate function of the contract is to enhance reproductive success by increasing inclusive fitness.

The above processes define personhood, a status based on biological processes that involve phenomena similar to those observed in imprinting for many species of animals. These processes capitalize on events in the stimulating environment encountered by developing organisms and are used to form social attachments. The focus shifts from automatic biological processes to what have been characterized as experience-expectant, experience-dependent, and activity-dependent systems.

A third set of principles defines moral agency: Principles governed by cognitive characteristics that make it possible for a person to attain a continuous concept of self, and understand ideas of causality and intentionality and the rules on which ethical systems depend. Moral agents are responsible to accept the duties required by the rules and laws society has adopted, and they must respect other moral agents, as well as look to the welfare of moral patients who are neither able to behave in accordance with social rules nor culpable when they violate them.

No single level of theory is adequate to guide us in our search for the morally permissible. Just as reality brings into play different principles when viewed at different levels, theories required to understand those realities must be framed using theories that vary qualitatively, and should become pluralistic when viewed in the different contexts within which they operate. Scientific methodologists contend that to frame science adequately, converging lines of evidence from a variety of sources should be used to establish the validity of theoretical constructs. Intersecting lines of theory also should be developed at multiple levels to support, rather than supplant, one another, and they should be adequate to allow emergent properties at more complex levels to be expressed and appreciated. A pluralistic theoretical approach is necessary to deal with issues as complex as the morality of reproduction, life, and death.

When I began writing I planned to produce one book that would discuss moral issues involved in human and nonhuman life and death. However, the development of basic issues regarding rules of argumentation, and theories of evolution, cognitive science, and moral philosophy required considerably more space than I thought they would, and it was necessary to bring a wide variety of evidence to bear on abstract principles. It was also necessary to discuss issues regarding what has been referred to as the naturalistic fallacy; these must be confronted when assuming a naturalistic stance, as I do. I also confronted slippery slope arguments and the problems of reductionism and genetic determinism. I considered it necessary to bring to the table a set of biological principles and a solid empirical base that seasoned philosophers should be made aware of, because they will be able to bring them to bear on discussions of critical issues regarding morality. In that first book I concentrated on issues in reproduction—the heart of evolutionary biology—and examined physiological and behavioral evidence regarding reproductive technologies and abortion in order to illuminate philosophical issues and to consider practical questions in bioethics.

The second book expanded the theoretical analyses begun in the first, and discussed death, suicide, euthanasia, and organ transplants, as well as the progress of, and ethical issues involved in, genetic screening and manipulation, and the progress of the Human Genome Project. Adequate treatment of these topics required discussion of issues in medical ethics, which led to an extended consideration of practical and ethical problems encountered in attempts to develop a national health care delivery system. The book became far too long to accommodate discussions of the status of nonhuman animals. The present book extended the discussion to that subject.

Concluding Thoughts

Throughout this book I have extensively referred to the ideas and conclusion of the two most prominent philosophers championing the welfare of animals: Tom Regan, who developed a theory of animal rights, and Peter Singer, whose preference utilitarianism formed the foundations for animal liberation. I challenged and argued against many of their positions, attempted to defeat many of their theories, and offered what I though was a more adequate view of the issues that should be considered when addressing the permissible use of animals by humans.

Many of my statements disputed their positions because their positions are clear and articulate, and represent dominant philosophical views that have directed thinking and a great deal of action. I want to emphasize that although much of my discussion was negative in tone, sometimes to the point of hostility, I have immense respect for the men and their beliefs. I respectfully disagreed with them in hope of promoting the kinds of discussions that can clarify issues regarding the values and dignities of life. It is out of respect for their formidable works that I devoted so much energy to arguing against them in the course of developing and defending my own positions.

I hope the theory and data brought to bear on critical issues in social policy will be of value to those who are charged with the responsibility to develop policies regarding the moral problems society faces. I consider it the responsibility of biological and social scientists to bring their peculiar talents and skills to bear on the solution of practical problems. I have done what I could toward achieving that goal.

This has been a long journey, and it has been exciting to work at a coherent approach adequate to the task of threading my way through the thicket of practical decisions that modern society must make. Although some of my conclusions can, will, and should be contested, on the whole I think my positions are defensible, even though they might have to be modified as counter-arguments are presented. I consider the fomentation of debate to be the reason we engage in dialogues regarding bioethics, as well as to expose eternal metaphysical and epistemological issues to examination in the light of biological and psychological realities.

The powers of modern biology and medical technology, along with their economic implications, make it necessary to engage in proactive discussions regarding the welfare of individuals. Such discussions are absolutely essential if we are to develop and maintain a just society, which most of us want. I fervently believe the Darwinian perspective is the vehicle that will move us toward an understanding of life's processes viewed from the rich context of the basics of organismic existence that any moral system must be framed to respect.

References

Adams, C. J. (1996). Caring about suffering: A feminist exploration. In J.Donovan & C. J. Adams (Eds.), *Beyond animal rights*. New York: Continuum Publishing, pp. 170–196.

Alcock, J. (1989). *Animal behavior* (4th ed.). Sunderland, MA: Sinauer Associates.

Alexander, R. D. (1987). *The biology of moral systems*. New York: Aldine de Gruyter.

Almond, B. (1993). Rights. In P. Singer (Ed.), *A companion to ethics*. Oxford: Basil Blackwell, pp. 259–269.

Als, H. (1995). The preterm infant: A model for the study of fetal brain expectation. In J.-P. Lecanuet, W.P. Fifer, N.A. Krasnegor, & W.P. Smotherman (Eds.), *Fetal development*. Hillsdale, NJ: Lawrence Erlbaum Associates, pp. 439–471.

American Psychological Association. (1986). Guidelines for ethical conduct in the care and use of animals. *Journal for the Experimental Analysis of Behavior*, 45, 127–132.

Animal rights handbook. (1990). Los Angeles: Living Planet Press.

Arluke, A. (1992). Trapped in a guilt cage. *New Scientist*, 134, #1815, 33–35.

Astington, J. (1993). *Developing theories of mind*. Cambridge: Harvard University Press.

Bahrick, L. E. (1988). Intermodal learning in infancy: Learning on the basis of two kinds of invariant relations in audible and visible events. *Child Development*, 59, 197–209.

Baillargeon, R. (1995). Physical reasoning in infancy. In M. S. Gazzaniga (Ed.), *The cognitive neurosciences*. Cambridge: MIT Press, pp. 181–204.

Baldwin, E. (1993). The case for animal research in psychology. *Journal of Social Issues*, 49, 121–131.

Barkow, J. H., Cosmides, L., & Tooby, J. (1992). *The adapted mind*. Oxford: Oxford University Press.

Baron-Cohen, S. (1995a). *Mindblindness*. Cambridge: MIT Press.

Baron-Cohen, S. (1995b). The eye detection detector (EDD) and the shared attention mechanism (SAM): Two cases for evolutionary psychology. In C. Moore & P. J. Dunham (Eds.), *Joint attention*. Hillsdale, NJ: Lawrence Erlbaum Associates, pp. 41–60.

Baron-Cohen, S. & Swettenham, J. (1996). The relationship between SAM and ToMM: Two hypotheses. In P. Carruthers & P. K. Smith (Eds.), *Theories of theories of mind*. Cambridge: Cambridge University Press, pp. 158–168.

Bateson, P. (1992). Do animals feel pain? *New Scientist*, 134, 1818, 30–33.

Baumeister, R. F. & Leary, M. R. (1995). The need to belong: Desire for interpersonal attachments as a fundamental human motivation. *Psychological Bulletin*, 117, 497–529.

Beck, B. (1995). Reintroduction, zoos, conservation, and animal welfare. In B. G. Norton, M. Hutchins, E. F. Stevens, & T. L. Maple (Eds.), *Ethics on the ark*. Washington, DC: Smithsonian Institution Press, pp. 155–163.

Becker, L. C. (1973). *On justifying moral judgments*. London: Routledge & Kegan Paul.

Benson, J. (1978). Duty and the beast. *Philosophy*, 53, 529–549.

Bentler, P. M. (1980). Multivariate analysis with latent variables: Causal modeling. *Annual Review of Psychology*, 31, 419–456.

Bertenthal, B. I., Proffitt, D. R., & Cutting, J. E. (1984). Infant sensitivity to figural coherence in biomechanical notions. *Journal of Experimental Child Psychology*, 37, 213–230.

Bettinger, R. L. (1991). *Hunter-gatherers: Archaeological and evolutionary theory*. New York: Plenum Press.

Bickerton, D. (1990). *Language and species*. Chicago: University of Chicago Press.

Birke, L. & Michael, M. (1992). Views from behind the barricade. *New Scientist*, 134, #1815, 29–32.

Blum, D. (1994). *The monkey wars*. New York: Oxford University Press.

Botham, P. & Purchase, I. (1992). Why laboratory rats are here to stay. *New Scientist*, 134, #1819, 29–30.

Bower, T. G. R. (1982). *Development in infancy* (revised ed.). San Francisco: W. H. Freeman.

Brandt, R. B. (1987). Public policy and life and death decisions regarding defective newborns. In R. C. McMillan, H. T. Engelhardt, & S. F. Spicker (Eds.), *Euthanasia and the newborn*. Dordrecht, Holland: D. Reidel, pp. 191–208.

Brennan, A. A. (1986). Ecological theory and value in nature. *Philosophical Inquiry*, 8, 66–96.

Brink, D. O. (1993). The separateness of persons, distributive norms, and moral theory. In R. G. Frey & C. W. Morris (Eds.), *Value, welfare, and morality*. Cambridge: Cambridge University Press, pp. 252–289.

Brown, H. I. (1977). *Perception, theory and commitment*. Chicago: University of Chicago Press.

Brunswik, E. (1952). The conceptual framework of psychology. In *International encyclopedia of unified science* (vol. 1). Chicago: University of Chicago Press, pp. 1–102.

Brunswik, E. (1956). *Perception and the representative design of psychological experiments*. Berkeley, CA: University of California Press.

Butterworth, G. (1995). Origins of mind in perception and action. In C. Moore & P. J. Dunham (Eds.), *Joint attention*. Hillsdale, NJ: Lawrence Erlbaum Associates, pp. 29–59.

Callicott, J. B. (1980). Animal liberation: A triangular affair. *Environmental Ethics* 2, 311–338.

Callicott, J. B. (1985). Review of Tom Regan, *The case for animal rights*. *Environmental Ethics*, 7, 365–372.

Callicott, J. B. (1989). Animal liberation and environmental ethics: Back together again. In J. B. Callicott (Ed.), *In defense of the land ethic*. Albany, NY: State University of New York Press, pp. 49–59.

Cann, R. L. (1995). Mitochondrial DNA and human evolution. In J.-P. Changeux & J. Chavaillon (Eds.), *Origins of the human brain*. Oxford: Oxford University Press, pp. 127–135.

Carey, S. & Spelke, E. (1994). Domain-specific knowledge and conceptual change. In L. A. Hirschfeld & S. A. Gelman (Eds.), *Mapping the mind*. Cambridge: Cambridge University Press, pp. 169–200.

Caro, T. M. & Hauser, M. D. (1992). Is there teaching in nonhuman animals? *Quarterly Review of Biology*, 67, 151–174.

Caron, A. J., Caron, R. F., & Carlson, V. R. (1979). Infant perception of the invariant shape of objects varying in slant. *Child Development*, 50, 716–721.

Carruthers, P. (1992). *The animals issue*. Cambridge: Cambridge University Press.

Carruthers, P. & Smith, P. K. (1996). Introduction. In P. Carruthers & P. K. Smith (Eds.), *Theories of theories of mind*. Cambridge: Cambridge University Press, pp. 1–8.

Cavalieri, P. & Singer, P. (1993). *The great ape project*. New York: St. Martin's Press.

Chagnon, N. A. (1992). *Yanomamo: The last days of Eden*. New York: Harcourt Brace Jovanovich.

Cheng, H., Cao, Y., & Olson, L. (1996). Spinal cord repair in adult paraplegic rats: Partial restoration of hind limb function. *Science*, 273, 510–513.

Cohen, C. (1986). The case for the use of animals in biomedical research. *New England Journal of Medicine*, 315, 865–870.

Cohen, J. (1988). *Statistical power analysis for the behavioral sciences* (2nd ed.). Hillsdale, NJ: Lawrence Erlbaum Associates.

Coile, D. C. & Miller N. E. (1984). How radical animal activists try to mislead humane people. *American Psychologist*, 39, 700–701.

Collard, A. (1989). *Rape of the wild* . . . Bloomington, IN: University of Indiana Press.

Condon, W. S. & Sander, L. (1974). Neonate movement is synchronized with adult speech: Interactional participation and language acquisition. *Science*, 183, 99–101.

Conway, W. (1995). Zoo conservation and ethical paradoxes. In B. G. Norton, M. Hutchins, E. F. Stevens, & T. L. Maple (Eds.), *Ethics on the Ark*. Washington, DC: Smithsonian Institution Press, pp. 1–9.

Copp, D. (1993). Reason and needs. In R. G. Frey & R. G. Morris (Eds.), *Value, welfare, and morality*. Cambridge: Cambridge University Press, pp. 112–137.

Crade, M. & Lovett, S. (1988). Fetal response to sound stimulation: Preliminary report exploring use of sound stimulation in routine obstetrical ultrasound examinations. *Journal of Ultrasound Medicine*, 7, 499–503.

Cronbach, L. J., Gleser, G. C., Nanda, H., & Rajaratnam, N. (1972). *The dependability of behavioral measurements*. New York: John Wiley.

Cronbach, L. J. & Meehl, P. E. (1955). Construct validity in psychological tests. *Psychological Bulletin*, 52, 288–302.

Cronin, H. (1991). *The ant and the peacock*. Cambridge: Cambridge University Press.

Curtin, D. (1996). Toward an ecological ethic of care. In J. Donovan & C. J. Adams (Eds.), *Beyond animal rights*. New York: Continuum Publishing, pp. 60–76.

Daly, M. & Wilson, M. (1988). *Homicide*. New York: Aldine de Gruyter.

Daniels, N. (Ed.). (1989). *On reading Rawls*. Stanford, CA: Stanford University Press.

Dannemiller, J. L. & Stephens, B. R. (1988). A critical test of infant pattern preference models. *Child Development*, 59, 210–216.

Darwin, C. (1859). *On the origin of species by means of natural selection*. New York: D. Appleton.

Darwin, C. (1871). *The descent of man*. New York: D. Appleton.

Darwin, C. (1887). *The autobiography of Charles Darwin*. London: John Murray.

Dawkins, M. S. (1990). From an animal's point of view: Motivation, fitness, and animal welfare. *Behavioral and Brain Sciences*, 13, 1–9.

DeCasper, A. J. & Fifer, W. P. (1980). Of human bonding: Newborns prefer their mothers' voices. *Science*, 208, 1174–1176.

DeGrazia, D. (1996). *Taking animals seriously*. Cambridge: Cambridge University Press.

Dennett, D. C. (1978). *Brainstorms*. Cambridge: MIT Press.

Dennett, D. C. (1991). *Consciousness explained*. Boston: Little, Brown.

Dennett, D. C. (1995). *Darwin's dangerous idea*. New York: Simon & Schuster.

Devine, P. E. (1978). The moral basis of vegetarianism. *Philosophy*, 53, 481–505.

DeWaal, C. S. (1996). Playing chicken. Report of the Center for Science in the Public Interest. http://www.cspinet.org/reports/polt.html.

de Waal, F. B. M. (1982). *Chimpanzee politics*. Baltimore: Johns Hopkins University Press.

de Waal, F. B. M. (1989). *Peacemaking among primates*. Cambridge: Harvard University Press.

de Waal, F. B. M. (1994). Overview—Culture and cognition. In R. W. Wrangham, W. C. McGrew, F. B. M. de Waal, & P. G. Heltne (Eds.), *Chimpanzee cultures*. Cambridge: Harvard University Press, pp. 263–265.

de Waal, F. B. M. (1996). *Good natured*. Cambridge: Harvard University Press.

Dewsbury, D. A. (1990). Early interactions between animal psychologists and animal activists and the founding of the APA committee on precautions in animal experimentation. *American Psychologist*, 45, 315–327.

Diamond, A. (1991). Neuropsychological insights into the meaning of object concept development. In S. Carey & R. Gelman (Eds.), *The epigenesis of mind*. Hillsdale, NJ: Lawrence Erlbaum Associates, pp. 67–110.

Diamond, J. (1992). *The third chimpanzee*. New York: HarperCollins.

Dodd, B. (1979). Lip reading in infants: Attention to speech presented in- and out-of-synchrony. *Cognitive Psychology*, 11, 478–484.

Donovan, J. (1993). Animal rights and feminist theory. In G. Gaard (Ed.), *Ecofeminism*. Philadelphia: Temple University Press, pp. 167–194.

Doran, D. M. & Hunt, K. D. (1994). Comparative locomotor behavior of chimpanzees and bonobos: Species and habitat differences. In R. W. Wrangham, W. C. McGrew, F. B. M. de Waal, & P. G. Heltne (Eds.), *Chimpanzee cultures*, Cambridge: Harvard University Press, pp. 93–108.

Dresser, R. (1988). Standards for animal research: Looking at the middle. *Journal of Medicine and Philosophy*, 13, 123–143.

Dunham, P. J. & Dunham, F. (1995). Optimal social structures and adaptive infant development. In C. Moore & P. J. Dunham (Eds.), *Joint attention*. Hillsdale, NJ: Lawrence Erlbaum Associates, pp. 159–188.

Dworkin, R. (1977). *Taking rights seriously*. Cambridge: Harvard University Press.

Dwyer, J. & Loew, F. M. (1994). Nutritional risks of vegan diets to women and children: Are they preventable? *Journal of Agricultural and Environmental Ethics*, 7, 87–109.

Eddy, T. J. Gallup, G. G., & Povinelli, D. J. (1993). Attribution of cognitive states to animals: Anthropomorphism in comparative perspective. *Journal of Social Issues*, 49, 87–101.

Ehrenfeld, D. (1995). Foreword. In B. G. Norton, M. Hutchins, E. F. Stevens, & T. L. Maple (Eds.), *Ethics on the ark*. Washington, DC: Smithsonian Institution Press, pp. xvii–xix.

Eimas, P. D. (1982). Speech perception: A view of the initial state and perceptual mechanisms. In J. Mehler, E. C. T. Walker, & M. Garrett (Eds.), *Perspectives on mental representation*. Hillsdale, NJ: Lawrence Erlbaum Associates, pp. 339–360.

Eimas, P. D. & Miller, J. L. (1992). Organization in the perception of speech by young infants. *Psychological Science*, 3, 340–345.

Eimas, P., Siqueland, E. R., Jusczyk, P. W., & Vigorito, J. (1971). Speech perception in infants. *Science*, 171, 303–306.

Eldredge, N. & Gould, S. J. (1972). Punctuated equilibria: An alternative to phyletic gradualism. In T. J. M. Schopf (Ed.), *Models in paleobiology*. San Francisco: Freeman, Cooper, pp. 82–115.

Elston, M. A. (1992). Victorian values and animal rights. *New Scientist*, 134, 1822, 28–31.

Emlen, S. T. (1993). Ethics and experimentation: Hard choices for the field ornithologist. *Auk*, 110, 406–409.

Etcoff, N. L. & Magee, J. J. (1992). Categorical perception of facial expressions. *Cognition*, 44, 227–240.

Feeney, D. M. (1987). Human rights and animal welfare. *American Psychologist*, 42, 593–599.

Feinberg, J. (1978). Human duties and animal rights. In R. K. Morris & M. W. Fox (Eds.), *On the fifth day*. Washington, DC: Acropolis Books, pp. 45–69.

Feinberg, J. (1980). Potentiality, development, and rights. In T. Regan (Ed.), *Matters of life and death*. New York: Random House, 1980. (Reprinted in J. Feinberg (Ed.). (1984). *The problem of abortion*. Belmont, CA: Wadsworth, pp. 145–150.)

Feinberg, J. (1984). *Harm to others*. Oxford: Oxford University Press.

Feinberg, J. (1989). Rawls and intuitionism. In N. Daniels (Ed.), *On reading Rawls*. Stanford, CA: Stanford University Press, pp. 108–123.

Fernald, A. (1992). Human maternal vocalizations to infants as biologically relevant signals: An evolutionary perspective. In J. H. Barkow, L. Cosmides, & J. Tooby (Eds.), *The adapted mind*. New York: Oxford University Press, pp. 391–428.

Fetzer, J. H. (1996). Ethics and evolution. In J. Hurd (Ed.), *Investigating the biological foundations of human morality*. Lewiston, NY: Edwin Mellen Press, pp. 223–242.

Feyerabend, P. (1975). *Against method*. London: Verso Press.

Fifer, W. P. & Moon, C. M. (1995). The effects of fetal experience with sound. In J.-P. Lecanuet, W. P. Fifer, N. A. Krasnegor, & W. P. Smotherman (Eds.), *Fetal development*. Hillsdale, NJ: Lawrence Erlbaum Associates, pp. 351–366.

Finsen, S. (1988). Sinking the research lifeboat. *Journal of Medicine and Philosophy*, 13, 197–212.

Forer, L. G. (1991). *Unequal protection: Women, children, and the elderly in court.* New York: W. W. Norton.

Fox, M. W. (1986). *Laboratory animal husbandry: Ethology, welfare, and experimental variables.* Albany, NY: State University of New York Press.

Fox, M. W. (1990). *Inhumane society.* New York: St. Martin's Press.

Francione, G. L. (1995). *Animals, property, and the law.* Philadelphia: Temple University Press.

Francione, G. L. (1996). *Rain without thunder.* Philadelphia: Temple University Press.

Frey, R. G. (1980). *Interests and rights.* Oxford: Oxford University Press.

Frey, R. G. (1983). *Rights, killing, and suffering.* Oxford: Basil Blackwell.

Frey, R. G. (1984a). Introduction: Utilitarianism and persons. In R. G. Frey (Ed.), *Utility and rights.* Minneapolis: University of Minnesota Press, pp. 3–19.

Frey, R. G. (1984b). Act-utilitarianism, consequentialism, and moral rights. In R. G. Frey (Ed.), *Utility and rights.* Minneapolis: University of Minnesota Press, pp. 61–85.

Frey, R. G. (1990). Animals, science, and morality. *Behavioral and Brain Sciences*, 13, 22.

Gallistel, C. R. (1981). Bell, Magendie, and the proposals to restrict the use of animals in neurobehavioral research. *American Psychologist*, 36, 357–360.

Gallup, G. G., Jr. & Suarez, S. D. (1985). Alternatives to the use of animals in psychological research. *American Psychologist*, 40, 1104–1111.

Gardner, R. A., Gardner, B. T., & Van Cantfort, E. (1989). *Teaching sign language to chimpanzees.* Albany, NY: State University of New York Press.

Gauthier, D. (1993). Value, reasons, and the sense justice. In R. G. Frey & R. G. Morris (Eds.), *Value, welfare, and morality.* Cambridge: Cambridge University Press, pp. 180–208.

Gavaghan, H. (1992). Animal experiments the American way. *New Scientist*, 134, 1821, 32–36.

Geary, D. (1995). Reflection of evolution and culture in children's cognition. *American Psychologists*, 50, 24–37.

Geist, V. (1995). Noah's ark II: Rescuing species and ecosystems. In B. G. Norton, M. Hutchins, E. F. Stevens, & T. L. Maple (Eds.), *Ethics on the ark.* Washington, DC: Smithsonian Institution Press, pp. 93–101.

George, K. P. (1994a). Discrimination and bias in the vegan ideal. *Journal of Agricultural and Environmental Ethics*, 7, 19–28.

George, K. P. (1994b). Use and abuse revisited: Response to Pluhar and Varner. *Journal of Agricultural and Environmental Ethics*, 7, 41–76.

Ghiselin, M. T. (1969). *The triumph of the Darwinian method*. Berkeley, CA: University of California Press.

Ghiselin, M. T. (1971). The individual in the Darwinian revolution. *New Literary History*, 3, 113–134.

Gigerenzer, G. & Hug, K. (1992). Domain-specific reasoning: Social contracts, cheating, and perspective change. *Cognition*, 43, 127–171.

Gilligan, C. (1982). *In a different voice*. Cambridge: Harvard University Press.

Goldschmidt, T. (1996). *Darwin's dreampond*. Cambridge: MIT Press.

Gomez, J-C. (1996). Non-human primate theories of (non-human primate) minds: Some issues concerning the origins of mind-reading. In P. Carruthers & P. K. Smith (Eds.), *Theories of theories of mind*. Cambridge: Cambridge University Press, pp. 330–343.

Goodin, R. E. (1993). Utility and the good. In R. Singer (Ed.), *A companion to ethics*. Oxford: Basil Blackwell, pp. 241–248.

Gopnik, A. & Meltzoff, A. N. (1997). *Words, thoughts, and theories*. Cambridge: MIT Press.

Gopnik, A. & Wellman, M. H. (1994). The theory theory. In P. Carruthers & P. K. Smith (Eds.), *Theories of theories of mind*. Cambridge: Cambridge University, pp. 257–293.

Goren, C. C., Sarty, M., & Wu, P. Y. K. (1975). Visual following and pattern discrimination of face-like stimuli by newborn infants. *Pediatrics*, 56, 544–549.

Gould, S. J. & Vrba, E. (1981). Exaptation: A missing term in the science of form. *Paleobiology*, 8, 4–15.

Grady, D. (1996). Research uses grow for virtual cadavers. *New York Times*, Oct. 8, B5.

Griffin J. (1993). On the winding road from good to right. In R. G. Frey & C. W. Morris (Eds.), *Value, welfare, and morality*. Cambridge: Cambridge University Press, pp. 158–179.

Gruen, L. (1993). Dismantling oppression: An analysis of the connection between women and animals. In G. Gaard (Ed.), *Ecofeminism*. Philadelphia: Temple University Press, pp. 60–90.

Hampson, J. (1989). Legislation and the changing consensus. In G. Langley (Ed.), *Animal experimentation: The consensus change*. New York: Chapman & Hall, pp. 219–251.

Hancocks, D. (1995). Lions and tigers and bears, oh no! In B. G. Norton, M. Hutchins, E. F. Stevens, & T. L. Maple (Eds.), *Ethics on the ark*. Washington, DC: Smithsonian Institution Press, pp. 31–37.

Hanson, N. R. (1969). *Perception and discovery*. San Francisco: Freeman, Cooper.

Hare, R. M. (1979). What is wrong with slavery. *Philosophy and Public Affairs*, 8, 103–121.

Hargrove, E. C. (1995). The role of zoos in the twenty-first century. In B. G. Norton, M. Hutchins, E. F. Stevens, & T. L. Maple (Eds.), *Ethics on the ark*. Washington, DC: Smithsonian Institution Press, pp. 13–19.

Harlow, H. F. (1949). The formation of learning sets. *Psychological Review*, 56, 51–56.

Harlow, H. F. (1953). Motivation as a factor in new responses. *Nebraska Symposium in Motivation*, Lincoln, NB: University of Nebraska Press, pp. 24–49.

Harner, M. (1977). The ecological basis for Aztec sacrifice. *American Ethnologist*, 4, 117–135.

Harris, J. (1992). *Wonderwoman and superman*. Oxford: Oxford University Press.

Harris, M. (1979). *Cultural materialism: The struggle for a science of culture*. New York: Random House.

Hauser, M. D. (1996). *The evolution of communication*. Cambridge: MIT Press.

Hazard, H. (1989). Current legislation initiatives in the USA. In G. Langley (Ed.), *Animal experimentation*. New York: Chapman & Hall, pp. 252–259.

Hebb, D. O. (1949). *The organization of behavior*. New York: John Wiley.

Held, R. (1982). Visual development: From resolution to perception. In J. Mehler, E. C. T. Walker, & M. Garrett (Eds.), *Perspectives on mental representation*. Hillsdale, NJ: Lawrence Erlbaum Associates, pp. 399–408.

Hepper, P. G. (1995). The behavior of the fetus as an indicator of neural functioning. In J.-P. Lecanuet, W. P. Fifer, N. A. Krasnegor, & W. P. Smotherman (Eds.), *Fetal development*. Hillsdale, NJ: Lawrence Erlbaum Associates, pp. 405–418.

Herzog, H. A., Jr. (1988). The moral status of mice. *American Psychologist*, 43, 473–474.

Hill, K. & Hurtado, A. M. (1996). *Ache life history*. New York: Aldine de Gruyter.

Hilleman, M. R. (1995). Viral vaccines in historical perspective. *Developments in Biological Standardization*, 84, 107–116.

Hilts, P. J. (1994). Research animals used less often. *New York Times*, March 3, A7.

Hilts, P. J. (1996). Love of numbers leads to chromosome 17. *New York Times*, September 10, B5.

Hinde, R. A. (1974). *Biological bases of human social behavior*. New York: McGraw-Hill.

Hinde, R. A. (1982). *Ethology: Its nature and relations with other sciences*. Oxford: Oxford University Press.

Hodos, W. (1983). Animal welfare considerations in neuroscience research. *Annals of the New York Academy of Sciences*, 406, 119–127.

Hollands, C. (1989). Trivial and questionable research on animals. In G. Langley (Ed.), *Animal experimentation*. New York: Chapman & Hall, pp. 118–143.

Holt, J. T., Thompson, M. E., Szabo, C., et al. (1996). Growth retardation and tumour inhibition by BRCA1. *Nature Genetics*, 12, 298–302.

Hull, C. L. (1943). *The principles of behavior*. New York: Appleton-Century-Crofts.

Hutchins, M., Dresser, B., & Wemmer, C. (1995). Ethical considerations in zoo and aquarium research. In B. G. Norton, M. Hutchins, E. F. Stevens, & T. L. Maple (Eds.), *Ethics on the ark*. Washington, DC: Smithsonian Institution Press, pp. 253–276.

Huttenlocher, P. R. (1990). Morphometric study of human cerebral cortex development. *Neuropsychologia*, 28, 517–527.

Huxley, T. H. (1894). *Evolution and ethics*. London: Macmillan.

James, D., Pillai, M., & Someleniec, J. (1995). Neurobehavioral development in the human fetus. In J.-P. Lecanuet, W. P. Fifer, N. A. Krasnegor, & W. P. Smotherman (Eds.), *Fetal development*. Hillsdale, NJ: Lawrence Erlbaum Associates, pp. 101–128.

Jamieson, D. (1990). Rights, justice, and duties to provide assistance: A critique of Regan's theory of rights. *Ethics,* 100, 349–362.

Jamieson, D. (1995a). Zoos revisited. In B. G. Norton, M. Hutchins, E. F. Stevens, & T. L. Maple (Eds.), *Ethics on the ark*. Washington, DC: Smithsonian Institution Press, pp. 52–66.

Jamieson, D. (1995b). Wildlife conservation and individual animal welfare. In B. G. Norton, M. Hutchins, E. F. Stevens, & T. L. Maple (Eds.), *Ethics on the ark*. Washington DC: Smithsonian Institution Press, pp. 69–73.

Jensen, R. A., Thompson, M.E., Letton, T.L., et al. (1996). BRCA1 is secreted and exhibits properties of a granin. *Nature Genetics*, 12, 303–308.

Johnson, M. H. (1990). Cortical maturation and the development of visual attention in early infancy. *Journal of Cognitive Neuroscience*, 2, 81–95.

Johnson, M. H., Dziurawiec, S., Ellis, H. D., & Morton, J. (1991). Newborns preferential tracking of faces and its subsequent decline. *Cognition*, 40, 1–19.

Johnson, M. H. & Morton, J. (1991). *Biology and cognitive development*. Oxford: Basil Blackwell.

Johnson, R. L. Rothman, A. L., Xie, J., et al. (1996). Human homolog of *patched*, a candidate gene for the basal cell nevus syndrome. *Science*, 272, 1668–1671.

Johnson, T. H. (1961). *Final harvest: Emily Dickinson's poems*. Boston: Little, Brown.

Joreskog, K. G. & Sorbom, D. (1984). *LISREL VI: Analysis of linear structural relationships by maximum likelihood and least square methods*. Chicago, Ill., SPSS Inc.

Jusczyk, P. W. (1982). Auditory versus phonetic coding of speech signals during infancy. In J. Mehler, E. C. T. Walker, & M. Garrett (Eds.), *Perspectives on mental representation*. Hillsdale, NJ: Lawrence Erlbaum Associates, pp. 361–388.

Kagan, S. (1988). The additive fallacy. *Ethics*, 99, 5–31.

Kahn, A. (1990). Linking sex and oat bran: That's science. *Los Angeles Times*, June 3, E1.

Kamm, F. M. (1993). *Morality, mortality* (Vol. I). Oxford: Oxford University Press.

Kaplan, R. M. (1993). Application of a general health policy model in the American health care crisis. *Journal of the Royal Society of Medicine*, 86, 277–281.

Kaplan, R. M. (1994). The Ziggy theorem: Toward an outcomes-focused health psychology. *American Psychologist*, 13, 451–460.

Keeley, L. H. (1996). *War before civilization*. New York: Oxford University Press.

Kekes, J. (1993). *The morality of pluralism*. Princeton, NJ: Princeton University Press.

Kheel, M. (1996). The liberation of nature: A circular affair. In *Beyond animal rights*. New York: Continuum Publishing, pp. 17 33.

Kilner, J. F. (1990). *Who lives? Who dies?* New Haven, CT: Yale University Press.

Kleinig, J. (1991). *Valuing life*. Princeton, NJ: Princeton University Press.

Koch, F. & Koch, G. (1985). *The molecular biology of poliovirus*. Vienna: Springer-Verlag.

Koontz, F. (1995). Wild animal acquisition ethics for zoo biologists. In B. G. Norton, M. Hutchins, E. F. Stevens, & T. L. Maple (Eds.), *Ethics on the ark*. Washington, DC: Smithsonian Institution Press, pp. 127–145.

Krechevsky, I. (1932). "Hypotheses" in rats. *Psychological Review*, 39, 516–532.

Krings, M., Stone, A., Schmitz, R. W., et al. (1997). Neanderthal DNA sequences and the origin of modern humans. *Cell*, 90, 19–30.

Kuhl, P. K. (1992). Infants' perception and representation of speech: Development of a new theory. In J. Ohala, T. Neary, B. Derwing, M. Hodge, & G. Giebe (Eds.), *Proceedings of the international conference on spoken language processing*. Edmonton, Alberta, Canada: University of Alberta Press, pp. 449–456.

Kuhl, P. K. & Meltzoff, A. N. (1988). Speech as an intermodal object of perception. In A. Yonas (Ed.), *Perceptual development in infancy*. Hillsdale, NJ: Lawrence Erlbaum Associates, pp. 235–256.

Kuhl, P. K., Williams, K. A., & Meltzoff, A. N. (1991). Cross-modal speech perception in adults and infants using nonspeech auditory stimuli. *Journal of Experimental Psychology: Human Perception and Performance*, 17, 829–840.

Kuhn, T. S. (1962). The structure of scientific revolutions. *International encyclopedia of unified science*, (Vol. 2, #2) Chicago, IL: University of Chicago Press.

Kummer, H., & Cords, M. (1991). Cues of ownership in longtailed macaques, *Macaca fascikularis*. *Animal Behavior* 42, 529–549.

Kymlicka, W. (1993). The social contract tradition. In P. Singer (ed.), *A companion to ethics*. Oxford: Basil Blackwell, pp. 186–196.

Lacy, R. (1995). Culling surplus animals for population management. In B. G. Norton, M. Hutchins, E. F. Stevens, & T. L. Maple (Eds.), *Ethics on the ark*. Washington, DC: Smithsonian Institution Press, pp. 187–194.

Lakatos, I. (1970). Falsification and the methodology of scientific research programmes. In I. Lakatos & A. Musgrave (Eds.), *Criticism and the growth of knowledge*. Cambridge: Cambridge University Press.

Langley, G. (1989). Plea for a sensitive science. In G. Langley (Ed.), *Animal experimentation: The consensus changes*. New York: Chapman & Hall, pp. 193–218.

Laplante, D. P., Orr, R. R., Neville, K., Vorkapich, L., & Sasso, D. (1996). Discrimination of stimulus rotation by newborns. *Infant Behavior and Development*, 19, 271–279.

Leahy, M. P. T. (1991). *Against liberation*. London: Routledge.

Lecanuet, J.-P., Granier-Deferre, C., & Busnel, M. C. (1995). Human fetal auditory perception. In J.-P. Lecanuet, W. P. Fifer, N. A. Krasnegor, & W. P. Smotherman (Eds.), *Fetal development*. Hillsdale, NJ: Lawrence Erlbaum Associates, pp. 239–262.

Lecours, A. R. (1982). Correlates of developmental behavior in brain maturation. In T. G. Bever (Ed.), *Regressions in mental development*. Hillsdale, NJ: Lawrence Erlbaum Associates, pp. 267–298.

Lee, R. B. (1979). *The !Kung San: Men, women, and work in a foraging society*. Cambridge: Cambridge University Press.

Leehey, S. C., Moskowitz-Cook, A., Brill, S., & Held, R. (1975). Orientational anisotropy in infant vision. *Science*, 190, 900–902.

Leopold, A. (1949). *A Sand County almanac*. Oxford: Oxford University Press.

Leslie, A. M. (1994). ToMM, ToBy, and agency: Core architecture and domain specificity. In L. A. Hirschfeld & S. A. Gelman (Eds.), *Mapping the mind*. Cambridge: Cambridge University Press, pp. 119–148.

Locke, J. (1993). *The child's path to spoken language*. Cambridge: Harvard University Press.

Loftin, R. (1995). Captive breeding of endangered species. In B. G. Norton, M. Hutchins, E. F. Stevens, & T. L. Maple (Eds.), *Ethics on the ark*. Washington, DC: Smithsonian Institution Press, pp. 164–180.

Lomasky, L. E. (1987). *Persons, rights, and the moral community*. New York: Oxford University Press.

Lorenz, K. (1943). Die angeborenen Formen moglicher Erfahrung. *Zeitschrift fur Tierpsychologie*, 5, 235–409.

Luke, B. (1996). Justice, caring, and animal liberation. In J. Donovan & C. J. Adams (Eds.), *Beyond animal rights*. New York: Continuum Publishing, pp. 77–102.

Mack, E. (1993). Agent-relativity of value, deontic restraints, and self-ownership. In R. G. Frey & C. W. Morris (Eds.), *Value, welfare, and morality.* Cambridge: Cambridge University Press, pp. 209–232.

MacKenzie, D. (1992). The laboratory rat's guide to Europe. *New Scientist,* 134, #1821, 29–31.

Mackie, J. L. (1984). Rights, utility, and universalization. In R. G. Frey (Ed.), *Utility and rights.* Minneapolis: University of Minnesota Press, pp. 86–105.

Macklin, R. (1988). Theoretical and applied ethics: A reply to skeptics. In D. M. Rosenthal & F. Shehadi (Eds.), *Applied ethics and ethical theory.* Salt Lake City, UT: University of Utah Press, pp. 50–70.

Makin, J. W. & Porter, R. H. (1989). Attractiveness of lactating females' breast odors to neonates. *Child Development,* 60, 803–810.

Malenky, R. K., Kuroda, S., Vineberg, E. O., & Wrangham, R. W. (1994). The significance of terrestrial herbaceous foods for bonobos, chimpanzees, and gorillas. In R. W. Wrangham, W. C. McGrew, F. B. M. De Waal, & P. G. Heltne (Eds.), *Chimpanzee cultures.* Cambridge: Harvard University Press, pp. 59–76.

Mangels, A. R. & Havala, S. (1994). Vegan diets for women, infants, and children. *Journal of Agricultural and Environmental Ethics,* 7, 111–122.

Maple, T. (1995). Toward a responsible zoo agenda. In B. G. Norton, M. Hutchins, E. F. Stevens, & T. L. Maple (Eds.), *Ethics on the ark.* Washington, DC: Smithsonian Institution Press, pp. 20–30.

Maratos, O. (1982). Trends in the development of imitation in early infancy. In T. G. Bever (Ed.), *Regressions in mental development.* Hillsdale, NJ: Lawrence Erlbaum Associates, pp. 81–101.

Martin, G. B. & Clark, R. D. (1982). Distress crying in neonates: Species and peer specificity. *Developmental Psychology,* 18, 3–9.

Masataka, N. (1996). Perception of motherese in a signed language by 6-month-old deaf infants. *Developmental Psychology,* 32, 874–879.

Maugh, T. H. (1995). 2nd breast cancer gene found. *San Francisco Chronicle,* Dec. 21, A20.

Mayr, E. (1970). *Population, species, and evolution.* Cambridge: Harvard University Press.

Mayr, E. (1982). *The growth of biological thought.* Cambridge: Harvard University Press.

Mayr, E. (1991). *One long argument.* Cambridge: Harvard University Press.

McConway, K. (1992). The number of subjects in animal behaviour experiments: Is Still still right? In M.S. Dawkins & M. Gosling (Eds.), *Ethics in research on animal behaviour.* London: Academic Press, pp. 35–38.

McGrew, W. C. (1994). Tools compared: The material of culture. In R. W. Wrangham, W. C. McGrew, F. B. M. de Waal, & P. G. Heltne (Eds.), *Chimpanzee cultures.* Cambridge: Harvard University Press, pp. 25–39,

Meehl, P. E. (1986). What social scientists don't understand. In D. W. Fiske & R. A. Shweder (Eds.), *Metatheory in social science*. Chicago: University of Chicago Press, (pp. 315–338).

Mehler, J. & Christophe, A. (1995). Maturation and learning of language in the first year of life. In M. S. Gazzaniga (Ed.), *The cognitive neurosciences*. Cambridge: MIT Press, pp. 943–954.

Mehler, J. & Dupoux, E. (1994). *What infants know*. Oxford: Basil Blackwell.

Meltzoff, A. H. (1988). The human infant as "homo imitans." In T. R. Zentall & B. G. Galef, Jr. (Eds.), *Social learning*. Hillsdale, NJ: Lawrence Erlbaum Associates, pp. 319–341.

Meltzoff, A. H. (1990). Foundations for developing a concept of self: The role of imitation in relating self to other and the value of social mirroring, social modeling, and self practice in infancy. In D. Cicchetti & M. Beeghly (Eds.), *The self in transition: Infancy to childhood*. Chicago: University of Chicago Press, pp. 139–164.

Meltzoff, A. H. (1995). What infant memory tells us about infantile amnesia: Long-term recall and deferred imitation. *Journal of Experimental Child Psychology, 59,* 497–515.

Meltzoff, A. N. (1996). The human infant as imitative generalist: A 20-year progress report on infant imitation with implications for comparative psychology. In C. M. Heyes & B. G. Galef, Jr. (Eds.), *Social learning in animals: The roots of culture*. New York: Academic Press, pp. 347–370.

Meltzoff, A. N. & Moore, M. K. (1977). Imitation of facial and manual gestures by human neonates. *Science, 198,* 75–78.

Meltzoff, A. N. & Moore, M. K. (1983). Newborn infants imitate adult facial gestures. *Child Development, 54,* 702–709.

Meltzoff, A. N. & Moore, M. K. (1989). Imitation in newborn infants: Exploring the range of gestures imitated and the underlying mechanisms. *Developmental Psychology, 25,* 954–962.

Meltzoff, A. N. & Moore, M. K. (1992). Early imitation within a functional framework: The importance of person identity, movement, and development. *Infant Behavior and Development, 15* 479–505.

Meltzoff, A. H. & Moore, M. K. (1994). Imitation, memory, and representation of persons in 6-week-old infants. *Infant Behavior and Development, 17,* 83–99.

Mench, J. & Tienhoven, A. van (1986). Farm animal welfare. *American Scientist, 74,* 598–603.

Midgley, M. (1983). *Animals and why they matter*. Athens, GA: University of Georgia Press.

Midgley, M. (1989). Are you an animal? In G. Langley (Ed.), *Animal experimentation*. New York: Chapman & Hall, pp. 1–18.

Milewski, A. E. (1989). Visual discrimination and detection of configurational invariance in 3-month-old infants. *Developmental Psychology, 15,* 357–363.

Miller, N. E. (1985). The value of behavioral research on animals. *American Psychologist,* 40, 423–440.

Miller, N. E. & Dollard, J. (1941). *Social learning and imitation.* New York: Yale University Press.

Millstone, E. (1989). Methods and practices of animal experimentation. In G. Langley (Ed.), *Animal experimentation.* New York: Chapman & Hall, pp. 72–87.

Moon, C., Cooper, R. P., & Fifer, W. P. (1993). Two-day-olds prefer their native language. *Infant Behavior and Development,* 16, 495–500.

Moon, C. & Fifer, W. (1990). Syllables as signals for 2-day-old infants. *Infant Behavior and Development,* 13, 377–390.

Morton, D. B. (1989). The scientist's responsibility for refinement: A guide to better animal welfare and better science. In G. Langley (Ed.), *Animal experimentation.* New York: Chapman & Hall, pp. 169–192.

Mowrer, O. H. (1960). *Learning theory and behavior.* New York: John Wiley.

Muroyama, Y. & Sugiyama, Y. (1994). Grooming relationships in two species of chimpanzees. In R. W. Wrangham, W. C. McGrew, F. B. M. De Waal, & P. G. Heltne (Eds.), *Chimpanzee cultures.* Cambridge, MA: Harvard University Press, pp. 169–180.

Nagel, T. (1979). The fragmentation of value. In T. Nagel (Ed.), *Mortal questions,* Cambridge: Cambridge University Press, pp. 128–141.

Narveson, J. (1987). On a case for animal rights. *Monist,* 70, 31–49.

Neville, H. J. (1995). Developmental specificity in neurocognitive development in humans. In M. S. Gazzaniga (Ed.), *The cognitive neurosciences.* Cambridge, MA: MIT Press, pp. 218–231.

Newcomer, C. E. (1990). Laws, regulations, and policies pertaining to the welfare of laboratory animals. In B. E. Rollin & M. L. Kesel (Eds.), *The experimental animal in biomedical research* (Vol. I). Boca Raton, FL: CRC Press, pp. 37–48.

Newport, E. (1991). Contrasting conceptions of the critical period for language. In S. Carey & R. Gelman (Eds.), *The epigenesis of mind.* Hillsdale, NJ: Lawrence Erlbaum Associates, pp. 111–130.

Nicoll, C. & Russell, S. (1990). Analysis of animal rights literature reveals the underlying motives of the movement: Ammunition for counter offensive by scientist [editorial]. *Endocrinology,* 127, 985–989.

Nicoll, C. S. & Russell, S. M. (1991). Mozart, Alexander the Great, and the animal rights/liberation philosophy. *Federation of the Associated Societies of Experimental Biology,* 5, 2888–2892.

Norton, B. G. (1987). *Why preserve natural variety?* Princeton, NJ: Princeton University Press.

Norton, B. G. (1995). Caring for nature: A broader look at animal stewardship. In B. G. Norton, M. Hutchins, E. F. Stevens, & T. L. Maple (Eds.), *Ethics on the ark.* Washington, DC: Smithsonian Institution Press, pp. 102–121.

Norton, B. G., Hutchins, M., Stevens, E. F., & Maple, T. L. (1995). *Ethics on the ark*. Washington, DC: Smithsonian Institution Press,

Nowakowski, R. S. (1987). Basic concepts of CNS development. *Child Development*, 58, 568–595.

O'Neill, P. & Petrinovich, L. in (in press). A cross-cultural study of moral intuitions. *Evolution and Human Behavior*.

Orlans, F. B. (1993). *In the name of science*. New York: Oxford University Press.

Patterson, F., & Gordon, W. (1993). The case for the personhood of gorillas. In P. Cavalieri & P. Singer (Eds.), *The great ape project*. New York: St. Martin's Press, pp. 58–77

Petrinovich, L. (1973). Darwin and the representative expression of reality. In P. Ekman (Ed.), *Darwin and facial expression*. New York: Academic Press, pp. 223–256.

Petrinovich, L. (1976). Molar reductionism. In L. Petrinovich & J. L. McGaugh (Eds.), *Knowing, thinking, and believing*. New York: Plenum Press, pp. 11–27.

Petrinovich, L. (1979). Probabilistic functionalism: A conception of research method. *American Psychologist*, 34, 373–390.

Petrinovich, L. (1981). A method for the study of development. In K. Immelmann, G. Barlow, L. Petrinovich, & M. Main (Eds.), *Behavioral development*. Cambridge: Cambridge University Press, pp. 90–130.

Petrinovich, L. (1989). Representative design and the quality of generalization. In L. W. Poon, D. C. Rubin, & B. A. Wilson (Eds.), *Everyday cognition in adulthood and late life*. Cambridge: Cambridge University Press, pp. 11–24.

Petrinovich, L. (1995). *Human evolution, reproduction, and morality*. New York: Plenum Press.

Petrinovich, L. (1996). *Living and dying well*. New York: Plenum Press.

Petrinovich, L. & O'Neill, P. (1996). Influence of wording and framing effects on moral intuitions. *Ethology and Sociobiology*, 17, 145–171.

Petrinovich, L., O'Neill, P., & Jorgensen, M. (1993). An empirical study of moral intuitions: Toward an evolutionary ethics. *Journal of Personality and Social Psychology*, 64, 467–478.

Pettit, P. (1993). Consequentialism. In P. Singer (Ed.), *A companion to ethics*. Oxford: Basil Blackwell, pp. 230–240.

Piaget, J. (1954). *The construction of reality in the child*. New York: Basic Books.

Pinker, S. (1994). *The language instinct*. New York: Morrow.

Pinker, S. (1995). Language acquisition. In L. Gleitman & M. Liberman (Eds.), *Language: An invitation to cognitive science* (vol. 1, 2nd ed.). Cambridge: MIT Press, pp. 135–182.

Plous, S. (1993). Psychological mechanisms in the human use of animals. *Journal of Social Issues*, 49, 11–52.

Pluhar, E. B. (1993). On vegetarianism, morality, and science. A counter reply. *Journal of Agricultural and Environmental Ethics*, 6, 185–213.

Pluhar, E. G. (1994). Vegetarianism, morality, and science revisited. *Journal of Agricultural and Environmental Ethics*, 7, 77–82.

Popper, K. R. (1959). *The logic of scientific discovery*. New York: Basic Books.

Popper, K. R. (1963). *Conjectures and refutations*. New York: Basic Books.

Porter, R. II., Makin, J. W., Davis, L. B., & Christensen, K. M. (1991). An assessment of the salient olfactory environment of formula-fed infants. *Physiology and Behavior*, 50, 907–911.

Povinelli, D. (1994). What chimpanzees (might) know about the mind. In R. W. Wrangham, W. C. McGrew, F. B. M. De Waal, & P. G. Heltne (Eds.), *Chimpanzee cultures*. Cambridge: Harvard University Press, pp. 285–300.

Povinelli, D. (1996). Chimpanzee theory of mind?: The long road to strong inference. In P. Carruthers & P. K. Smith, *Theories of theories of mind*. Cambridge: Cambridge University Press, pp. 293–329.

Povinelli, D. J. & Eddy, T. J. (1996). What young chimpanzees know about seeing. *Monographs of the Society for Research in Child Development*, 61, #3.

Prechtl, H. F. R. (1982). Regressions and transformations during neurological development. In T. G. Bever (Ed.), *Regressions in mental development*. Hillsdale, NJ: Lawrence Erlbaum Associates, pp. 103–115.

Premack, D. (1986). *Gavagai! Or the future history of the animal language controversy*. Cambridge: MIT Press.

Premack, D. & Premack, A. J. (1994). Moral belief: Form versus content. In L. A. Hirschfeld & S. A. Gelman (Eds.), *Mapping the mind*. Cambridge: Cambridge University Press, pp. 149–168.

Premack, D. & Premack, J. (1995). Origins of human social competence. In M. S. Gazzaniga (Ed.), *The cognitive neurosciences*. Cambridge: MIT Press, pp. 205–218.

Rachels, J. (1990). *Created from animals*. Oxford: Oxford University Press.

Rachels, J. (1993). Why Darwinians should support equal treatment for other apes. In P. Cavalieri & P. Singer (Eds.), *The great ape project*. New York: St. Martin's Press, pp. 152–157.

Rakic, P. (1995). Corticogenesis in human and nonhuman primates. In M. S. Gazzaniga (Ed.), *The cognitive neurosciences*. Cambridge: MIT Press, pp. 127–146.

Rakic, P., Bourgeois, J.-P., Eckenhoff, M. E., Zecevic, N., & Goldman-Rakic, P. S. (1986). Concurrent overproduction of synapses in diverse regions of the primate cerebral cortex. *Science*, 232, 232–235.

Rawls, J. (1971). *A theory of justice*. Cambridge: Harvard University Press.

Read, P.P. (1974). *Alive*. New York: J. B. Lippincott.

Regan, T. (1975). The moral basis of vegetarianism. *Canadian Journal of Philoso-*

phy, 5, 181–214. (Reprinted in T. Regan (Ed.). 1982. *All that dwell therein*. Berkeley, CA: University of California Press, pp. 3–39.)

Regan, T. (1979). An examination and defense of one argument concerning animal rights. *Inquiry*, 22, #1–2. (Reprinted in T. Regan (Ed.). 1982. *All that dwell therein*. Berkeley, CA: University of California Press, pp. 113–147.)

Regan, T. (1980). Animal rights, human wrongs. *Environmental Ethics*, 2, 99–120. (Reprinted in T. Regan (Ed.). 1982. *All that dwell therein*. Berkeley, CA: University of California Press, pp. 75–101.)

Regan, T. (1983). *The case for animal rights*. Berkeley, CA: University of California Press.

Regan, T. (1989). Ill-gotten gains. In G. Langley (Ed.), *Animal experimentation*. New York: Chapman & Hall, pp. 19–41.

Regan, T. (1995). Are zoos morally defensible? In B. G. Norton, M. Hutchins, E. F. Stevens, & T. L. Maple (Eds.), *Ethics on the ark*. Washington, DC: Smithsonian Institution Press, pp. 38–51.

Reissland, N. (1988). Neonatal imitation in the first hour of life. Observations in rural Nepal. *Developmental Psychology*, 24, 464–469

Richards, R. J. (1996). Review of Lewis Petrinovich, *Human evolution, reproduction, and morality*. *Quarterly Review of Biology*, 71, 559–560.

Rodd, R. (1990). *Biology, ethics and animals*. Oxford: Oxford University Press.

Rodman, J. (1977). I. The liberation of nature? *Inquiry*, 20, 83–131.

Rollin, B. E. (1989). *The unheeded cry*. Oxford: Oxford University Press.

Rollin, B. E. (1992). *Animal rights and human morality*. Buffalo, NY: Prometheus Books.

Rollin, B. E. (1995). *Farm animal welfare*. Ames, IA: Iowa State University Press.

Rolston, H. III. (1992). Disvalues in nature. *Monist*, 75, 250–278.

Ronca, A. E. & Alberts, J. R. (1995). Maternal contributions to fetal experience and the transition from prenatal to postnatal life. In J.-P. Lecanuet, W. P. Fifer, N. A. Krasnegor, & W. P. Smotherman (Eds.), *Fetal development*. Hillsdale, NJ: Lawrence Erlbaum Associates, pp. 331–350.

Rowan, A. N. (1984). *Of mice, models, and men*. Albany, NY: State University of New York Press.

Rowan, A. N. & Rollin, B. E. (1983). Animal research—for and against: A philosophical, social, and historical perspective. *Perspectives in Biology and Medicine*, 27, 1–17.

Ruesch, H. (1979). *Vivisection is scientific fraud*. Los Angeles: Civis-Hans Ruesch Foundation.

Rumbaugh, D. M. (Ed.). (1977). *Language leaning by a chimpanzee: The LANA project*. New York: Academic Press.

Rumbaugh, D. M., Savage-Rumbaugh, E. S., & Sevcik, R. A. (1994). Biobehavioral roots of language: A comparative perspective of chimpanzee, child, and culture. In R. W. Wrangham, W. C. McGrew, F. B. M. de Waal, & P. G. Heltne (Eds.), *Chimpanzee cultures.* Cambridge: Harvard University Press, pp. 319–334.

Russell, S. M., & Nicoll, C. S. (1996). A dissection of the chapter "Tools for research" in Peter Singer's *Animal liberation. Proceedings of the Society for Experimental Biology and Medicine*, 211, 109–138.

Ryder, R. D. (1970). *Speciesism.* Privately printed leaflet, Oxford, (cited in Ryder, 1989, p. 338)

Ryder, R. D. (1989). *Animal revolution.* Oxford: Basil Blackwell.

Sanday, P. R. (1986). *Divine hunger: Cannibalism as a cultural system.* Cambridge: Cambridge University Press.

Savage-Rumbaugh, E. S. (1986). *Ape language: From conditioned response to symbol.* New York: Columbia University Press.

Schaal, B., Orgeur, P., & Rognon, C. (1995). Human fetal auditory perception. In J.-P. Lecanuet, W. P. Fifer, N. A. Krasnegor, & W. P. Smotherman (Eds.), *Fetal development.* Hillsdale, NJ: Lawrence Erlbaum Associates, pp. 205–262.

Sharpe, R. (1989). Animal experiments—A failed technology. In G. Langley (Ed.), *Animal experimentation.* New York: Chapman & Hall, pp. 88–117.

Shatz, C. J. (1992). The developing brain. *Scientific American*, 267, 60–67.

Shepherd, G. M. (1988). *Neurobiology* (2nd ed.). Oxford: Oxford University Press.

Simpson, A. W. B. (1984). *Cannibalism and the common law.* Chicago: University of Chicago Press.

Singer, P. (1975). *Animal liberation.* New York: Avon Books—Discus Printing.

Singer, P. (1979). *Practical ethics.* Cambridge: Cambridge University Press.

Singer, P. (1981). *The expanding circle.* New York: Farrar, Straus & Giroux.

Singer, P. (1987). Animal liberation or animal rights? *Monist*, 70, 3–14.

Singer, P. (1990a). *Animal liberation* (revised ed.). New York: Avon Books.

Singer, P. (1990b). The significance of animal suffering. Ethics and animals. *Behavioral and Brain Sciences*, 13, 9–12, 45–49.

Singer, P. (1993). *Practical ethics.* (2nd ed.). Cambridge: Cambridge University Press.

Singer, P. (1996). Ethics and the limits of scientific freedom. *Monist*, 79, 218–229.

Skinner, B. F. (1950). Are theories of learning necessary? *Psychological Review*, 57, 193–216.

Slater, A. M. (1993). Visual perceptual abilities at birth: Implications for face perception. In B. de Boysson-Bardies, S. de Schonen, P. Jusczyk, P. McNeilage, & J. Morton, *Developmental neurocognition: Speech and face processing in the first year of life*. Dordecht, The Netherlands: Kluwer Academic Publishers, pp. 125–134.

Slicer, D. (1991). Your daughter or your dog? A feminist assessment of the animal research issue. *Hypatia*, 6, 108–124.

Smart, J. J. C. (1973). An outline of a system of utilitarian ethics. In *Utilitarianism: For and against*. Cambridge: Cambridge University Press, pp. 1–74.

Smith, J. A. & Boyd, K. M. (1991). *Lives in the balance*. Oxford: Oxford University Press.

Smotherman, W. P. & Robinson, S. R. (1995). Tracing developmental trajectories into the prenatal period. In J.-P. Lecanuet, W. P. Fifer, N. A. Krasnegor, & W. P. Smotherman (Eds.), *Fetal development*. Hillsdale, NJ: Lawrence Erlbaum Associates, pp. 15–32.

Sober, E. (1986). Philosophical problems for environmentalism. In B. Norton (Ed.), *The preservation of species: The value of biological diversity*. Princeton, NJ: Princeton University Press, pp. 173–195.

Sorabji, R. (1993). *Animal minds and human morals*. Ithaca, NY: Cornell University Press.

Spelke, E. S., Vishton, P., & von Hofsten, C. (1995). Object perception, object-directed action, and physical knowledge in infancy. In M. S. Gazzaniga (Ed.), *The cognitive neurosciences*. Cambridge: MIT Press, pp. 165–180.

Spencer, H. (1887). *Factors of organic evolution*. London: Williams & Norgate.

Sperber, D. (1994). The modularity of thought and the epidemiology of representations. In L. A. Hirschfeld & S. A. Gelman (Eds.), *Mapping the mind*. Cambridge: Cambridge University Press, pp. 39–67.

Sperling, S. (1988). *Animal liberators*. Berkeley, CA: University of California Press.

Stephens, M. (1989). Replacing animal experiments. In G. Langley (Ed.), *Animal experimentation*. New York: Chapman & Hall, pp. 144–168.

Stewart, G. R. (1960). *Ordeal by hunger*. Boston: Houghton Mifflin. (Reprinted in 1960, Lincoln, NE: University of Nebraska Press.)

Still, A. W. (1982). On the number of subjects used in animal behaviour experiments. *Animal Behaviour*, 30, 873–880.

Stringer, C. & Gamble, C. (1993). *In search of the Neanderthals*. New York: Thames & Hudson.

Stromswold, K. (1995). The cognitive and neural bases of language acquisition. In M. S. Gazzaniga (Ed.), *The cognitive neurosciences*. Cambridge: MIT Press, pp. 855–870.

Sumner, L. W. (1981). *Abortion and moral theory*. Princeton, NJ: Princeton University Press.

Sumner, L. W. (1984). Rights denaturalized. In R. G. Frey (Ed.), *Utility and rights*. Minneapolis: University of Minnesota Press, pp. 20–41.

Sumner, L. W. (1988). Animal welfare and animal rights. *Journal of Medicine and Philosophy*, 13, 159–176.

Suppress. (1991). Pasadena, CA: Supress, Inc.

Swisher, C. C. III, Rinks, W. J.,-Anton, S. C., et al. (1996). Latest *Homo erectus* of Java: Potential contemporaneity with *Homo sapiens* in southeast Asia. *Science*, 274, 1870–1874.

Tannenbaum, J. (1995). Animals and the law: Cruelty, property, rights . . . Or how the law makes up in common sense what it may lack in metaphysics. In A. Mack (Ed.), *In the company of animals*. Social Research, 62, #3, pp. 539–607.

Tattersall, I. (1995). *The fossil trail*. Oxford: Oxford University Press.

Taylor, P. W. (1986). *Respect for nature*. Princeton, NJ: Princeton University Press.

Terrace, H. S. (1979). *Nim*. New York: Knopf.

Thomas, D. (1971). *The poems of Dylan Thomas*. New York: New Directions Publishing Corp., pp. 49–50.

Thomson, J. J. (1990). *The realm of rights*. Cambridge: Harvard University Press.

Tinklepaugh, L. (1928). An experimental study of representative factors in monkeys. *Journal of Comparative Psychology*, 8, 197–236.

Tolman, E. C. (1932). *Purposive behavior in animals and men*. New York: Appleton-Century-Crofts.

Tolman, E. C. (1959). Principles of purposive behaviorism. In S. Koch (Ed.), *Psychology: A study of a science*, Vol. 2. New York: McGraw-Hill, pp. 92–157.

Tomasello, M. (1994a). The question of chimpanzee culture. In R. W. Wrangham, W. C. McGrew, F. B. M. De Waal, & P. G. Heltne (Eds.), *Chimpanzee cultures*. Cambridge: Harvard University Press, pp. 301–318.

Tomasello, M. (1995). Joint attention as social cognition. In C. Moore & P. J. Dunham (Eds.), *Joint attention*. Hillsdale, NJ: Lawrence Erlbaum Associates, pp. 103–130.

Tomasello, M., Kruger, A. C., & Ratner, H. H. (1993). Cultural learning. *Behavioral and Brain Sciences*, 16, 495–511.

Tooby, J. & Cosmides, L. (1992). The psychological foundations of culture. In J. H. Barkow, L. Cosmides, & J. Tooby (Eds.), *The adapted mind*. New York: Oxford University Press, pp. 19–136.

Tooby, J. & Cosmides, L. (1995). Introduction. In M. Gazzaniga (Ed.), *The cognitive neurosciences*. Cambridge: MIT Press, pp. 1181–1183.

Tooley, M. (1983). *Abortion and infanticide*. Oxford: Oxford University Press.

Trevarthen, C. (1982). Basic patterns of psychogenetic change in infancy. In T. G. Bever (Ed.), *Regressions in mental development*. Hillsdale, NJ: Lawrence Erlbaum Associates, pp. 7–46.

van Hoof, J. A. R. A. M. (1994). Understanding chimpanzee understanding. In R. W. Wrangham, W. C. McGrew, F. B. M. De Waal, & P. G. Heltne (Eds.), *Chimpanzee cultures*. Cambridge: Harvard University Press, pp. 267–284.

van Wezel, A. L. (1981). Present state and developments in the production of inactivated poliomyelitis vaccine. *International Symposium on Reassessment of Inactivated Poliomyelitis Vaccine, Developments in Biological Standardization*, 47, 7–13.

Varner, G. E. (1994a). What's wrong with animal by-products? *Journal of Agricultural and Environmental Ethics*, 7, 7–17.

Varner, G. E. (1994b). In defense of the vegan ideal. *Journal of Agricultural and Environmental Ethics*, 7, 29–40.

Vrijenhoek, R. (1995). Natural processes, individuals, and units of conservation. In B. G. Norton, M. Hutchins, E. F. Stevens, & T. L. Maple (Eds.), *Ethics on the ark*. Washington, DC: Smithsonian Institution Press, pp. 74–92.

Wall, P. (1992). Neglected benefits of animal research. *New Scientist*, 134, #1817, 30–31.

Wallman, J. (1992). *Aping language*. Cambridge: Cambridge University Press.

Walton, D. (1992). *The place of emotion in argument*. University Park, PA: University of Pennsylvania Press.

Walton, G. E. & Bower, T. G. R. (1993). Newborns form "prototypes" in less than 1 minute. *Psychological Science*, 4, 203–205.

Wang, X. T. (1996a). Domain-specific rationality in human choices: Violations of utility axioms and social contexts. *Cognition*, 60, 31–63.

Wang, X. T. (1996b). Evolutionary hypotheses of risk-sensitive choice: Age differences and perspective change. *Ethology and Sociobiology*, 17, 1–15.

Wang, X. T. & Johnston, V. S. (1995). Perceived social context and risk preference: A re-examination of framing effects in a life-death decision problem. *Journal of Behavioral Decision Making*, 8, 279–293.

Wanpo, H., Clochon, R., et al. (1995). Early *Homo* and associated artefacts from Asia. *Nature*, 378, 275–278.

Werker, J. F. (1989). Becoming a native listener. *American Scientist*, 77, 54–59.

Wertheimer, M. (1961). Psychomotor coordination of auditory and visual space at birth. *Science*, 134, 1692.

White, T. D. (1992). *Prehistoric cannibalism*. Princeton, NJ: Princeton University Press.

Williams, G. W. (1966). *Adaptation and natural selection*. Princeton, NJ: Princeton University Press.

Williams, G. W. (1989). A sociological expansion of *Evolution and ethics*. In J. Paradis & G. C. Williams (Eds.), *Evolution and ethics*. Princeton, NJ: Princeton University Press, pp. 179–214.

Wilson, E. O. (1975). *Sociobiology: The new synthesis.* Cambridge: Harvard University Press.

Wilson, E. O. (1984). *Biophilia.* Cambridge: Harvard University Press.

Wilson, E. O. (1992). *The diversity of life.* Cambridge: Harvard University Press.

Wilson, E. O. (1993). Biophilia and the conservation ethic. In S. R. Kellert & E. O. Wilson (Eds.), *The biophilia hypothesis.* Washington, DC: Island Press, pp. 31–41.

Wilson, E. O. (1994). *Naturalist.* Washington, DC: Island Press.

Wilson, J. Q. (1993). *The moral sense.* New York: Free Press.

Woodward, J. & Goodstein, D. (1996). Conduct, misconduct and the structure of science. *Scientific American, 84,* 479–490.

Wooster, R., Bignell, G., Lancaster, J., et al. (1995). Identification of the breast cancer susceptibility gene BRCA2. *Nature, 378,* 789–792.

Wrangham, R. W., De Waal, F. B. M., & McGrew, W. C. (1994). The challenge of behavioral diversity. In R. W. Wrangham, W. C. McGrew, F. B. M. De Waal, & P. G. Heltne (Eds.), *Chimpanzee cultures.* Cambridge: Harvard University Press, pp. 1–18.

Wrangham, R. W. & Peterson, D. (1996). *Demonic males.* New York: Houghton Mifflin.

Wuichel, J. & Norton, B. (1995). Differing conceptions of animal welfare. In B. G. Norton, M. Hutchins, E. F. Stevens, & T. L. Maple (Eds.), *Ethics on the ark.* Washington, DC: Smithsonian Institution Press, pp. 235–250.

Wynn, K. (1992). Addition and subtraction by human infants. *Nature, 358,* 749–750.

Young, W. (1996). Spinal cord regeneration. *Science, 273,* 451.

Zheng Yi. (1996). *Scarlet memorial.* Boulder, CO: Westview Press.

Name Index

Subject Index